Harty's **Endodontics in Clinical Practice**
Fourth edition

Harty's Endodontics in Clinical Practice

Fourth edition

T. R. Pitt Ford
BDS, PhD (University of London), FDS RCPS Glasgow

Reader in Endodontology, United Medical and Dental Schools,
University of London, UK

wright

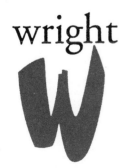

Wright
An imprint of Butterworth-Heinemann
Linacre House, Jordan Hill, Oxford OX2 8DP
A division of Reed Educational and Professional Publishing Ltd

 A member of the Reed Elsevier plc group

OXFORD BOSTON JOHANNESBURG
MELBOURNE NEW DELHI SINGAPORE

First published 1976
Second edition 1982
Third edition 1990
Fourth edition 1997
Reprinted 1997

British Library Cataloguing in Publication Data
Harty, F. J. (Frederick John), 1927–
    Harty's endodontics in clinical practice – 4th ed.
    1. Endodontics
    I. Title   II. Ford, Pitt.   III. Endodontics in clinical practice
    617.6'342

ISBN 0 7236 1020 7

Library of Congress Cataloguing in Publication Data
Harty's endodontics in clinical practice. – 4th ed./[edited by]
    T. R. Pitt Ford.
    p.   cm.
    Rev. ed. of: Endodontics in clinical practice/[edited by] F. J.
    Harty. 3rd ed. 1990.
    Includes bibliographical references and index.
    ISBN 0 7236 1020 7
    1. Endodontics.   I. Pitt Ford, T. R.   II. Harty, F. J.
    III. Endodontics in clinical practice.
    [DNLM: 1. Endodontics.   WU 230 H3371]
    RK351.E535
    617.6'342–dc20

                                        96–30102
                                        CIP

Typeset by BC Typesetting, Bristol BS15 5YD
Printed and bound in Great Britain by The Bath Press

Contents

Contributors

P.M.H. Dummer BDS PhD
Professor
Department of Restorative Dentistry
Dental School
University of Wales College of Medicine
Cardiff, Wales

A.L. Frank DDS
Professor
Department of Endodontics
Loma Linda University
Loma Linda
California, USA

J.L. Gutmann DDS
Professor
Department of Restorative Sciences
Baylor College of Dentistry
Texas A&M University System
Dallas
Texas, USA

R. Ibbetson BDS MSc FDS RCS
Consultant
Department of Continuing Education
Eastman Dental Institute
University of London
London, England

D.A. McGowan MDS PhD FDS RCS
FFD RCSI FDS RCPS
Professor of Oral Surgery
Glasgow Dental Hospital and School
University of Glasgow
Glasgow, Scotland

T.M. Odor BDS MSc
Research Fellow
Department of Conservative Dentistry
United Medical and Dental Schools
University of London
London, England

D. Ørstavik cand odont dr odont
Senior Scientist
Scandinavian Institute of Dental Materials
Haslum, Norway

S. Patel BDS FDS RCS
Department of Paediatric Dentistry
Eastman Dental Institute
University of London
London, England

T.R. Pitt Ford BDS PhD FDS RCPS
Reader in Endodontology
United Medical and Dental Schools
University of London
London, England

D.C. Rule BDS FDS RCS DOrth RCS
MCCD RCS
Consultant
Department of Paediatric Dentistry
Eastman Dental Institute
University of London
London, England

E.M. Saunders BDS PhD
Senior Lecturer
Department of Conservative Dentistry
Dental School
University of Dundee
Dundee, Scotland

W.P. Saunders BDS PhD FDS RCS
FDS RCPS MRD
Professor of Endodontology
Glasgow Dental Hospital and School
University of Glasgow
Glasgow, Scotland

R.T. Walker RD BDS MSc PhD FDS RCPS
Professor of Conservative Dentistry
University of West Indies
Trinidad and Tobago

J. Webber BDS MS
Practice limited to endodontics
Lister House Dental Practice
London, England

Preface

Since the last edition of this book, Fred Harty retired from active dental practice, and he therefore decided to invite a colleague to produce the new edition of this long-established clinical handbook. Unfortunately, he tragically died before completion of the book, which is now dedicated to his memory.

This book is intended *inter alia* as an undergraduate text for dental students in the UK, and over the last 6 years the dental course has been lengthened to strengthen the scientific basis of dentistry. This has not necessarily resulted in more teaching in the traditional clinical dental subjects; however, students are now more analytical and ready to question clinical procedures that are not based on sound principles. New graduates in the UK are required to undergo a formal period of training in dental practice, and this presents an opportunity to translate the teaching given in dental school into everyday clinical practice, and should result in more competent dental practitioners in the future.

Recognized specialist practice in endodontics is now set to happen in the UK, after much patient negotiation with the authorities. It should be of particular benefit to patients, who will be able to be referred to specially trained practitioners for difficult or unusual endodontic procedures. As there will never be a sufficient number of specialists to treat more than the most difficult cases, there is still a major place for undergraduates to be taught practical endodontics; indeed, most endodontic treatment will be carried out in general dental practice. Therefore, it is essential that general dental practitioners keep up to date, and this book is primarily intended to help them to do so, by supporting what they learn on short continuing education courses. The authorities in the UK now stress the importance of continuing education, and it is no longer acceptable for practitioners to rely on their teaching at dental school. Many treatment procedures taught even 20 years ago have radically altered.

The book has been thoroughly revised and a number of new authors have been brought in to write up-to-date authoritative chapters and to give the book international appeal. It is not intended that the book should be a substitute for many large well-established textbooks, but there is a need for a handbook to help busy practitioners to update themselves. An accusation is sometimes made that endodontists are excellent at filling root canals, but they lack the knowledge of subsequent restoration of the dentition. This criticism is unjustified; however, to counter it, a new chapter on the restoration of root filled teeth has been added. Further, the new training for specialist endodontists in the UK will have a substantial component of restorative dentistry to address this issue. To make the book more easily read by busy practitioners, the Harvard system of referencing has been replaced by a numerical system.

I would like to express my thanks to all the contributors who have tirelessly given of their time and expertise to create this new edition. I would also like to acknowledge the patience of my wife and family, together with the help of Butterworth-Heinemann in bringing this book to fruition.

T.R. Pitt Ford

1

Introduction, history and scope

T.R. Pitt Ford

Introduction	**Tissue response to root canal infection**
Modern endodontics	**Quality assurance**
Scope of endodontics	**Recent developments**
Role of microorganisms	**References**

Introduction

Endodontic treatment can simply be defined as the precautions taken to maintain the health of the vital pulp in a tooth, or the treatment of a damaged or necrotic pulp in a tooth to allow the tooth to remain functional in the dental arch. This concept of treating the pulp of the tooth to preserve the tooth itself is a relatively modern development in the history of dentistry and it may be useful to review, very briefly, the history of pulp treatment in order to appreciate better modern views on endodontic treatment. Toothache has been a scourge to humanity from the earliest times. Both the Chinese and the Egyptians left records describing caries and alveolar abscesses. The Chinese considered that these abscesses were caused by a white worm with a black head which lived within the tooth. The 'worm theory' was current until the middle of the 18th century, when doubts were raised [16], but they could not be expressed forcibly because senior figures still believed in the worm theory [9]. The Chinese treatment for an abscessed tooth was aimed at killing the worm with a preparation that contained arsenic. The use of this drug was taught in most dental schools as recently as the 1950s, in spite of the realization that it was self-limiting and that extensive tissue destruction occurred if

minute amounts of the drug leaked into the soft tissues.

Pulpal treatment during Greek and Roman times was aimed at destroying the pulp by cauterization with a hot needle or boiling oil, or with a mixture of opium and *Hyoscyamus*. At the end of the first century, it was realized that pain could be relieved by drilling into the pulp chamber to obtain drainage. In spite of modern 'wonder drugs' there is still no better method of relieving the pain of an abscessed tooth than drainage.

Endodontic knowledge remained static until the 16th century when pulpal anatomy was described. Before the latter part of the 19th century, root canal therapy consisted of alleviating pulpal pain and the main function of the opened root canal was to provide retention for a dowel crown [6,7]. At the same time bridgework became popular and many dental schools taught that no tooth should be used as an abutment unless it was first devitalized [41]. Root canal therapy became commonplace partly for these reasons and also because the discovery of cocaine led to painless pulp extirpation. The injection of 4% cocaine as a mandibular nerve block was first reported in 1884 [7,43]; and 20 years later the first synthetic local anaesthetic, procaine, was produced. At this time reports of endodontic surgery appear [18]. Shortly after the discovery of X-rays by Roentgen in 1895, the first radiograph of teeth was taken [6,15,17]. This further popularized root canal therapy and gave the treatment respectability.

About the same time dental manufacturers began to produce special instruments which were used primarily to remove pulp tissue or clean debris from the canal. There was no concept of filling the root canals since the object of the procedure was to provide retention for a post crown.

By 1910 root canal therapy had reached its zenith and no self-respecting dentist would extract a tooth. Every root stump was retained and a crown constructed. Sinus tracts often appeared and were treated by various ineffective methods for many years. The connection between the sinus tract and the pulpless tooth was known but no one acted upon it.

In 1911 William Hunter [8,22] attacked 'American dentistry' and blamed bridgework for several diseases of unknown aetiology. He obtained recovery from these conditions in a few patients by extracting their teeth. It is interesting to note that he did not condemn root canal therapy itself, but rather the ill-fitting bridgework and the sepsis that surrounded it. About this time bacteriology became established and the findings of bacteriologists added fuel to the fire of Hunter's condemnations. Radiography, which at first helped the dentist, now gave irrefutable evidence of disease surrounding the roots of pulpless teeth.

Whilst the theory of focal infection was not enunciated by Billings [4] until 1918, Hunter's condemnations started a reaction to root canal therapy, and the wholesale removal of both non-vital and perfectly healthy teeth began. The blame for obscure diseases was placed on the dentition and, as dentists could not refute this theory, countless mouths were mutilated. Naturally not all dentists accepted this wholesale dental destruction. Some, particularly in continental Europe, continued to save teeth in spite of the focal sepsis theory.

It is difficult to know why continental dentists disregarded this theory and one explanation may be that continental patients equated the loss of teeth with a loss of virility and therefore did not allow their dentists to mutilate their dentitions. Alternatively it could be that continental dentists were not so readily swayed by fashion as were their Anglo-Saxon colleagues.

Modern endodontics

The re-emergence of endodontics as a respectable branch of dental science began in the 1930s [14,34]. The occurrence and degree of bacteraemia during tooth extraction were shown to depend on the severity of periodontal disease and the amount of tissue damage at operation. The incongruity between bacteriological findings in the treatment of chronic oral infection and the histological picture was demonstrated. If the gingival sulcus was cauterized before extraction, microorganisms could not be demonstrated in the blood stream immediately postoperatively.

Gradually, the concept that a 'dead' tooth was not necessarily infected began to be accepted. Further, it was realized that the function and usefulness of the tooth depended on the integrity of the periodontal tissues and not on the vitality of the pulp [28]. Another important advance was the formulation of the 'hollow tube' theory [42], which was later questioned in research using sterile polyethylene tube implants in rats [52,53]. The tissue surrounding the lumina of clean, disinfected tubes, which were closed at one end, was relatively free of inflammation and displayed a normal capacity for repair. When such tubes were filled with sterile autoclaved muscle or muscle contaminated with Gram-negative cocci, the inflammatory reaction was only severe around the openings of the tubes containing contaminated muscle. These findings changed the emphasis of the 'hollow tube' theory, and stress is now placed on the microbial contents of the tube. If the tube contains microorganisms then the potential for repair is far less favourable than when the lumen of the tube is clean and sterile [54]. This situation is likely to be found in most root canals requiring treatment.

The concept that 'apical seal' was important led to the search for filling and sealing materials which are stable, non-irritant and provide a perfect seal at the apical foramen. With the more recent realization of the importance of coronal leakage [44,45], total obturation of the root canal space has assumed much greater importance.

Until relatively recently, endodontists were preoccupied with the perceived effects of various potent drugs on the microorganisms within the root canal rather than effective cleaning, shaping and filling of the canal space. This preoccupation diverted attention from the more pertinent problem of the effect of such drugs on the adjacent tissues. Antiseptics that kill bacteria are toxic to living tissue and act for a short period [5]; the most effective method of eliminating bacteria from root canals is instrumentation combined with irrigation.

Scope of endodontics

The extent of the subject has altered considerably in the last 50 years. Formerly, endodontic treatment confined itself to root canal filling techniques by conventional methods; even endodontic surgery, which is an extension of these methods, was considered to be in the field of oral surgery. Modern endodontics has a much wider field [2] and includes the following:

1. Diagnosis of oral pain.
2. Protection of the healthy pulp from disease or injury.
3. Pulp capping (both indirect and direct).
4. Pulpotomy (both conventional and partial).
5. Pulpectomy.
6. Root canal treatment of infected root canals.
7. Surgical endodontics, which includes apicectomy, hemisection, root amputation and replantation.

Role of microorganisms

The Chinese considered that dental abscesses were caused by small organisms, worms, which were held responsible until the 18th century. At the end of the 19th century Miller [29] was demonstrating the role of bacteria in root canal infection, and noted that different microorganisms were found in the root canal compared with the open pulp chamber. Shortly afterwards, systematic culturing of root canals was undertaken [36]. Unfortunately, these methods, which were potentially so valuable for improving root canal treatment, were used to condemn much of the dentistry done at the time [22]. During the 1930s microbiological techniques were used to re-establish the scientific basis of root canal treatment; however, techniques at that time only readily identified aerobic bacteria, and led to confusing results in later clinical studies [3,46]. This resulted in clinicians being complacent about the role of microorganisms, and performing treatment simply as a technical exercise.

The development of anaerobic culturing allowed many unknown microorganisms present in root canals to be grown [30]. This rapidly led to the demonstration of the majority of canal microorganisms being anaerobes [25,47], and the realization that canals previously considered sterile contained anaerobes alone. Further, when traumatized teeth were examined, there was a close correlation between the presence of anaerobic bacteria in the root canal and a periapical radiolucency [47]. This was later demonstrated experimentally in teeth where the pulp tissue had been removed; only in those where the pulp was infected did periapical inflammation occur [31]. Anaerobic culturing of root canals is not a technique for everyday clinical use; however, the research has given rational explanations for pulp disease and its treatment [48]. With rapid increase in knowledge, the anaerobic root canal bacteria are continually being reclassified. Only a few years ago *Bacteroides* were being reported as major pathogens of root canals [20], yet they have already been reclassified into two new genera, *Prevotella* and *Porphyromonas*, according to their ability to ferment carbohydrate [48]. Classification is now based on biochemical tests and is rapidly being dominated by molecular biologists. Bacteria, which previously could not be cultured and so were considered absent, are now being found with increasing frequency, and it is likely that the flora of root canals will appear very different in a few years as knowledge expands.

Most root canal infections contain a mixture of bacteria [12,13,47], and it has been shown that the relative proportions of different bacteria are determined by environmental conditions [13]. If a mixture of bacteria is inoculated into root canals at a fixed proportion, their relative numbers change over time, with a decline in aerobes and an increase in anaerobes [13]. Further, it has been established that combinations of bacteria are more likely to survive than inocula of single species, e.g. *Prevotella oralis* [12]. It is clear that one species can produce substances that others can metabolize in order to survive [48].

Bacteria are normally confined to the root canal system in pulpless teeth [32] and it is unusual for periapical lesions to contain bacteria unless there is an acute abscess. At the orifice of the root canal a large number of inflammatory cells are normally found and they prevent the bacteria from entering the tissues [38].

Tissue response to root canal infection

The presence of bacteria, their byproducts or damaged tissue in the root canal can cause periradicular inflammation, typically at the apical foramen but also around the foramina of any lateral or accessory canals, or at a fracture. The periradicular inflammation prevents the spread of infection from the tooth into the alveolar bone, otherwise osteomyelitis would result. The inflammatory lesion contains numerous inflammatory cells, e.g. polymorphonuclear leukocytes, macrophages, lymphocytes and plasma cells. The interaction between these cells and the antigenic substances from the root canal results in the release of a large number of inflammatory mediators. The inflammatory mediators include neuropeptides, the complement system, lysozymes and metabolites of arachidonic acid [49]. Prostaglandins and leukotrienes play an important role in the development of periradicular lesions [27,50].

As long as antigens emerge from canal foramina, there will be a continuing inflammatory response, mediated in a number of different ways. This is a very dynamic response to rapidly multiplying bacteria in the root canal, and may not be readily apparent to the clinician observing a radiograph or a histologist examining a slide of fixed cells. Effective elimination of the microorganisms allows inflammation to subside and healing to occur.

Quality assurance

The general public across the world now expect professional people to deliver a high standard of service; dentistry, and in particular endodontic treatment, is no exception. The European Society of Endodontology has recently issued quality guidelines for endodontic treatment [11]. It is essential that dental practices have a quality control system to ensure that each step in history, diagnosis and treatment is carried out in a logical and consistent manner. This is to ensure a high standard of care and treatment. Patients are increasingly well-informed and will not tolerate poor standards, e.g. in sterilization procedures, or out-of-date views.

Those dentists who have undertaken further training to become specialists are expected to achieve consistently high standards in diagnosis and treatment. However, general practitioners cannot continue to practise in the way they were taught at dental school many years ago; they must keep up to date and offer referral to an appropriate specialist when the treatment required is beyond their skill. This change has already occurred in the USA and is spreading to other countries.

Almost all endodontic procedures can be carried out with a predictably high rate of success. It has long been reported that root canal treatment has a success rate of over 90% [21,23,26]. It is essential that individual practitioners achieve similar rates of success, and that their treatment conforms to published guidelines. Success can be measured in different ways and it is insufficient to rely on clinical evidence alone; the use of radiography for follow-up is essential [19].

Recent developments

Pulpal damage in the main is caused by dental caries, infection consequent to trauma or infection as a result of operative dentistry. With a reduced incidence of dental caries, greater emphasis on preventing sports injuries and preparation of smaller cavities combined with better restorative materials in operative dentistry, the number of teeth with damaged pulps should decline. This will probably not result in lower demand for endodontic treatment, as patient expectations will continue to increase. The degree to which adhesive restorative materials will be successful in preventing pulpal damage in clinical practice is another unquantifiable variable.

Diagnosis of pulp disease is on occasions difficult, and hopes of new equipment to facilitate knowledge of the state of the pulp have not yet been realized clinically, although research into laser Doppler flowmetry, which assesses blood flow, as opposed to established methods of stimulating neural activity, continues [24,33,35]. Most research has involved young teeth with large pulps, and it may be challenging to develop equipment that produces good signals from a pulp which has receded in a tooth which may be heavily restored.

Research into new radiographic imaging systems is still progressing [37], but as yet no simple-to-use and clinically reliable system is available. When one is produced with a simplified and more comfortable sensor, it is likely to be expensive. Simultaneously, recent advances in film technology have achieved the maintenance of radiograph quality with a substantial reduction in radiation exposure [40]. The many problems experienced with present radiographic methods can to a large extent be eliminated by accurate technique.

Preparation of root canals has not altered substantially in recent years. Most of the short-cut approaches have not stood the test of time. File manufacturers have begun to produce instruments with safe tips that will not ledge preparations so easily. This has probably allowed canal preparation techniques to incorporate some limited rotation of files, which has for so long been considered incorrect. Developments are occurring with different materials for files, file sizes and tapers, but it is too early to say whether they will have a profound effect on canal preparation. There have been no recent major changes in canal obturation, although research is concerned with developing yet more ways to introduce heated gutta-percha into the canal system.

There has been a quiet revolution in endodontic surgery. Apart from a reduction in indications, because root canal retreatment is more predictably successful than root-end surgery [1], root-end preparation and obturation have altered. Gone is the indiscriminate use of a bur to cut the root-end cavity, and in its place is ultrasonic preparation with specially shaped tips that clean and shape the end of the root canal much more effectively and safely. The use of amalgam for root-end filling has ceased, with zinc oxide–eugenol materials being in vogue [10,39], and exciting developments occurring in alternative materials [51].

The importance of good coronal restoration of root filled teeth has been highlighted [45], and this is facilitated by the use of adhesive materials where appropriate, the placement of suitable bases and well-fitting restorations.

Endodontic referral practice is undertaking more root canal retreatment because of technical deficiencies in the original treatment. In many cases this is difficult and challenging but success can be very rewarding, particularly when the alternative is extraction. It is perhaps encouraging that many more patients are refusing to allow a tooth with an exposed or infected pulp to be extracted, but instead ask for it to be saved by root canal treatment, which in most cases is better for oral health.

References

1. ALLEN RK, NEWTON CW, BROWN CE (1989) A statistical analysis of surgical and nonsurgical endodontic retreatment cases. *Journal of Endodontics* **15**, 261–266.
2. AMERICAN ASSOCIATION OF ENDODONTISTS (1994) *Glossary – Contemporary Terminology for Endodontics*, 5th edn. Chicago, IL, USA: American Association of Endodontists.
3. BENDER IB, SELTZER S, TURKENKOPF S (1964) To culture or not to culture? *Oral Surgery, Oral Medicine, Oral Pathology* **18**, 527–540.

4. BILLINGS F (1918) *Focal Infection*. New York, NY, USA: Appleton.

5. CHONG BS, PITT FORD TR (1992) The role of intracanal medication in root canal treatment. *International Endodontic Journal* **25**, 97–106.

6. CRUSE WP, BELLIZZI R (1980) A historic review of endodontics, 1689–1963, Part 1. *Journal of Endodontics* **6**, 495–499.

7. CRUSE WP, BELLIZZI R (1980) A historic review of endodontics, 1689–1963, Part 2. *Journal of Endodontics* **6**, 532–535.

8. CRUSE WP, BELLIZZI R (1980) A historic review of endodontics, 1689–1963, Part 3. *Journal of Endodontics* **6**, 576–580.

9. CURSON I (1965) History and endodontics. *Dental Practitioner and Dental Record* **15**, 435–439.

10. DORN SO, GARTNER AH (1990) Retrograde filling materials: a retrospective success–failure study of amalgam, EBA, and IRM. *Journal of Endodontics* **16**, 391–393.

11. EUROPEAN SOCIETY OF ENDODONTOLOGY (1994) Concensus report of the European Society of Endodontology on quality guidelines for endodontic treatment. *International Endodontic Journal* **27**, 115–124.

12. FABRICIUS L, DAHLEN G, HOLM SE, MÖLLER AJR (1982) Influence of combinations of oral bacteria on periapical tissues of monkeys. *Scandinavian Journal of Dental Research* **90**, 200–206.

13. FABRICIUS L, DAHLEN G, ÖHMAN AE, MÖLLER AJR (1982) Predominant indigenous oral bacteria isolated from infected root canals after varied times of closure. *Scandinavian Journal of Dental Research* **90**, 134–144.

14. FISH EW, MACLEAN I (1936) The distribution of oral streptococci in the tissues. *British Dental Journal* **61**, 336–362.

15. GROSSMAN LI (1976) Endodontics 1776–1976: a bicentennial history against the background of general dentistry. *Journal of the American Dental Association* **93**, 78–87.

16. GUERINI V (1909) *History of Dentistry*. Philadelphia, PA, USA: Lea and Febiger.

17. GUTMANN JL (1987) History. In: Cohen S, Burns RC. (eds) *Pathways of the Pulp*, 4th edn, pp 756–782. St Louis, MO, USA; Mosby-Year Book.

18. GUTMANN JL, HARRISON JW (1991) *Surgical Endodontics*, pp. 3–41. Boston, MA, USA: Blackwell Scientific Publications.

19. GUTMANN JL, PITT FORD TR (1992) Problems in the assessment of success and failure. In: Gutmann JL, Dumsha TC, Lovdahl PE, Hovland EJ (eds) *Problem Solving in Endodontics. Prevention, Identification and Management*, 2nd edn, pp. 1–11. St Louis, MO, USA; Mosby-Year Book.

20. HAAPASALO M (1989) *Bacteroides* spp. in dental root canal infections. *Endodontics and Dental Traumatology* **5**, 1–10.

21. HARTY FJ, PARKINS BJ, WENGRAF AM (1970) Success rate in root canal therapy – a retrospective study of conventional cases. *British Dental Journal* **128**, 65–70.

22. HUNTER W (1911) The role of sepsis and antisepsis in medicine. *Lancet* **1**, 79–86.

23. INGLE JI, BAKLAND LK (1994) *Endodontics*, 4th edn, pp. 21–44. Malvern, PA, USA: Williams & Wilkins.

24. INGOLFSSON AER, TRONSTAD L, RIVA CE (1994) Reliability of laser Doppler flowmetry in testing vitality of human teeth. *Endodontics and Dental Traumatology* **10**, 185–187.

25. KANTZ WE, HENRY CA (1974) Isolation and classification of anaerobic bacteria from intact chambers of non-vital teeth in man. *Archives of Oral Biology* **19**, 91–96.

26. KEREKES K, TRONSTAD L (1979) Long-term results of endodontic treatment performed with a standardized technique. *Journal of Endodontics* **5**, 83–90.

27. MCNICHOLAS S, TORABINEJAD M, BLANKENSHIP J, BAKLAND L (1991) The concentration of prostaglandin E_2 in human periradicular lesions. *Journal of Endodontics* **17**, 97–100.

28. MARSHALL JA (1928) The relation to pulp-canal therapy of certain anatomical characteristics of dentin and cementum. *Dental Cosmos* **70**, 253–263.

29. MILLER WD (1894) An introduction to the study of the bacterio-pathology of the dental pulp. *Dental Cosmos* **36**, 505–528.

30. MÖLLER AJR (1966) Microbiological examination of root canals and periapical tissues of human teeth, pp. 1–380. Thesis. Gothenberg, Sweden: Akademiforlaget.

31. MÖLLER AJR, FABRICIUS L, DAHLEN G, ÖHMAN AE, HEYDEN G (1981) Influence on periapical tissues of indigenous oral bacteria and necrotic pulp tissue in monkeys. *Scandinavian Journal of Dental Research* **89**, 475–484.

32. NAIR PNR (1987) Light and electron microscopic studies of root canal flora and periapical lesions. *Journal of Endodontics* **13**, 29–39.

33. ODOR TM, PITT FORD TR (1996) Effect of wavelength and bandwidth on the clinical reliability of laser Doppler recordings. *Endodontics and Dental Traumatology* **12**, 9–15.

34. OKELL CC, ELLIOTT SD (1935) Bacteraemia and oral sepsis with special reference to the aetiology of subacute endocarditis. *Lancet* **2**, 869–872.

35. OLGART L, GAZELIUS B, LINDH-STROMBERG U (1988) Laser Doppler flowmetry in assessing vitality in luxated permanent teeth. *International Endodontic Journal* **21**, 300–306.

36. ONDERDONK TW (1901) Treatment of unfilled root canals. *International Dental Journal* **22**, 20–22.

37. ONG EY, PITT FORD TR (1995) Comparison of Radiovisiography with radiographic film in root length determination. *International Endodontic Journal* **28**, 25–29.

38. PITT FORD TR (1982) The effects on the periapical tissues of bacterial contamination of the filled root canal. *International Endodontic Journal* **15**, 16–22.

39. PITT FORD TR, ANDREASEN JO, DORN SO, KARIYAWASAM SP (1994) Effect of IRM root end fillings on

healing after replantation. *Journal of Endodontics* **20**, 381–385.

40. POWELL-CULLINGFORD AW, PITT FORD TR (1993) The use of E–speed film for root canal length determination. *International Endodontic Journal* **26**, 268–272.

41. PRINZ H (1945) *Dental Chronology. A Record of the More Important Historic Events in the Evolution of Dentistry.* London, UK: Kimpton.

42. RICKERT UG, DIXON CM (1931) The controlling of root surgery. Paris, France: Eighth International Dental Congress. **IIIa**, pp 15–22.

43. ROBERTS DH, SOWRAY JH (1987) *Local Analgesia in Dentistry*, 3rd edn, pp. 1–4. Oxford, UK: Wright.

44. SAUNDERS WP, SAUNDERS EM (1990) Assessment of leakage in the restored pulp chamber of endodontically treated multirooted teeth. *International Endodontic Journal* **23**, 28–33.

45. SAUNDERS WP, SAUNDERS EM (1994) Coronal leakage as a cause of failure in root-canal therapy: a review. *Endodontics and Dental Traumatology* **10**, 105–108.

46. SELTZER S, TURKENKOPF S, VITO A, GREEN D, BENDER IB (1964) A histologic evaluation of periapical repair following positive and negative root canal cultures. *Oral Surgery, Oral Medicine, Oral Pathology* **17**, 507–532.

47. SUNDQVIST G (1976) Bacteriological studies of necrotic dental pulps, pp. 1–94. Thesis. Umea, Sweden: University of Umea.

48. SUNDQVIST G (1994) Taxonomy, ecology, and pathogenicity of the root canal flora. *Oral Surgery, Oral Medicine, Oral Pathology* **78**, 522–530.

49. TORABINEJAD M (1994) Mediators of acute and chronic periradicular lesions. *Oral Surgery, Oral Medicine, Oral Pathology* **78**, 511–521.

50. TORABINEJAD M, COTTI E, JUNG T (1992) Concentration of leukotriene B_4 in symptomatic and asymptomatic periapical lesions. *Journal of Endodontics* **18**, 205–208.

51. TORABINEJAD M, HONG CU, LEE SJ, MONSEF M, PITT FORD TR (1995) Investigation of mineral trioxide aggregate for root-end filling in dogs. *Journal of Endodontics* **21**, 603–608.

52. TORNECK CD (1966) Reaction of rat connective tissue to polyethylene tube implants. Part I. *Oral Surgery, Oral Medicine, Oral Pathology* **21**, 379–387.

53. TORNECK CD (1967) Reaction of rat connective tissue to polyethylene tube implants. Part II. *Oral Surgery, Oral Medicine, Oral Pathology* **24**, 674–683.

54. WU MK, MOORER WR, WESSELINK PR (1989) Capacity of anaerobic bacteria enclosed in a simulated root canal to induce inflammation. *International Endodontic Journal* **22**, 269–277.

2

General and systemic aspects of endodontics

D.A. McGowan

Introduction

It might be questioned whether there are any systemic aspects of endodontology worthy of serious consideration. However, periapical infection can occasionally cause serious systemic upset, and the success of endodontic treatment may also be modified by general factors. With more predictable modern endodontic techniques, and greater understanding of the underlying microbiology and antibiotic therapy, a compromised medical status is becoming less of a contraindication to endodontic treatment. However, it is important that this is undertaken by a competent operator and with the appropriate precautions, together with any necessary advice from the patient's physician.

An underlying medical problem may explain an incomplete and less prompt response to treatment than expected. In the case of infective endocarditis, there is convincing evidence of a connection between dental treatment and infection, although it is weakly expressed in root canal treatment.

The dentist is largely dependent on the medical history to identify systemic disease or therapy which may be significant, although if endodontic treatment is not urgent, doubtful information can be checked with the patient's medical practitioner. Many patients have systemic disorders, which are well-controlled by therapy and therefore unlikely to influence the outcome of dental treatment, but the therapy itself may raise problems such as drug interactions. Comprehensive and sensible treatment planning, based on a careful analysis of the information gathered from thorough examination and history taking, is the patient's best protection from harm, and the dentist's best protection from criticism, legal or otherwise.

The fear of transmission of human immunodeficiency virus (HIV) or hepatitis viruses has highlighted the fact that up-to-date guidelines for cross-infection control must be as rigorously applied in endodontics as in any other aspect of the dentist's work [5].

Differential diagnosis of dental pain

The diagnosis of pulpal pain is a common-place task for the experienced dentist and is discussed in detail in Chapter 4, but the differential diagnosis of pain in the teeth, jaws and face is wider than is sometimes appreciated. Pain may be referred from a distant origin, it may have an unusual local cause, or it may even be of psychogenic origin in the absence of organic disease, and may be modified by apparently unrelated factors. These wider aspects must be constantly borne in mind and carefully considered, especially if the pattern of presentation is unusual, the examination findings are sparse or conflicting, or if pain persists in spite of apparently successful treatment.

The essence of good clinical practice is a methodical and disciplined approach: with history, followed by examination, followed by radiography, followed by analysis and conclusion. This is not a novel approach, but how often is one guilty of a quick glance at a radiograph and jumping to a conclusion – usually right, but sometimes embarrassingly wrong!

Pain history

A thorough pain history will point to a diagnosis in most cases, or at least suggest areas where investigation may be most fruitful. The patient should be asked to describe the pain without being asked leading questions (Table 2.1).

Examination

Visual examination of a patient commences with his or her entry to the surgery, and observation of the general demeanour can be revealing. Observation of the face with special reference to symmetry, particularly of the cheeks, the mandibular angle region and the nasolabial folds, can give a clue to the early recognition of swelling, and a glance in a mirror by the patient may confirm the suspicion. Observation of the patient's face in conversation can also alert the clinician to quite subtle neurological deficit or simply guarding of tender areas. Flinching from examination may be a more accurate indication of tenderness than response to questioning during examination. The observation of mandibular movements is the essential preliminary to examination of temporomandibular joint function.

It would be tedious to list all the features of a comprehensive examination of the teeth and jaws, but it is perhaps worth stressing that the soft tissues of the cheeks, palate, tongue and floor of the mouth can also yield vital information. The necessity or desirability of detailed occlusal examination depends on the circumstances of practice, and there are wide differences of opinion as to the significance of minor variations from the theoretical norm. However, there is no disputing the prevalence of symptoms arising from dysfunction of the temporomandibular apparatus, and their importance in the differential diagnosis of orofacial pain. The maxillary sinus as a cause of pain is considered below.

Table 2.1 Pain history

Description	Describe the pain in your own words.
Duration	How long have you been having pain?
	Have you had pain like this before?
Site	Where exactly is your pain?
	Does it spread anywhere else?
Nature	What does it feel like?
	Is it a sharp pain or a dull pain?
Periodicity	When do you get the pain?
	Does it come and go?
	Is there any particular pattern to the pain?
Associated symptoms	Do you notice anything else wrong?
Precipitating	
or relieving factors	Does anything make it worse?
	Does anything make it better?
	What painkillers have you taken, and to what effect?

Thermal or electrical stimulation of suspect teeth, differential local anaesthetic injections and removal of restorations all have their place in diagnosis, and radiography is essential, but all these techniques must supplement history and examination, and never supplant them.

Psychogenic pain

The orofacial region (including the teeth) is a common site for the expression of pain or discomfort as a manifestation of psychiatric disease or disorder. It may represent anything from a plea for help in unhappiness to a symptom of frank psychosis, or more commonly, neurosis. The dentist should avoid being manipulated by the patient, or perhaps even by the patient's family, into offering inappropriate treatment when the diagnosis is uncertain and the evidence conflicting. It is hard to refuse treatment and to seem unsympathetic, but the likelihood of further escalating demands should be borne in mind. It is sometimes wiser to delay active treatment and to advise that spontaneous improvement may occur or, even if there should be deterioration, that location of the source should be easier and hence diagnosis assisted. The watchword is: 'The treatment shall do the patient no harm'. The dental practitioner has the opportunity to refer the patient for a second opinion where the diagnosis continues to be elusive.

Patients with psychogenic facial pain commonly exhibit certain characteristics which may help recognition of the problem. The reported duration of the pain, prior to seeking treatment, is often longer than might reasonably be expected, and the stated severity is out of proportion to the distress, disturbance of life or self-therapy. There may be an obvious family or social gain for the sufferer. The pain may not follow anatomical boundaries and may characteristically be described as 'gripping' in nature. It does not in itself disturb sleep, though there may be a coincident disturbance of sleep pattern. Other chronic pain conditions such as headache, low back pain and abdominal or pelvic pain are frequently present, and there have often been recent distressing life events, such as bereavement, divorce or job loss. Psychiatric

treatment may be curative, or at least supportive, and any embarrassment about direct referral may be eased by using a dental specialist or general medical practitioner as an intermediary.

Maxillary sinus

The close proximity of the maxillary sinuses to the upper teeth can lead to diagnostic confusion and the risk of surgical penetration [20]. The distinction between toothache and sinusitis can be difficult unless there is either obvious dental disease or a typical acute or recurrent sinusitis with nasal discharge. Acute sinusitis rarely occurs without preceding symptoms of 'a cold', and tenderness to pressure of a whole quadrant of teeth is characteristic. Periapical infection of premolar or molar teeth may on occasions lead to purulent discharge into the sinus, and indeed it is remarkable that this is not more common. Penetration of the sinus wall or even the sinus lining by endodontic instruments, or during periradicular surgery, may lead to acute sinusitis from bacterial contamination and, though spontaneous resolution of symptoms may follow, prescription of an antibiotic and ephedrine nasal drops is prudent.

Small communications will usually heal spontaneously, and in the case of periradicular surgery the replacement of the surgical flap is sufficient to seal the opening. The identity of microorganisms involved in sinus infection is often unclear, but broad-spectrum antibiotics, e.g. doxycycline, are favoured; doxycycline is conveniently administered in a single daily 200 mg dose. Alternatively, amoxycillin, which is of proven benefit in periapical infection, may be preferred. It is customary to maintain treatment for 5 days, though, since sinus contamination is transient, one or two large doses of amoxycillin may be just as effective. If there is poor sinus drainage, e.g. a history of chronic sinusitis, nasal drops (0.5% ephedrine) should be prescribed. Inhalations such as menthol and eucalyptus have a soothing effect.

A connection between sinus disease and root canal treatment has been reported in a single study in Austria [3]. A number of patients suffering from aspergillosis of the maxillary sinus had previously had root canal treatment using zinc oxide-based cements, which have been shown to promote cultures of *Aspergillus*.

Systemic disease and endodontics

Systemic conditions rarely contraindicate endodontic treatment, but some problems are worth considering. Disabled or debilitated patients cannot be expected readily to tolerate complex and lengthy treatment procedures, but even in severe ill-health, some patients have a strong desire to retain their natural teeth, and the dentist's duty is to try to respond. Even in terminal illness simple treatment can be a great aid to comfort, masticatory function and morale. Good decision-making is dependent on frank and thoughtful discussion with the patient and his or her medical advisers. In some conditions, for example, cardiac abnormalities, endodontic treatment should only be carried out if a high standard of treatment can be achieved, and referral may be indicated.

Both the patient's general prognosis and the prognosis for the tooth being treated must be considered, and it may be necessary to choose the radical option of extraction. In chronic disease subject to cyclical remission, whether it be spontaneous or in response to therapy, it is obviously sensible to time dental intervention to coincide with optimum physical state.

This is particularly true of haematological disorders, such as leukaemia, especially if the patient receives periodic transfusion or cycles of chemotherapy. Sufferers from haemorrhagic diatheses will not require factor replacement or antifibrinolytic therapy for root canal treatment alone, but will do so if endodontic surgery is needed. When it is being planned, the patient's haematologist should be consulted so that the patient can be adequately prepared.

An object of root canal treatment is resolution of periapical inflammation, and when the capacity for healing is reduced, then the response to treatment might be expected to be disappointing. There is, however, no hard evidence to show that the presence of systemic disease has a major influence on the healing of periapical lesions. Claims that diabetes or steroid medication are important have not been substantiated, and opinion now seems to favour a more positive approach to treatment even in immuno-compromised patients [13]. Progressive narrowing of pulp chambers and root canals in patients receiving substantial doses of corticosteroids following renal transplantation has been observed [23]; the effect was monitored radiographically and appeared to be due to excessive dentine formation. As infection of transplanted kidneys is caused by different organisms from infective endocarditis, there would not appear to be a need for antibiotic prophylaxis [14].

Endodontics and infective endocarditis

In the last decade, recommendations on prevention of infective endocarditis following dentistry have become much more straightforward and practical, and an international consensus appears to be developing. A major influence has been the reports of a working party of the British Society for Antimicrobial Chemotherapy [6–8,10]. The working party suggested that the only dental treatment procedures likely to produce significant bacteraemia were 'extractions, or scaling, or surgery involving the gingival tissues'. The exclusion of endodontic procedures was deliberate, as it was felt that *significant* bacteraemia would not arise from manipulation of instruments within the root canal, and that experimental studies [1,2,4] indicated that only by deliberately prolonged and exaggerated disturbance of the periapical tissues with an instrument passed through the apical foramen, or in the course of open periradicular surgery, could detectable bacteraemia be produced.

The working party was well aware of the variety of clinical practice, and presented its conclusions as general advice which would, and should, be modified in individual circumstances by a thoughtful clinician. It might be prudent to use antibiotic prophylaxis for endodontic manipulation in the presence of acute periapical infection or gross periodontal disease with mobility. The antibiotic regime recommended – a single 3 g dose of amoxycillin taken orally under supervision 1 h before treatment – was intended to be a simple way of producing a reliably high and prolonged blood level of a penicillin and it has certainly proved acceptable to the dental profession in the UK [16]. A second dose, 6–8 hours later, is recommended on the basis of animal experimental studies [22] and provides extra assurance with minimal inconvenience for high-risk patients. In case of hypersensitivity to penicillins or exposure more than once in the preceding month, clindamycin 600 mg is now advised, replacing erythromycin, which frequently produced nausea and vomiting in the doses formerly recommended. The working party has repeatedly invited reports of apparent failure of the regimes advised, but so far there has been little response.

There is general agreement that prophylaxis should be targeted on these patients with enhanced susceptibility to endocardial infection [10]. While there are subtle variations in the degree of risk associated with different predisposing cardiac lesions, it is sufficient for the dentist to regard as 'at risk' all patients with known rheumatic or congenital heart disease, or with murmurs associated with cardiac disease, or who have undergone valve replacement, or who have previously suffered an attack of infective endocarditis. Where there is a clear history of an episode of rheumatic fever and where this can be confirmed from records or by consultation with a physician, then the patient should be treated as 'at risk'. For all at-risk patients it is essential that endodontic treatment is carried out to a high standard to eliminate the root canal as a possible source of subsequent bacteraemia. Patients who have undergone coronary arterial bypass grafting are not at risk of endocarditis [10].

It is important to maintain optimum periodontal and dental health in patients at risk of endocarditis. Where treatment is required a simple method of reducing bacteraemia is use of a 0.2% chlorhexidine mouthwash preoperatively. The fewer live bacteria released into the circulation, the smaller is the likely risk of infection.

Periradicular surgery obviously falls within the definition of 'other surgery involving the gingival tissues', and so antibiotic cover is indicated, but there are other considerations in at-risk patients. Surgery should only be undertaken where it is clearly indicated (Chapter 9). Where appropriate root canal cleaning, shaping and filling, followed by periradicular surgery, can be undertaken in a single visit instead of over a number of episodes, each requiring antibiotic cover. Salvage procedures for teeth with poor prognosis (e.g. perforations) are inadvisable in at-risk patients. Replantation of avulsed teeth can be attempted in at-risk patients provided that the procedure is done under antibiotic cover, the tooth splinted and the endodontic follow-up is carried out by an experienced operator.

Endodontics in patients with prosthetic hip joints

The alleged connection between dental disease or treatment and late infection in patients who have undergone hip joint replacement is spurious [21]. There is no special risk to such patients from any form of dental treatment, and certainly not from endodontic procedures [9].

Use of antibiotics in endodontics

Antibiotics or other antimicrobial drugs kill susceptible bacteria or arrest their multiplication, and so allow the natural defence processes to combat infection, and healing to progress (Table 2.2). They neither directly relieve pain nor reduce swelling, nor do they compensate for inaccurate diagnosis. They should not be used to treat pulpitis, but reserved to control a spreading cellulitis or a periapical abscess in conjunction with drainage. Overuse should be avoided to prevent resistant strains of organisms developing.

The institution of drainage and the mechanical elimination of pus are the prime purposes of opening a root canal in an abscessed tooth. There are occasions when the ideal treatment is not feasible or is unsuccessful, and in such circumstances use of an

Table 2.2 Useful antibacterial drugs

Phenoxymethylpenicillin capsules, 250 mg
One or two 6-hourly at least 30 min before food for
4–7 days

Amoxycillin capsules, 250 mg
One or two 8-hourly for 4–7 days

Amoxycillin oral powder, 3 g sachet
3 g repeated after 8 h; also first choice for prophylaxis
of infective endocarditis

Erythromycin tablets, 250 mg
One or two 6-hourly for 4–7 days; prophylaxis of infective
endocarditis: 1.5 g (erythromycin stearate) 1 h before
operation and 500 mg 6 h later

Metronidazole tablets, 200 mg
One 8-hourly for 5 days

antibiotic is justified. The clinician must not allow the patient to dictate inappropriate prescription. In debilitated or immunocompromised patients, a case can be made for more liberal use of antibiotics.

Ideally, the choice of an antibiotic should be based on the results of identification and sensitivity testing of the microorganisms responsible for the infection, but this is seldom feasible in practice. The necessary laboratory procedures depend mainly on culture techniques, which require at least 24 h to produce meaningful results; anaerobic culturing is necessary as the majority of root canal pathogens are anaerobes [25]. Direct microscopy of stained samples yields little more information than general knowledge of the most prevalent pathogens. Fortunately, most of the bacteria likely to be associated with dentoalveolar infection are still sensitive to penicillins [18]. Amoxycillin may be preferred because of its efficient absorption after oral administration, and there is some evidence that two 3 g doses, 8 h apart, may be as effective as the traditional 5-day course of phenoxymethylpenicillin 250 mg four times a day [19]. For patients hypersensitive to penicillins, erythromycin (250 mg four times a day for 5 days) is a rational choice.

As strict anaerobes are important pathogens in dentoalveolar infection, so metronidazole has a place in therapy, especially where response to penicillin, amoxycillin or erythromycin is poor. Metronidazole (200 mg three times a day for 5 days) can be used either alone or in conjunction with the first-choice drug. A potential hazard of the use of wide-spectrum antibiotics is interference with absorption of the oestrogen component of combined oral contraceptives, with consequent loss of effect. Women taking such preparations concurrently should be advised not to rely on this method of contraception alone for 1 month after the end of the antibiotic course [15].

Control of pain and anxiety

Pain and anxiety control are central to successful endodontic treatment. The drugs available for local analgesia and for sedation are both safe and effective but, as with any potent therapeutic agent, need to be employed with skill and discretion, particularly in patients who are taking other medication regularly [24]. A whole spectrum of techniques of control of pain and anxiety are applicable in endodontics as in other dental treatment (Table 2.3). These range from simple persuasion and a comforting and sympathetic manner, through sedation to full general anaesthesia, and every patient will require some support. Local anaesthetic techniques are well-established, and 2–4 ml lignocaine 2% with 1 : 80 000 adrenaline is a safe and effective preparation for all patients [11]. An aspirating syringe system should be used to help avoid inadvertent intravascular injection. Only in very rare cases where true allergy to lignocaine is proven need an alternative solution, e.g. prilocaine, be used.

General anaesthesia is beyond the scope of this chapter but conscious sedation using either an inhaled mixture of nitrous oxide and oxygen, or intravenous administration of midazolam, is a safe and effective way of overcoming anxiety and allowing the nervous but cooperative patient to accept treatment. Such techniques should only rarely be required for root canal treatment; periradicular surgery may more often require sedation. If a patient cannot tolerate root canal treatment without sedation at each visit, then the treatment plan should perhaps be simplified.

Table 2.3 Useful analgesics

Mild to moderate pain
Aspirin tablets, 300 mg (or aspirin tablets dispersible, 300 mg)
One to three every 4–6 h as necessary, maximum 4 g/day

Paracetamol tablets, 500 mg
One to two every 6 h as necessary, maximum 4 g/day

Ibuprofen tablets, 200 mg
One to two every 4–6 h as necessary, preferably after food, maximum 2.4 g/day

Moderate to severe pain
Dihydrocodeine tablets, 30 mg
30 mg every 4–6 h as necessary, after food, maximum 1.8 g/day

Pentazocine tablets, 25 mg
Two every 3–4 h after food, maximum 3 g/day

Severe pain
Pethidine tablets, 25 mg
Two to four every 4 h, maximum 6 g/day

Analgesics

Analgesics may be used to treat existing pain, or to reduce afterpain following surgery as a prophylactic measure prior to the local anaesthetic wearing off. Analgesics administered preoperatively are useful in reducing postoperative pain [17]. Aspirin and paracetamol remain the most effective and widely used remedies for local pain of mild to moderate severity. The contraindications to aspirin in patients with peptic ulceration or bleeding diatheses are well-known, but in addition it is now not advised in children for fear of causing Reye's syndrome. When paracetamol is used, it is essential to warn patients not to exceed the daily maximum dose of 4 g, because of the risk of severe and sometimes fatal liver damage. Other non-steroidal anti-inflammatory drugs (NSAIDs) such as diflunisal or ibuprofen may be used if preferred, though any advantage over the longer established drugs has yet to be clearly established.

Dihydrocodeine tartrate and pentazocine are used to combat more severe pain, but both frequently cause unpleasant side-effects, including dizziness and nausea, and their effectiveness is rather unpredictable. On the rare occasions that severe pain persists, then pethidine 50 mg, one or two tablets 4-hourly, can be given and the patient's condition reviewed the next day. Pethidine is a controlled drug, with special legal requirements for safe storage and prescription, so for this reason dihydrocodeine is more frequently used by dentists.

Local treatment, such as drainage and irrigation of a root canal, grinding a tooth free of occlusal contact, replacement of a failed temporary filling following root canal cleaning, or irrigation of a surgical wound, is a far more effective way of dealing with pain than the indiscriminate use of analgesics.

Dental Practitioners' Formulary

This formulary [12], which is published together with the *British National Formulary* jointly by the British Dental Association, British Medical Association and the Royal Pharmaceutical Society of Great Britain, is a succinct and authoritative guide to prescribing for the dentist and is regularly updated. It is an indispensable source of advice and a mine of information which should be at hand in every surgery. The sections on antibiotics and analgesics are particularly valuable, as are the tables of potential drug interactions and the section on medical emergencies in dental practice. For further information on medical complications in dentistry, the reader is referred to *Medical Problems in Dentistry* [24].

References

1. BAUMGARTNER JC, HEGGERS JP, HARRISON JW (1976) The incidence of bacteremias related to endodontic procedures. I. Nonsurgical endodontics. *Journal of Endodontics* **2**, 135–140.
2. BAUMGARTNER JC, HEGGERS JP, HARRISON JW (1977) Incidence of bacteremias related to endodontic procedures. II. Surgical endodontics. *Journal of Endodontics* **3**, 399–402.
3. BECK-MANNAGETTA J, NECEK D (1986) Radiologic findings in aspergillosis of the maxillary sinus. *Oral Surgery, Oral Medicine, Oral Pathology* **62**, 345–349.

4. BENDER IB, SELTZER S, TASHMAN S, MELOFF G (1963) Dental procedures in patients with rheumatic heart disease. *Oral Surgery, Oral Medicine, Oral Pathology* **16,** 466–473.

5. BRITISH DENTAL ASSOCIATION (1988) The control of cross–infection in dentistry. *British Dental Journal* **165,** 353–354.

6. BRITISH SOCIETY FOR ANTIMICROBIAL CHEMOTHERAPY (1982) The antibiotic prophylaxis of infective endocarditis. *Lancet* **2,** 1323–1326.

7. BRITISH SOCIETY FOR ANTIMICROBIAL CHEMOTHERAPY (1986) Prophylaxis of infective endocarditis. *Lancet* **1,** 1267.

8. BRITISH SOCIETY FOR ANTIMICROBIAL CHEMOTHERAPY (1990) Antibiotic prophylaxis of infective endocarditis. *Lancet* **335,** 88–89.

9. BRITISH SOCIETY FOR ANTIMICROBIAL CHEMOTHERAPY (1992) Case against antibiotic prophylaxis for dental treatment of patients with joint prostheses. *Lancet* **339,** 301.

10. BRITISH SOCIETY FOR ANTIMICROBIAL CHEMOTHERAPY (1992) Antibiotic prophylaxis and infective endocarditis. *Lancet* **339,** 1292–1293.

11. CAWSON RA, CURSON I, WHITTINGTON DR (1983) The hazards of dental local anaesthetics. *British Dental Journal* **154,** 253–258.

12. *DENTAL PRACTITIONERS' FORMULARY* (1992–1994) London: British Medical Association.

13. DEPAOLA LG, PETERSON DE, OVERHOLSER CD ET AL. (1986) Dental care for patients receiving chemotherapy. *Journal of the American Dental Association* **112,** 198–203.

14. FRENCH GL (1993) Ask the expert. *Pediatric Nephrology* **7,** 346.

15. GIBSON J, MCGOWAN DA (1994) Oral contraceptives and antibiotics: important considerations for dental practice. *British Dental Journal* **177,** 419–422.

16. HOLBROOK WP, HIGGINS B, SHAW TRD (1987) Recent changes in antibiotic prophylactic measures taken by dentists against infective endocarditis. *Journal of Antimicrobial Chemotherapy* **20,** 439–446.

17. JACKSON DL, MOORE PA, HARGREAVES KM (1989) Preoperative nonsteroidal anti-inflammatory medication for the prevention of postoperative dental pain. *Journal of the American Dental Association* **119,** 641–647.

18. LEWIS MAO, MACFARLANE TW, MCGOWAN DA (1988) Reliability of sensitivity testing of primary culture of acute dentoalveolar abscess. *Oral Microbiology and Immunology* **3,** 177–180.

19. LEWIS MAO, MCGOWAN DA, MACFARLANE TW (1986) Short-course high-dosage amoxycillin in the treatment of acute dento–alveolar abscess. *British Dental Journal* **161,** 299–302.

20. MCGOWAN DA, BAXTER PW, JAMES J (1993) *The Maxillary Sinus and its Dental Implications.* Oxford: Butterworth–Heinemann.

21. MCGOWAN DA, HENDREY ML (1985) Is antibiotic prophylaxis required for dental patients with joint replacements? *British Dental Journal* **158,** 336–338.

22. MCGOWAN DA, NAIR S, MACFARLANE TW, MACKENZIE D (1983) Prophylaxis of experimental endocarditis in rabbits using one or two doses of amoxycillin. *British Dental Journal* **155,** 88–90.

23. NASSTROM K, FORSBERG B, PETERSSON A, WESTESSON PL (1985) Narrowing of the dental pulp chamber in patients with renal diseases. *Oral Surgery, Oral Medicine, Oral Pathology* **59,** 242–246.

24. SCULLY C, CAWSON RA (1993) *Medical Problems in Dentistry,* 3rd edn. Oxford: Butterworth-Heinemann.

25. SUNDQVIST G (1994) Taxonomy, ecology, and pathogenicity of the root canal flora. *Oral Surgery, Oral Medicine, Oral Pathology* **78,** 522–530.

3

Pulp space anatomy and access cavities

R.T. Walker

Introduction

The major factors involved in the development of pulpal and periradicular disease are loss of integrity of coronal tooth substance and the entry of microorganisms into the dentine and pulp space. The chemomechanical removal of microorganisms, their substrate and products from the dentine and pulp space is the first aim of root canal treatment, with the second being the three-dimensional obliteration and sealing of the pulp space to prevent bacterial re-contamination.

A clear understanding of the anatomy of human teeth becomes an essential prerequisite to achieving the objectives of access, thorough cleaning, disinfection and obturation of the pulp space. Many of the problems encountered during endodontic treatment occur because of an inadequate understanding of the pulp space anatomy of teeth.

Both students and clinicians alike need to familiarize themselves with the irregularities, complexities and aberrations which are likely to occur within the pulp space. The importance of developing a visual picture of the expected locations and numbers of canals in a particular tooth cannot be overstressed.

Clinical radiographs show the forms of roots and pulp canals in two planes only. A third plane exists in a buccolingual direction. The pulp space volume is always much greater than the normal clinical radiograph would suggest. The internal anatomy of human teeth has been studied by many investigators who have provided a valuable insight into the size, shape and form of the pulp space. Methods of study have included replication techniques [9,18,27,57], ground sections [3,22,54], clearing techniques [30,38, 46,51,75] and radiography [5,29,34,35,42,43,

50,52,60,89]. Present-day knowledge of pulp space anatomy is based on research findings and individual case reports.

Nomenclature

Anatomically, the dental pulp space is surrounded by dentine to form the pulp–dentine complex. Dentine forms the bulk of the mineralized tissue of the tooth. The dentinal tubules, which are interconnected, make up 20–30% of the total volume of dentine [19,28]. The number of tubules per square millimetre more than doubles and the area occupied by tubules increases threefold from the dentine near the amelodentinal junction to that near the pulp [14]. These differences have a significant clinical effect on the permeability of dentine. It is now realized that the dentinal tubules are an important reservoir of microorganisms when pulpal necrosis occurs [45]. Exposure of infected tubules during root-end resection may serve as a direct route of contamination from unclean root canals into the periradicular tissues [23,65].

The *pulp space* is divided into two parts: the *pulp chamber* which is usually described as that portion within the crown, and the *pulp* or *root canal* which lies within the confines of the root. The pulp chamber is a single cavity, the dimensions of which vary according to the outline of the crown and the structure of the roots. Thus, if the crown has well-developed cusps the pulp chamber projects into well-developed *pulp horns*. In multi-rooted teeth the depth of the pulp chamber depends upon the position of the root furcation and may extend beyond the anatomical crown. In young teeth the outline of the pulp chamber resembles the shape of the exterior of the dentine. With age the dentinal tubules and the pulp chamber become reduced in size by the laying down of *peritubular dentine, secondary dentine* and *irritation dentine*, particularly in areas where there has been caries, attrition, abrasion and exposure to operative treatment (Figure 3.1). The pulp chamber may then become irregular in outline. There is a gradual decrease with age in pulp space volume and the number of nerves, blood vessels and cells within, but an increase in the fibrous and mineral components. The rate at

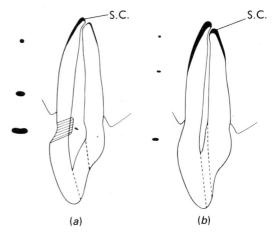

Figure 3.1 Alteration of pulp size with age. (a) Tooth of young adult; large pulp chamber with irritation dentine under tubules affected by cervical abrasion; small amount of secondary cementum (SC) at apex. (b) Tooth of older patient showing smaller pulp space and greater amounts of SC which have altered the relationship of the apical constriction to the foramen. Access cavities are indicated by dashed lines. To the left: cross-sections of the root canals are shown at selected levels.

which pulps age varies from one tooth to another, and from one patient to another. Calcific changes can lead to the pulp space appearing entirely obliterated radiographically. A residual canal, although radiographically unidentified, may remain within the root and be the route for bacteria to reach the apex and cause a periradicular radiolucency.

The pulp or root canals are continuous with the pulp chamber and normally their greatest diameter is at the pulp chamber level. Because roots tend to taper towards their apex, the canals also have a tapering form which ends in constricted openings at the root end, the *apical foramina*, which rarely open at the exact anatomical apex of the tooth. During root development the pulpal and periodontal tissues become separated, maintaining neural and vascular connections through the apical foramina.

The pulp space is complex and canals may divide and rejoin, and possess forms which are considerably more involved than many textbooks of anatomy imply. Many roots have additional canals and a variety of canal configurations. Eight separate pulp space configurations have been identified [75] (Figure 3.2). Generally, roots have a single

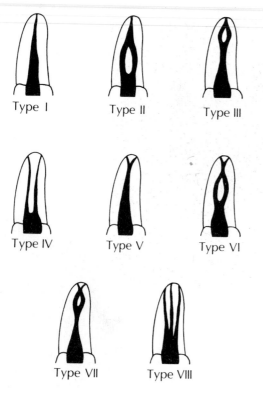

Figure 3.2 Types of canal configuration.

canal and single apical foramen (type I); however it is not uncommon for other canal complexities to be present and exit the root as one, two or three apical canals (types II–VIII).

Variations in the morphology of the dental pulp are caused by genetic and environmental influences. The canal configurations of human teeth are not only of clinical significance, but may be of great importance in understanding human evolution and contemporary biological variation. For example, a high frequency of single-rooted teeth with two canals suggests that the single-rooted condition represents a fusion, occurring in the relatively recent past, of two original roots.

Since roots tend to be broader buccolingually than they are mesiodistally, the pulp space is similar and oval in cross-section. The diameter of the root canal decreases towards the apical foramen and reaches its narrowest point 1.0–1.5 mm from the foramen. This point, the *apical constriction*, lies within dentine just prior to the first layers of cementum and is the narrowest point to which the canal tapers.

During root development the apical part of the pulp is described as being 'open' or having a 'blunderbuss' appearance. As the tooth matures the funnel-shaped foramen closes and constricts to a normal root shape with a small apical foramen. The position of the apical foramen may also alter relative to the root apex with the deposition of secondary cementum (Figure 3.1).

Accessory and lateral canals

The pulpal and periodontal tissues not only maintain connection through the apical foramina but also through *accessory* and *lateral* canals. A lateral canal can be found anywhere along the length of a root and tends to be at right angles to the main root canal. Accessory canals usually branch off the main root canal somewhere in the apical region. The presence of lateral canals in the furcation areas of molar teeth is well-documented and their incidence is high. Patent lateral canals are present in the coronal or middle third of 59% of molars [37]; 76% of molars have openings in the furcation [8]. It has been shown using a vascular injection technique that these auxiliary canals often had a greater diameter than the apical foramina, and the blood vessels passing through them often had a greater diameter than those in the apical foramina [32]. The accessory and lateral canals may be demonstrated by histological examination (Figure 3.3), clearing techniques (Figure 3.4), and clinical radiographs (Figure 3.5). The presence of these canals in teeth with diseased pulps allows an interchange of inflammatory breakdown products between the pulp space and the periradicular tissues which may influence the outcome of root canal treatment and the maintenance of periodontal health.

Location of apical foramina

The majority of endodontists consider that the apical extent of canal preparation should be determined by the position of the apical constriction in the region of the dentine–cementum junction (Figure 3.6). Provided that this point is not passed, the periradicular

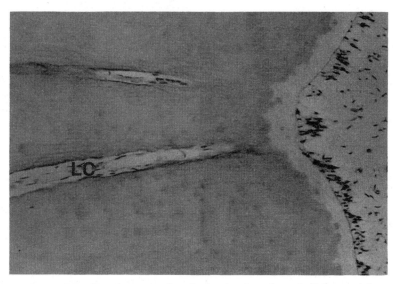

Figure 3.3 Histological section of tooth showing lateral canals (LC) containing vital tissue; the main part of the pulp is to the right.

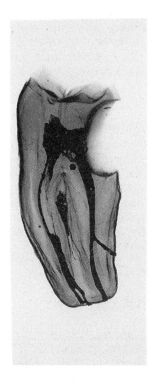

Figure 3.4 Cleared mandibular molar with a lateral canal in the distal root.

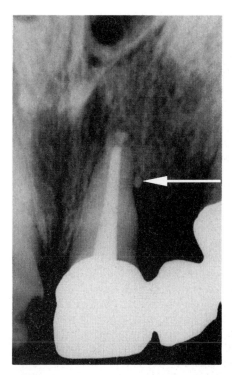

Figure 3.5 Radiograph of root-filled incisor showing sealer in a lateral canal and excess in the periradicular tissues (arrow).

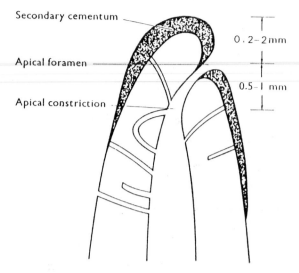

Secondary cementum

Apical foramen

Apical constriction

0.2–2 mm

0.5–1 mm

Figure 3.6 Diagrammatic section through apical third of root. The position of the apical foramen varies with age and may be 0.2–2.0 mm from the anatomical apex. The apical constriction may be 0.5–1.0 mm from the foramen.

tissues are not damaged during canal preparation and obturation.

Studies indicate that the apical foramina rarely coincide in position with the anatomical apex. According to various radiographic and morphological studies of different teeth [2,7,12,15,20,21,31,33,36,71], the average distance between the apical foramen and the most apical end of the root ranged between 0.2 and 2.0 mm. Furthermore, the apical constriction tends to occur about 0.5–1 mm from the apical foramen [12]. Ideally the apical constriction should be used as a natural 'stop' in root canal treatment, and the integrity of the constriction should be maintained during treatment if complications are to be avoided.

Pulp space anatomy and race

Racial variations in tooth form have interested descriptive and comparative anatomists, anthropologists, biologists, palaeontologists and dentists. These variations have not been totally explored because investigators have concentrated their efforts on the systematic description of dental crown morphology. The diverse aspects of root form and canal anatomy of human teeth have not received the same attention.

Variations in root form and number are likely to have a direct influence upon the configuration of the root canals in affected teeth. A variation which has received some attention is the three-rooted mandibular first molar. Surveys of population groups of Mongoloid origin indicate a high prevalence [47,67,69,70]. The prevalence of other Mongoloid root traits has not been studied to the same extent. Their projected influence upon pulp space anatomy is only now being realized. In clinical practice it is not always possible to make positive identification of these variations from radiographs, and there is a very definite need for clinicians to be made aware of the frequency of racially determined forms.

The descriptions of the frequently occurring root and canal forms of permanent teeth are based largely on studies conducted in Europe and North America, and relate to teeth of predominantly Caucasoid origin. Endodontic texts tend not to deal with the racial differences in root morphology or indeed the influences that known racial variations in root form may have upon the canal configurations of such teeth. In clinical practice, expectations are based upon the guidance that these texts give. The information presented may not be wholly applicable to teeth not of Caucasoid origin. For example, the average lengths of teeth, around which there is wide spread, apply to Caucasoid populations. Practitioners who regularly treat Negroid and Mongoloid populations are aware that these values do not coincide with their own clinical experience. Further studies of the morphology of samples of teeth of non-Caucasoid origin are required to establish the frequency of racially determined root and canal variations that may exist.

Pulp space anatomy and access cavities

Each line drawing (Figures 3.7–3.29) accompanying the description of pulp space anatomy represents, from left to right:

1. Longitudinal mesiodistal section, viewed from the lingual in anterior teeth and from the buccal in posterior teeth.

2. Longitudinal buccolingual section viewed from the mesial, and also the axial angulation of the tooth relative to the horizontal occlusal plane.
3. Horizontal sections through the root(s): (above) 3 mm from apex; (below) at the cervical level.
4. Incisal or occlusal view.

The outline of the access cavity is shown as a dashed line. The size of the pulp cavity is shown shortly after completion of root formation as a shaded area, and in old age by a black area. Each line drawing is accompanied by photographs of cleared specimens to give an insight into the variations of canal form which exist in the adult dentition.

Maxillary central and lateral incisors

The outlines and pulp cavities of these teeth are similar (Figures 3.7 and 3.8). Central incisors are larger, and on average 23 mm long. Lateral incisors are shorter with an average length of 21–22 mm. The canal form is usually type I, and it is extremely rare for these teeth to have more than one root or more than one root canal. Where abnormalities do occur they seem to affect the maxillary lateral incisor which may present with an extra root, second root canal, dens invaginatus, gemination or fusion [26,53,56,64].

The pulp chamber, when viewed labiopalatally, is seen to be pointed towards the incisal

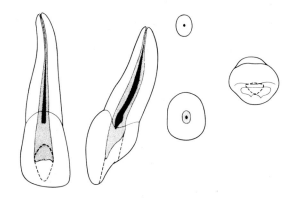

Figure 3.8 Maxillary lateral incisor with a type I configuration.

and widest at the cervical level. Mesiodistally both pulp chambers follow the general outline of their crowns and are thus widest at their incisal levels. The central incisors of young patients normally have three pulp horns. Lateral incisors usually have two pulp horns, and the incisal outline of the pulp chamber tends to be more rounded than that of central incisors.

The root canal differs greatly in outline when viewed mesiodistally and buccopalatally. The former view generally shows a fine straight canal that is seen on a radiograph. Buccopalatally the canal is very much wider and often shows a constriction just apical to the cervix; this view is rarely seen on radiographs and it is as well to remember that all canals have this third dimension when they are being accessed, shaped and filled. The canal is tapered with an oval or irregular cross-section cervically which becomes round near the apex. There is generally very little apical curvature in central incisors and where it is present it is usually distal or labial. However, the apex of lateral incisors is often curved, generally in a distal direction.

As the teeth age the anatomy of the pulp space alters with the deposition of secondary dentine. The roof of the pulp chamber recedes, in some cases to the cervical level, and the canal appears very narrow mesiodistally on a radiograph. However, if it is remembered that the diameter labiopalatally is much greater than that mesiodistally, it is often possible to negotiate a canal which appears very fine or non-existent on a pre-operative radiograph.

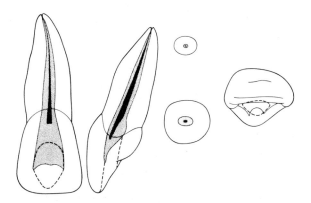

Figure 3.7 Maxillary central incisor with a type I configuration.

Maxillary canine

This is the longest tooth (average 26.5 mm). It seldom has more than one root canal; the pulp chamber is quite narrow, and since there is only one pulp horn it is pointed incisally. The general shape of the pulp space is similar to the central and lateral incisors, but as the root is much wider labiopalatally the pulp space follows this outline and is much wider in this plane than mesiodistally (Figure 3.9).

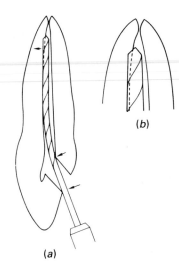

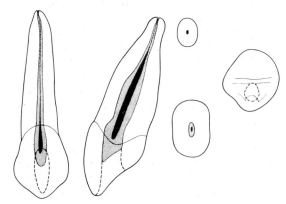

Figure 3.9 Maxillary canine with a type I configuration.

The type I root canal is oval and does not begin to become circular in cross-section until the apical third. The apical constriction is not as well-defined as in the central and lateral incisors. This, together with the fact that the root apex is often tapered and very thin, makes canal length measurement difficult. The canal is usually straight but may show a distal apical curvature, and less frequently a labial curvature; the curvature depends on the movement of the tooth during eruption.

Access cavities to maxillary incisors and canines

Access cavities in anterior teeth will vary in size and shape according to the dimension of the pulp. They should be designed so that instruments can reach the apical third of the root without bending, or binding against the walls of the access cavity or root canal. An access cavity that is too small and close to the cingulum leads to severe stresses in the instrument with binding against the access cavity walls and possible ledge formation apically (Figure 3.10).

Figure 3.10 (a) The access cavity is too small and close to the cingulum, therefore instruments do not lie passively in the canal and may ledge apically. It also hinders cleaning of the pulp chamber and near the apex. (b) Enlargement of the apex showing labial ledge and uninstrumented palatal side.

Ideally, the access cavity should extend far enough incisally to allow the unimpeded progress of the instrument to the apical part of the canal. Sometimes the incisal edge and/or the labial surface must be involved if access is to be adequate. At first sight, this incisolabial involvement would seem to be contraindicated for aesthetic reasons; however, if treatment is not carried out satisfactorily the tooth will have a poor prognosis. Modern bleaching and techniques for bonding restorative materials facilitate the maintenance of the aesthetic and physical requirements of these teeth without resorting to post-retained crowns.

As the pulp is broader incisally than it is cervically the outline should be triangular and must extend far enough mesially and distally to include the pulp horns (Figure 3.11). Once adequate access has been made into the pulp chamber the cervical constriction should be removed by files or Gates-Glidden burs to make instrumentation of the apical part easier.

Correct access-cavity design is particularly important in the older patient because the pulp space is more difficult to find, and narrow root canals require the use of fine instruments which can break if bent excessively. Since the roof of the pulp chamber is

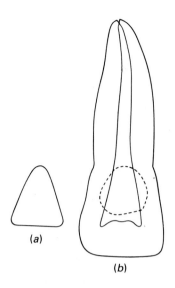

(a)

(b)

Figure 3.11 (a) The correct outline of the access cavity. (b) The dashed line indicates incorrect access.

narrow and often at the cervical level, it is wise to begin the access cavity rather closer to the incisal edge than normal so that the pulp chamber can be approached in a straight line. This approach has the advantage of minimizing tooth destruction.

Maxillary first premolar

This tooth is generally considered to be two-rooted with two canals. The frequency of single-rooted maxillary first premolars ranges from 31% to 39% in Caucasians [6,9,43,76]. In people of Mongoloid origin the frequency

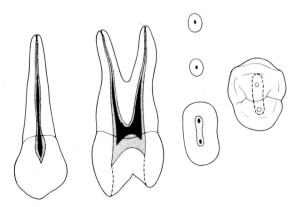

Figure 3.12 Maxillary first premolar with two roots.

of maxillary first premolars with one root is in excess of 60% [44,48,80,81]. In one study [9], 6% were reported to have three roots. A typical Caucasoid specimen has two well-developed fully formed roots which normally begin in the middle third of the root (Figure 3.12). The single-rooted condition prevalent in Mongoloid people represents a fusion of what were, in the distant past, two separate roots.

Irrespective of race, this tooth normally has two canals, and in the case of single-rooted specimens these canals may open through a common apical foramen. Many types of canal configuration are to be found in this tooth (Figure 3.13) and the presence of lateral canals, particularly in the apical region can be as high as 49% [76]. The three-rooted variety tends to have three canals and three apical foramina, two located buccally and one palatally.

Generally the average length of first pre-molars is 21 mm, that is, just shorter than second premolars. The pulp chamber is wide buccopalatally with two distinct pulp horns. In mesiodistal view the pulp chamber is much narrower. The floor is rounded with the highest point in the centre and generally just apical to the level of the cervix. The orifices into the root canals are funnel-shaped and lie buccally and palatally. As the tooth ages the dimensions of the pulp chamber do not alter appreciably, except in a cervico-occlusal direction. Secondary dentine is deposited on the roof of the pulp chamber and this has the effect of bringing the roof very much closer to the floor. The floor level remains apical to the cervix and the thickened roof may reach apical to the cervix. The root canals are normally separate, and very rarely blend into the ribbon-like type of canal frequently seen in the second premolar. They are usually fairly straight with a round cross-section.

Maxillary second premolar

The maxillary second premolar tends to be single-rooted. The type I canal form is preva-lent; however, over 25% of these teeth may present as types II and III, and a further 25% may have types IV–VII forms with two canals at the apex [77,80]. Thus the archetype maxil-

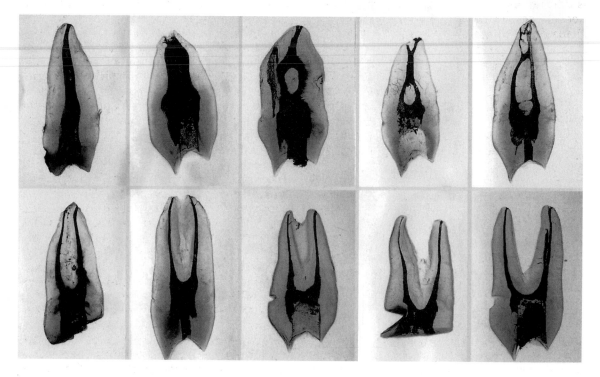

Figure 3.13 Cleared teeth showing various canal configurations in maxillary first premolars.

lary second premolar may be envisaged as having one root with a single canal (Figure 3.14). Very infrequently two roots may be present, and while the outward appearance may be similar to the first premolar, the floor of the pulp chamber is well apical to the cervix. The average length of the second pre-

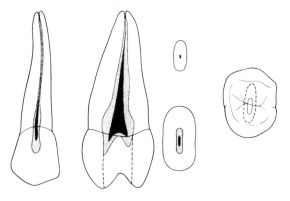

Figure 3.14 Maxillary second premolar with type I canal configuration

molar is slightly longer than the first at 21.5 mm.

The pulp chamber is wide buccopalatally and has two well-defined pulp horns. The root canal is wide buccopalatally and narrow mesiodistally. It tapers apically but rarely develops a circular cross-section except for the apical 2–3 mm. Often the root of this single-rooted tooth branches into two sections in the middle third of the root. These branches almost invariably join to form a common canal which has a relatively large foramen. The canal is usually straight but the apex may curve to the distal and less frequently to the buccal. As the tooth matures the roof of the pulp chamber recedes away from the crown.

Access cavities to maxillary premolars

Access should always be through the occlusal surface. Existing approximal or cervical cavities are unsatisfactory because saliva control is difficult and endodontic instruments would need to be bent to negotiate the canals. The shape of the access cavity is ovoid in a bucco-lingual direction. In the case of the first pre-molar the orifices of the root canal are readily visible as they lie just apical to the cervix. The second premolar root canal is ribbon-shaped and, because it lies well apical to the cervix, may not be readily visible. In preparing an access cavity, an inexperienced operator may incorrectly assume that the pulp horns are the canal orifices.

Maxillary first molar

Maxillary first molars are generally three-rooted with four root canals (Figure 3.15). The additional canal is located in the mesio-buccal root. The canal form of the mesio-buccal root has been thoroughly investigated. Studies *in vitro* indicate that a second canal is present in 55–74% of teeth [34,49,50,51, 54,63,72]. Canal configuration is usually type II (Figure 3.16); however, the presence of a type IV form with two separate apical foramina has been reported to be as high as 48% [50]. Studies *in vivo* have produced much lower figures for the prevalence of the second mesiobuccal canal, and show the diffi-culty in locating the extra canal. In clinical studies mesiobuccal roots with two canals could only be demonstrated in 18–50% [1,25,51,54,58,85]. The palatal and distobuccal roots usually present a type I configuration. In Caucasians, the length of this tooth is 22 mm, the palatal root being slightly longer than the buccal roots. In Mongoloid teeth

there is a tendency for the roots to be closer together and the average length slightly shorter.

The pulp chamber is quadrilateral in shape and wider buccopalatally than mesiodistally. It has four pulp horns, of which the mesio-buccal is the longest and sharpest in outline. The distobuccal pulp horn is smaller than the mesiobuccal but larger than the two palatal pulp horns. The floor of the pulp chamber is normally just apical to the cervix, and is rounded and convex towards the occlusal. The orifices of the main pulp canals are funnel-shaped and lie in the middle of the appropriate root. The minor mesiobuccal canal, if present, lies on a line joining the main mesiobuccal and palatal canal orifices. If this line is divided into thirds the minor mesiobuccal canal is found near the first division adjacent to the main mesiobuccal canal (Figure 3.15). Further, the transverse cross-sectional shape of the pulp chamber 1 mm above the pulpal floor is trapezoidal in 81% of teeth [63]. For this reason the mesio-buccal canal opening is closer to the buccal wall than is the distobuccal orifice. The disto-buccal root (and hence the opening into the root canal) is closer to the middle of the tooth than to the distal wall. The palatal root canal orifice lies in the middle of the palatal root and is normally easy to identify.

The cross-section of the root canals varies considerably. The mesiobuccal canals are usually the most difficult to instrument because they leave the pulp chamber in a mesial direction. The minor mesiobuccal canal is generally very fine and tortuous and usually joins the main canal. The orifice to this canal may be concealed by a dentine

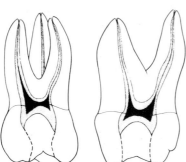 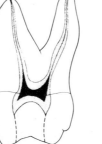 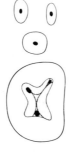 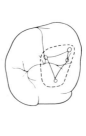

Figure 3.15 Maxillary first molar.

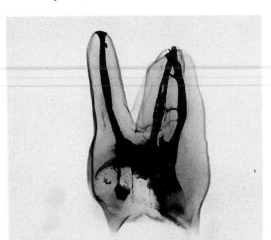

Figure 3.16 Cleared maxillary first molar with a type II canal configuration in the mesiobuccal root.

ficial tooth substance or restorative materials, and to complete the access cavity with a round bur in a low-speed handpiece. It is also important to measure on a preoperative radiograph, taken by the paralleling technique, the distance from cusp tips to roof of the pulp chamber. This distance may be marked on the bur as a depth gauge.

The variable nature of the pulp space anatomy of the maxillary first molar has received emphasis in recent clinical case reports. The occurrence of teeth with two palatal roots and multiple palatal canals has been reported [4,10,24,59,62,87].

ledge, which may need to be removed to detect the orifice [66]. As both mesiobuccal canals lie in a buccopalatal plane they are often superimposed on the preoperative radiograph. A further complication occurs because the mesiobuccal root often curves distopalatally in the apical third of the root. The distobuccal canal is the shortest and finest of the three canals and leaves the pulp chamber in a distal direction. It is ovoid in shape and again narrower mesiodistally. It tapers towards the apex and becomes circular in cross-section. The canal normally curves mesially in the apical half of the root. The palatal canal is the largest and longest of the three canals and leaves the pulp chamber as a round canal which gradually tapers apically. In 50% of roots it is not straight but curves buccally in the apical 4–5 mm. This curvature is not apparent on a clinical radiograph.

As the tooth ages the canals become much finer, and the canal orifices more difficult to find. Secondary dentine is deposited chiefly on the roof of the pulp chamber and to a lesser degree on the floor and walls. Thus the pulp chamber becomes very narrow between roof and floor. This may lead to problems during access cavity preparation for it is relatively easy (particularly with high-speed handpieces) to perforate the floor of the pulp chamber, even into the periodontal ligament. To prevent this accident it is wise to restrict the use of high-speed handpieces to super-

Maxillary second molar

The maxillary second molar is usually a smaller replica of the first molar (Figure 3.17). The roots are less divergent, and fusion between two roots is much more frequent than in the maxillary first molar. Teeth with three canals and three apical foramina are prevalent, and the average length is 21 mm.

Root fusion has been demonstrated in 45–55% of Caucasoid maxillary second molars [16,79], while in Mongoloid groups this figure may be within the range 65–85% [47,69,80]. Where root fusion does occur, canals and their orifices are much closer together (Figure 3.18), or they became confluent to produce the developmental phenomenon of a C-shaped canal [13].

Maxillary third molar

The maxillary third molar displays a great deal of variability. It may possess three separate roots, but more often fusion occurs partially or completely. The pulp space anatomy is unpredictable and these teeth may only have one or two canals. Root canal treatment, for reasons of access and anatomical variation, may therefore not always be practicable.

Access cavities to maxillary molars

The traditional access cavity outline for maxillary teeth is normally in the mesial two-thirds

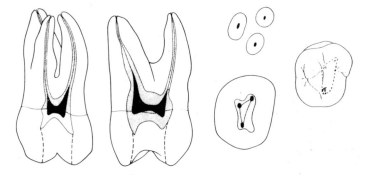

Figure 3.17 Maxillary second molar.

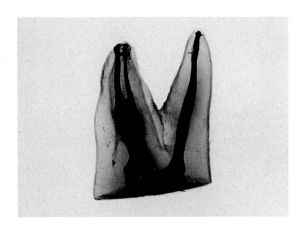

Figure 3.18 Cleared maxillary second molar with fused buccal roots.

of the occlusal surface leaving the oblique ridge intact, and is triangular with the base of the triangle towards the buccal, and the apex palatally. It has been suggested that this traditional shape should be modified in the case of the first molar to a trapezoid shape [85]. Because the distobuccal canal is not as close to the buccal surface as the mesiobuccal canal, less tooth needs to be removed from this area. The occlusal half of the access cavity should be similar in design to an inlay cavity. The walls should not be undercut but should flare occlusally to prevent the accidental forcing of the temporary filling into the pulp chamber during mastication, and thus prevent leakage occurring between visits.

Mandibular central and lateral incisors

The pulp space anatomy of mandibular incisors has been studied by many investigators, whose methods were various, and their results appear to be inconsistent. Methods of study have included replication techniques [18,27], ground sections [3,22], clearing techniques [30,38,46,73,75] and radiography [5,29,35,42,50,52].

Both teeth have an average length of 21 mm, although the central incisor may be a little shorter than the lateral incisor. The root canal morphology may be placed into one of three configurations [5]:

1. *Type I* – a single main canal extending from the pulp chamber to the apical foramen (Figure 3.19).
2. *Type II/III* – two main root canals which merge in the middle or apical third of the root into a single canal with one apical foramen (Figure 3.20).
3. *Type IV* – two main canals which remain distinct throughout the length of the tooth and exit through two major apical foramina (Figure 3.21).

All studies indicate that the type I canal form is most prevalent, types II and III less prevalent, and type IV least prevalent. The presence of two canals has been recorded to be as high as 41% [5]; however, the highest recorded figure for two separate apical foramina (type IV) is 5% [52]. There is some

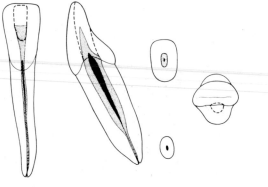

Figure 3.19 Mandibular central incisor with a type I canal configuration.

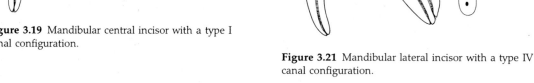

Figure 3.21 Mandibular lateral incisor with a type IV canal configuration.

evidence to suggest that there is a lower frequency of two canals in mandibular central and lateral incisors in Mongoloid people [82].

The pulp chamber is a smaller replica of the upper incisors. It is pointed incisally with three pulp horns which are not well developed, is oval in cross-section, and wider labiolingually than it is mesiodistally. When the tooth has a single root canal it is normally straight but may curve to the distal and less often to the labial. It does not begin to constrict until the middle third of the root when it becomes circular in outline. The tooth ages similarly to the upper incisors, and the incisal portion of the pulp chamber may recede to a level apical to the cervix.

Mandibular canine

This tooth resembles the maxillary canine, although its dimensions are smaller. It rarely has two roots and the average length is 22.5 mm. The type I canal form is most prevalent (Figure 3.22); the frequency of two canals is 14% [29]. However, fewer than 6% of mandibular canines display the type IV canal form with two separate apical foramina [50,73].

Access cavities to mandibular incisors and canines

Essentially these cavities are identical to those in maxillary incisors. However, because of the more pronounced labial curvature of the crown and because the canals (particularly in

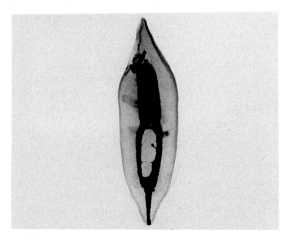

Figure 3.20 Cleared mandibular central incisor with a type II canal configuration.

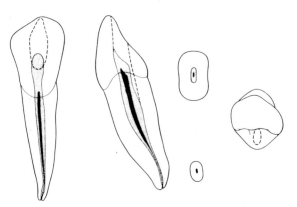

Figure 3.22 Mandibular canine with a type I canal configuration.

older patients) are so fine, it is sometimes necessary to involve the incisal edge and, on occasions, the labial surface of the tooth so that instruments may reach the apical 2–3 mm without being bent.

Mandibular premolars

These teeth are usually single rooted; however, the mandibular first premolar may occasionally present with a division of roots in the apical half. The type I canal configuration is the most prevalent (Figure 3.23). Where two canals are present they are more prevalent in the first premolar and may involve up to one-third of teeth [50,68,74,80]. Where division of canals is recognized, the tendency is for them to remain separate to produce a type IV/V form (Figure 3.24). The type II/III forms are seen in less than 5% of these teeth (Figure 3.25). The highest reported frequency of a second canal in second premolars is 11% [89]. Less than 2% of first premolars have three canals [50,74,80,89]. The presence of multiple canals has been reported [11,55,86].

In one of three reports to make reference to race, Black Americans had nearly three times as many mandibular first premolars with more than one canal than white patients [68]. A study of mandibular first premolars in the southern Chinese population of Hong Kong would also seem to indicate a high prevalence of teeth with more than one canal [80].

The pulp chamber is wide buccolingually, and while there are two pulp horns, only the

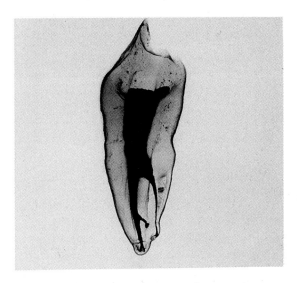

Figure 3.24 Cleared mandibular first premolar with a type IV canal configuration and a lateral canal.

buccal is well developed. The lingual pulp horn is very slight in the first premolar and better developed in the second premolar. The canals of these two teeth are similar, although smaller than the canines, and are thus wide buccolingually until they reach the middle third of the root, when they constrict to a circular cross-section or divide.

Access cavities to mandibular premolars

This is essentially similar to maxillary premolars and must be through the occlusal surface. In the first premolar with two canals

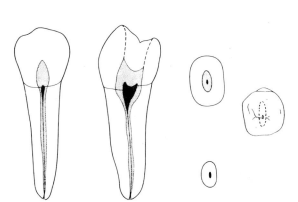

Figure 3.23 Mandibular second premolar with a type I canal configuration.

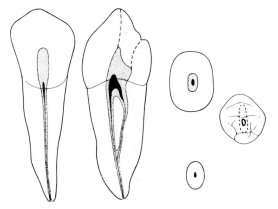

Figure 3.25 Mandibular first premolar with a type II canal configuration.

it may be necessary to extend the cavity on to the labial surface, if unimpeded straight-line access is to be obtained [41].

Mandibular first molar

The mandibular first molar usually has two roots – a mesial and a distal. The latter is smaller and usually rounder than the mesial. There is a Mongoloid variation in which there exists a supernumerary distolingual root. The frequency of this trait ranges from 6 to 44% [83]. The two-rooted molar usually has a canal configuration of three canals (Figure 3.26), and the average length is 21 mm. Two canals are usually located in the mesial root with one in the distal. The mesial root in 40–45% of cases has only one apical foramen [50,57,78]. The single distal canal is usually larger and more oval in cross-section than the mesial canals, and in 60% of cases emerges on the distal side of the root surface short of the anatomical apex [61].

The incidence of two distal canals in mandibular first molars has been reported as 38% [57]. The tendency for the mandibular first molar in Mongoloid people to have three roots would appear to have a direct influence upon the frequency of the second distal canal which approaches half of these teeth [83]. Specimens with three canals in the mesial root [17] and a total of five canals have also been observed (Figure 3.27).

The pulp chamber is wider mesially than it is distally and may have five pulp horns, the lingual pulp horns being longer and more pointed. The floor is rounded and convex toward the occlusal and lies just apical to the cervix. The root canals leave the pulp chamber through funnel-shaped openings, of which the mesial tend to be much finer than the distal. Of the two mesial canals, the mesiobuccal is the difficult canal to instrument because of its tortuous path. It leaves the pulp chamber in a mesial direction, which alters to a distal direction in the middle third of the root. The mesiolingual canal is slightly larger in cross-section and generally follows a much straighter course, although it may curve mesially towards the apical part. These canals may have a latticework arrangement of connections along their length (Figure 3.28). When a second distal canal is present on the distolingual aspect it tends to curve towards the buccal. With age the pulp chamber recedes from the occlusal surface and the canals become constricted.

Mandibular second molar

In Caucasoid populations the mandibular second molar presents as a smaller version of the mandibular first molar with an average length of 20 mm. The mesial root has two canals and, unlike the first molar, there is usually only one distal canal. The mesial canals tend to fuse in the apical third to give rise to one main apical foramen (Figure 3.29).

Recent studies [39,40,84,88] have highlighted the tendency for mandibular second molars to have fused roots in 33-52% of the Chinese. The fusion gives rise to a horse-

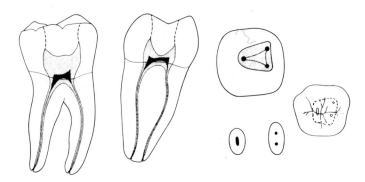

Figure 3.26 Mandibular first molar, with a type IV canal configuration in the mesial root (second from left).

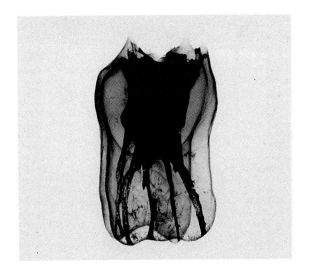

Figure 3.27 Cleared mandibular first molar viewed from the mesial aspect showing five canals.

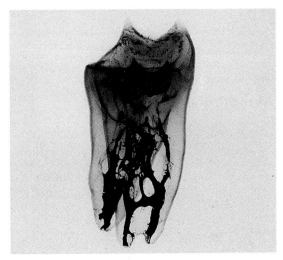

Figure 3.28 Cleared mandibular first molar viewed from the mesiobuccal aspect showing connections between the mesial canals.

shoe shape when the roots are viewed in cross-section. Where there is incomplete separation of roots there may also be incomplete division of canals giving rise to the C-shaped canal, which increases the likelihood of canal interconnections and unpredictably placed canal orifices. One such orifice has now been termed the median buccal canal orifice [88], which leads to the median buccal canal (Figure 3.30). A review of the clinical records of patients at Washington University indicated an 8% occurrence of this anomaly [13] – a figure considerably less than that for Chinese patients.

Mandibular third molar

This tooth is often malformed with numerous and/or poorly developed cusps. It generally has as many root canals as there are cusps. The root canals are generally larger than in other molars, probably because the tooth develops later in life. The roots and thus the pulp canals are short and poorly developed. Nevertheless, it is generally less difficult to carry out root canal treatment on mandibular third molars than maxillary third molars because access is easier due to the mesial inclination of these teeth and also because

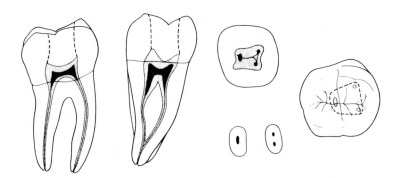

Figure 3.29 Mandibular second molar, with a type II canal configuration in the mesial root (second from left).

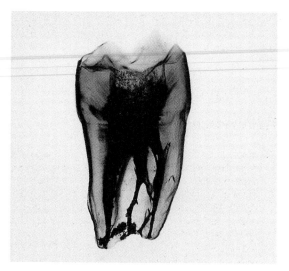

Figure 3.30 Cleared mandibular second molar with fused roots viewed from the buccal aspect showing the median buccal canal.

pulpal anatomy is likely to be similar to the second molar; however, aberrant forms do exist.

Access cavities to mandibular molars

The prevalence of the second distal canal in mandibular first molars necessitates a rectangular outline. Care should always to taken to remove the roof of the pulp chamber completely without causing damage to the floor of the pulp chamber. Where improved visual identification of canal orifices is required the access cavity may be extended. The walls of the access cavity should diverge towards the occlusal to resist masticatory forces and prevent dislodgement of the temporary restoration. Where canal abnormalities are suspected the access cavity may require enlargement and/or modification.

Pulp space anatomy of primary teeth

The object of endodontic therapy in primary teeth is to preserve the tooth in function. The techniques used to achieve this differ from those in permanent teeth.

The pulp cavities in primary teeth have certain common characteristics:

1. Proportionally they are much larger than in permanent teeth.
2. The enamel and dentine surrounding the pulp cavities are much thinner than in permanent teeth.
3. There is no clear demarcation between the pulp chamber and the root canals.
4. The pulp canals are more slender and tapering, and are longer in proportion to the crown, than the corresponding permanent teeth.
5. Multirooted primary teeth show a greater degree of interconnecting branches between pulp canals.
6. The pulp horns of primary molars are more pointed than suggested by cusp anatomy.

Primary incisors and canines

The pulp chambers of both maxillary and mandibular incisors and canines follow closely their crown outlines. However, the pulp tissue is much closer to the surface of the tooth, and the pulp horns are not as sharp and pronounced as in permanent teeth (Figure 3.31). The pulp canals are wide and tapering and there is no clear demarcation between pulp chamber and root canal. The canals may terminate in an apical delta. Occasionally the canals of lower incisors may be divided into two branches by a mesiodistal wall of dentine.

Maxillary primary incisors are 16 mm long, while the laterals are slightly shorter. Mandibular central incisors are 14 mm, and lateral incisors 15 mm. The canines are the longest primary teeth, (maxillary 19 mm, and mandibular 17 mm). As the root apices undergo resorption because of the developing permanent tooth, the roots are frequently shorter in older children.

Primary molars

As in the permanent dentition the maxillary molars are three-rooted whilst the mandibular molars only have two roots (Figure 3.31). The pulp chambers are large in relation to tooth size, and the pulp horns are well developed, particularly in the second molars. From a restorative point of view it is as well

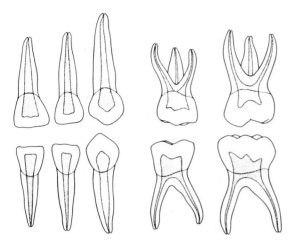

Figure 3.31 Pulpal anatomy of the primary teeth.

to remember that the tip of the pulp horns may be as close as 2 mm from the enamel surface, and thus great care must be taken in preparing cavities in these teeth if pulpal exposure is to be avoided. Because of the relatively large size of the pulp chamber there is relatively less hard tissue protecting the pulp.

The furcation of the roots is also very much closer to the cervical area of the crown and thus excessive instrumentation of the floor of the pulp chamber may lead to perforation. Mandibular molars normally have two root canals in each root, and the mesiobuccal root canal of the maxillary molars sometimes divides into two. Thus primary molars frequently have four canals.

Apical closure

While calcification and cementum deposition at the apex continue throughout life, apices can be considered to be fully formed several years after eruption, and approximate ages are shown in Table 3.1.

Table 3.1 Ages when root apices are considered fully formed

Tooth type	Age (years)
Primary incisor	2
Primary canine and molar	3
Permanent first molar	9
Permanent central incisor	10
Permanent lateral incisor	11
Permanent premolar	15
Permanent second molar	17
Permanent third molar	21

References

1. ADACHI Y (1978) The incidence and the location of secondary mesio-buccal canals in maxillary molars. *Japanese Journal of Conservative Dentistry* **21,** 65–72.
2. ALTMAN M, GUTTUSO J, SEIDBERG BH, LANGELAND K (1970) Apical root canal anatomy of human maxillary central incisors. *Oral Surgery, Oral Medicine, Oral Pathology* **30**, 694–699.
3. BARRETT MT (1925) The internal anatomy of the teeth with special reference to the pulp with its branches. *Dental Cosmos* **67**, 581–592.
4. BEATTY RG (1984) A five-canal maxillary first molar. *Journal of Endodontics* **10**, 156–157.
5. BENJAMIN KA, DOWSON J (1974) Incidence of two root canals in human mandibular incisor teeth. *Oral Surgery, Oral Medicine, Oral Pathology* **38**, 122–126.
6. BERNABA JM, MADEIRA MC, HETEM S (1965) Contribuicao para o estudo morfologico de raizes e canais do primeiro premolar superior humano. *Arquivos do Centro de Estudos da Faculdade Odontologia da UFMG* **2**, 81–92.
7. BURCH JG, HULEN S (1972) The relationship of the apical foramen to the anatomic apex of the tooth root. *Oral Surgery, Oral Medicine, Oral Pathology* **34**, 262–268.
8. BURCH JG, HULEN S (1974) A study of the presence of accessory foramina and topography of molar furcations. *Oral Surgery, Oral Medicine, Oral Pathology* **38**, 451–455.
9. CARNS EJ, SKIDMORE AE (1973) Configurations and deviations of root canals of maxillary first premolars. *Oral Surgery, Oral Medicine, Oral Pathology* **36**, 880–886.
10. CECIC P, HARTWELL G, BELLIZZI R (1982) The multiple root canal system in the maxillary first molar: a case report. *Journal of Endodontics* **8**, 113–115.
11. CHAN K, YEW SC, CHAO SY (1992) Mandibular premolar with three root canals – two case reports. *International Endodontic Journal* **25**, 261–264.
12. CHAPMAN CE (1969) A microscopic study of the apical region of human anterior teeth. *Journal of the British Endodontic Society* **3**, 52–58.
13. COOKE HG, COX FL (1979) C-shaped canal configurations in mandibular molars. *Journal of the American Dental Association* **99**, 836–839.
14. DOURDA AO, MOULE AJ, YOUNG WG (1994) A morphometric analysis of the cross-sectional area of dentine occupied by dentinal tubules in human third molar teeth. *International Endodontic Journal* **27**, 184–189.

15. DUMMER PMH, MCGINN JH, REES DG (1984) The position and topography of the apical canal constriction and apical foramen. *International Endodontic Journal* **17**, 192–198.

16. FABIAN H (1928) *Spezielle Anatomie des Gebisses.* Leipzig, Germany: Werner Klinkhardt.

17. FABRA-CAMPOS H (1989) Three canals in the mesial root of mandibular first permanent molars: a clinical study. *International Endodontic Journal* **22**, 39–43.

18. FISCHER G (1907) Uber die feinere Anatomie der Wurzelkanäle menschlicher Zähne. *Zahne Deutsche Monatsschrift für Zahnheilkunde* **25**, 544–552.

19. GARBEROGLIO R, BRÄNNSTRÖM M (1976) Scanning electron microscopic investigation of human dentinal tubules. *Archives of Oral Biology* **21**, 355–362.

20. GREEN D (1956) A stereomicroscopic study of the root apices of 400 maxillary and mandibular anterior teeth. *Oral Surgery, Oral Medicine, Oral Pathology* **9**, 1224–1232.

21. GREEN D (1960) Stereomicroscopic study of 700 root apices of maxillary and mandibular posterior teeth. *Oral Surgery, Oral Medicine, Oral Pathology* **13**, 728–733.

22. GREEN D (1973) Double canals in single roots. *Oral Surgery, Oral Medicine, Oral Pathology* **35**, 689–696.

23. GUTMANN JL, PITT FORD TR (1993) Management of the resected root end: a clinical review. *International Endodontic Journal* **26**, 273–283.

24. HARRIS WE (1980) Unusual root canal anatomy in a maxillary molar. *Journal of Endodontics* **6**, 573–575.

25. HARTWELL G, BELLIZZI R (1982) Clinical investigation of *in vivo* endodontically treated mandibular and maxillary molars. *Journal of Endodontics* **8**, 555–557.

26. HENRY PJ (1970) Two rooted central incisor. *Oral Surgery, Oral Medicine, Oral Pathology* **30**, 380.

27. HESS WL (1917) Zur Anatomie der Wurzelkanale des menschlicher Gebisses mit Beruechsichtigung der feineren Verzweigungen am Foramen apicale. *Schweizer Vierteljahrschrift fur Zahnheilkunde* **27**, 1–52.

28. HOPPE WF, STUBEN J (1965) Uber die messung des volumens der dentinkanälchen und über das Verhältnis des kanalvolumens zum gesamtdentinvolumen. *Stomata* **18**, 38–45.

29. KAFFE I, KAUFMAN A, LITTNER M, LAZARSON A (1985) Radiographic study of the root canal system of mandibular anterior teeth. *International Endodontic Journal* **18**, 253–259.

30. KELLER O (1928) Untersuchurgen zur Anatomie der wurzelkanale des menschlichen Gebisses nach dem Aufhellungsverfahren. *Schweizer Monatsschrift fur Zahnheilkunde* **38**, 635–657.

31. KEREKES K, TRONSTAD L (1977) Morphometric observations on root canals of human anterior teeth. *Journal of Endodontics* **3**, 24–29.

32. KRAMER IRH (1960) The vascular architecture of the human dental pulp. *Archives of Oral Biology* **2**, 177–189.

33. KUTTLER Y (1955) Microscopic investigation of root apices. *Journal of the American Dental Association* **50**, 544–552.

34. LANE AJ (1974) The course and incidence of multiple canals in the mesio-buccal root of the maxillary first molar. *Journal of the British Endodontic Society* **7**, 9–11.

35. LAWS AJ (1971) Prevalence of canal irregularities in mandibular incisors: a radiographic study. *New Zealand Dental Journal* **67**, 181–186.

36. LEVY AB, GLATT L (1970) Deviation of the apical foramen from the radiographic apex. *Journal of the New Jersey State Dental Society* **41**, 12–13.

37. LOWMAN JV, BURKE RS, PELLEU GB (1973) Patent accessory canals: incidence in molar furcation region. *Oral Surgery, Oral Medicine, Oral Pathology* **36**, 580–584.

38. MADEIRA MC, HETEM S (1973) Incidence of bifurcations in mandibular incisors. *Oral Surgery, Oral Medicine, Oral Pathology* **36**, 589–591.

39. MANNING SA (1990) Root canal anatomy of mandibular second molars. Part I. *International Endodontic Journal* **23**, 34–39.

40. MANNING SA (1990) Root canal anatomy of mandibular second molars. Part II C-shaped canals. *International Endodontic Journal* **23**, 40–45.

41. MILLER VDG (1980) An investigation of endodontic access cavity design in mandibular premolar and incisor teeth. MSc Project Report, University of London.

42. MIYOSHI S, FUJIWARA J, TSUJI Y, NAKATA T, YAMAMOTO K (1977) Bifurcated root canals and crown diameter. *Journal of Dental Research* **56**, 1425.

43. MUELLER AH (1933) Anatomy of the root canals of the incisors, cuspids, and bicuspids of the permanent teeth. *Journal of the American Dental Association* **20**, 1361–1386.

44. NELSON CT (1938) The teeth of the Indians of Pecos Pueblo. *American Journal of Physical Anthropology* **23**, 261–293.

45. OGUNTEBI BR (1994) Dentine tubule infection and endodontic therapy implications. *International Endodontic Journal* **27**, 218–222.

46. OKUMURA T (1927) Anatomy of the root canals. *Journal of the American Dental Association* **14**, 632–639.

47. PEDERSON PO (1949) The East Greenland Eskimo dentition. Numerical variations and anatomy. *Meddelelser om Gronland* BD 142, no. 3.

48. PINEDA F (1959) Investigacion de la forma, numero y direccion radiculares sobre 4252 dientes. *Revista de la Asociacion Dental Mexicana* **16**, 241–253.

49. PINEDA F (1973) Roentgenographic investigation of the mesiobuccal root of the maxillary first molar. *Oral Surgery, Oral Medicine, Oral Pathology* **36**, 253–260.

50. PINEDA F, KUTTLER Y (1972) Mesiodistal and buccolingual roentgenographic investigation of 7,275 root canals. *Oral Surgery, Oral Medicine, Oral Pathology* **33**, 101–110.

51. POMERANZ HH, FISHELBERG G (1974) The secondary mesiobuccal canal of maxillary molars. *Journal of the American Dental Association* **88**, 119–124.

52. RANKINE-WILSON RW, HENRY P (1965) The bifurcated root canal in lower anterior teeth. *Journal of the American Dental Association* **70,** 1162–1165.

53. REID JS, SAUNDERS WP, MACDONALD DG (1993) Maxillary permanent incisors with two root canals: a report of two cases. *International Endodontic Journal* **26,** 246–250.

54. SEIDBERG BH, ALTMAN M, GUTTUSO J, SUSON M (1973) Frequency of two mesiobuccal root canals in maxillary permanent first molars. *Journal of the American Dental Association* **87,** 852–856.

55. SERMAN NJ, HASSELGREN G (1992) The radiographic incidence of multiple roots and canals in human mandibular premolars. *International Endodontic Journal* **25,** 234–237.

56. SHAFER WG, HINE MK, LEVY BM (1983) *A Textbook of Oral Pathology,* 4th edn, pp. 38–45. Philadelphia, PA, USA: Saunders

57. SKIDMORE AE, BJORNDAL AM (1971) Root canal morphology of the human mandibular first molar. *Oral Surgery, Oral Medicine, Oral Pathology* **32,** 778–784.

58. SLOWEY RR (1974) Radiographic aids in the detection of extra root canals. *Oral Surgery, Oral Medicine, Oral Pathology* **37,** 762–772.

59. STONE LH, STRONER WF (1981) Maxillary molars demonstrating more than one palatal root canal. *Oral Surgery, Oral Medicine, Oral Pathology* **51,** 649–652.

60. SYKARAS S, ECONOMOU P (1970) Root canal morphology of the mesiobuccal root of the maxillary first molar. *Odontostomatologica Procodos* **24,** 99–107.

61. TAMSE A, LITTNER MM, KAFFE I, MOSKONA D, GAVISH A (1988) Morphological and radiographic study of the apical foramen in distal roots of mandibular molars. Part 1. The location of the apical foramen on various root aspects. *International Endodontic Journal* **21,** 205–210.

62. THEWS ME, KEMP WB, JONES CR (1979) Aberrations in palatal root and root canal morphology of two maxillary first molars. *Journal of Endodontics* **5,** 94–96.

63. THOMAS RP, MOULE AJ, BRYANT R (1993) Root canal morphology of maxillary permanent first molar teeth at various ages. *International Endodontic Journal* **26,** 257–267.

64. THOMPSON BH, PORTELL FR, HARTWELL GR (1985) Two root canals in a maxillary lateral incisor. *Journal of Endodontics* **11,** 353–355.

65. TIDMARSH BG, ARROWSMITH MG (1989) Dentinal tubules at the root ends of apicected teeth: a scanning electron microscopic study. *International Endodontic Journal* **22,** 184–189.

66. TING PCS, NGA L (1992) Clinical detection of minor mesiobuccal canal of maxillary first molars. *International Endodontic Journal* **25,** 304–306.

67. TRATMAN EK (1938) Three rooted lower molars in man and their racial distribution. *British Dental Journal* **64,** 264–274.

68. TROPE M, ELFENBEIN L, TRONSTAD L (1986) Mandibular premolars with more than one root canal in different race groups. *Journal of Endodontics* **12,** 343–345.

69. TURNER CG (1967) The dentition of the Arctic peoples PhD thesis. Madison, WI, USA: University of Wisconsin.

70. TURNER CG (1971) Three rooted mandibular first permanent molars and the question of American Indian origins. *American Journal of Physical Anthropology* **34,** 229–241.

71. VANDE VOORDE HE, BJORNDAHL AM (1969) Estimating endodontic 'working length' with paralleling radiographs. *Oral Surgery, Oral Medicine, Oral Pathology* **27,** 106–110.

72. VERTUCCI FJ (1974) The endodontic significance of the mesiobuccal root of the maxillary first molar. *US Navy Medicine* **63,** 29–31.

73. VERTUCCI FJ (1974) Root canal anatomy of the mandibular anterior teeth. *Journal of the American Dental Association* **89,** 369–371.

74. VERTUCCI FJ (1978) Root canal morphology of mandibular premolars. *Journal of the American Dental Association* **97,** 47–50.

75. VERTUCCI FJ (1984) Root canal anatomy of the human permanent teeth. *Oral Surgery, Oral Medicine, Oral Pathology* **58,** 589–599.

76. VERTUCCI FJ, GEGAUFF A (1979) Root canal morphology of the maxillary first premolar. *Journal of the American Dental Association* **99,** 194–198.

77. VERTUCCI F, SEELIG A, GILLIS R (1974) Root canal morphology of the human maxillary second premolar. *Oral Surgery, Oral Medicine, Oral Pathology* **38,** 456–464.

78. VERTUCCI FJ, WILLIAMS RG (1974) Root canal anatomy of the mandibular first molar. *Journal of the New Jersey Dental Association* **45,** 27–28.

79. VISSER JB (1943) Uber Wurzelverschmelzungen an den oberen Molaren des menschlichen Gebisses. *Acta Neerlandica Morphologica* **5,** 1–10.

80. WALKER RT (1987) A comparative investigation of the root number and canal anatomy of permanent teeth in a southern Chinese population. PhD thesis, University of Hong Kong.

81. WALKER RT (1987) Root form and canal anatomy of maxillary first premolars in a southern Chinese population. *Endodontics and Dental Traumatology* **3,** 130–134.

82. WALKER RT (1988) The root canal anatomy of mandibular incisors in a southern Chinese population. *International Endodontic Journal* **21,** 218–223.

83. WALKER RT (1988) The root form and canal anatomy of mandibular first molars in a southern Chinese population. *Endodontics and Dental Traumatology* **4,** 19–22.

84. WALKER RT (1988) Root form and canal anatomy of mandibular second molars in a southern Chinese population. *Journal of Endodontics* **14,** 325–329.

85. WELLER RN, HARTWELL GR (1989) The impact of improved access and searching techniques on

detection of the mesio-lingual canal in maxillary molars. *Journal of Endodontics* **15,** 82–83.

86. WONG M (1991) Four root canals in a mandibular second premolar. *Journal of Endodontics* **17,** 125–126.

87. WONG M (1991) Maxillary first molar with three palatal canals. *Journal of Endodontics* **17,** 298–299.

88. YANG ZP, YANG SF, LIN YC, SHAY JC, CHI CY (1988) C-shaped root canals in mandibular second molars in a Chinese population. *Endodontics and Dental Traumatology* **4,** 160–163.

89. ZILLICH R, DOWSON J (1973) Root canal morphology of the mandibular first and second premolars. *Oral Surgery, Oral Medicine, Oral Pathology* **36,** 738–744.

4

The dental pulp

T.R. Pitt Ford

Introduction

The student of endodontics should be aware that the best root filling is healthy pulp tissue; and he, or she, should know how it can be damaged, what can be done to prevent damage, and the appropriate treatment. It should not be assumed that every damaged pulp must be extirpated and that pulpal conservation is an unsatisfactory procedure.

The dental pulp is in the centre of the tooth and is the tissue from which the dentine was formed during tooth development. It remains throughout life and provides nourishment for the odontoblasts which line its surface. These odontoblasts have long processes which extend approximately one-third as far as the amelodentinal junction [11]. The tubules beyond the odontoblast processes are normally patent and filled with tissue fluid. When irritants are applied to the distal ends of the dentinal tubules, the odontoblasts will form more dentine, within the pulp as irritation dentine, within tubules as peritubular dentine, or lead to the occlusion of tubules by mineralized deposits as tubular sclerosis.

The pulp and dentine can thus be regarded as one interconnected tissue – the dentino-pulpal complex. This is normally protected from irritation by an intact layer of enamel. When enamel is destroyed by caries, erosion or operative procedures, the pulp is at risk. In a young patient the tubules are wider and the pulp closer to the surface, so a similarly sized breach of enamel will have a greater effect on the pulp than one in an older patient. The more the area of exposed dentine, the greater is the effect on the pulp, therefore the potential damage of crown preparations and large cavities is greater than that of small cavities.

Pulpal response to irritants

The pulpal response to irritation is inflammation and formation of hard tissues, irritation dentine and tubular sclerosis; these hard tissues attempt to wall off the irritants from the pulp which will then cease to be inflamed.

It has been shown that if buccal cavities are prepared in otherwise sound teeth and the cavities left open to salivary contamination, the pulp underneath the exposed tubules becomes inflamed [55]. Furthermore, when severe irritants, namely microorganisms in carious dentine, are placed on the cavity floor under a restoration, the pulpal reaction is always severe. If the irritant is removed and a restoration with a lining (base) placed, the pulpal inflammation subsides and irritation dentine is formed [56]. Thus it has been demonstrated experimentally that damaged pulps have the capacity to recover.

Diagnosis of pulpal damage

The dentist who intends to restore a broken-down or decayed tooth needs to determine whether the pulp of the tooth is dead, dying or alive, in order for treatment to be successful. There is as yet no routine test which directly indicates the vitality of the pulp. Currently available tests assess the function of pulpal nerves, by the application of electric current or a rapid change in temperature. Several studies have reported on the experimental use of laser Doppler flowmetry to measure blood flow in teeth [37,59,61], but the technique is not yet at the stage for simple routine clinical use.

In teeth with damaged pulps, because pulpal inflammation is often localized, the response to thermal or electric testing may come from the significant amount of remaining normal pulp; this indicates a healthier state than exists. When the pulp does not respond to testing, it cannot always be assumed to be dead, for the pulp may have formed large amounts of irritation dentine and retreated sufficiently far from the stimulus not to respond. The correlation between histological findings and the results of pulp tests is satisfactory at a crude level but is poor when exacerbating or relieving factors, or the nature of the pain are correlated [28,50,72]. In view of this poor correlation, clinicians have rejected previous complex histopathological classifications and developed a simple clinical classification of the state of the pulp:

1. Normal pulp.
2. Reversible pulpitis.
3. Irreversible pulpitis.
4. Pulpal necrosis.

The reader should be aware that inflammatory changes in the pulp can be localized; for example, a pulp horn may display a microabscess while the opposite pulp horn is normal and uninflamed. These marked variations within a single pulp are in contrast to descriptions found in some older textbooks and obviously hinder diagnosis. The view that increased pulpal pressure causes strangulation of the vessels in the apical part of the root, because the tooth provides a rigid closed system, is an oversimplification as there are physiological mechanisms to prevent this [41,46,83].

Pulpitis which causes symptoms is regarded as *acute*, whereas if it is symptomless it is classified as *chronic*; these descriptions refer to the incidence of pain, not the type of inflammatory cells found at histological examination. Pain may range from short sharp bouts, through a continuous dull ache, to a severe throbbing pain. The pain may arise by stimulation such as drinking a cold liquid or be spontaneous. Its character and occurrence usually change with time as the pulpal disease progresses. A patient may give a history of initially short bouts of pain stimulated by drinking cold liquids, that developed into a continuous dull ache; when she rang to ask for the appointment the tooth was throbbing, but now that she is sitting in the dental chair the pain has gone. It is very likely that the pulp initially exhibited reversible inflammation, which progressed to irreversible inflammation, but the pulp has now become necrotic.

Often the dentist will be restoring symptomless teeth but some will be causing pain. In either case it is necessary to determine the state of the pulp before commencing restorative treatment. If in doubt a period of observation may be appropriate, but if advanced restorative treatment is planned and the pulp is suspect, root canal treatment may be indicated rather than risk the embarrassment of needing to perform this later, when careful diagnosis would have revealed the state of the pulp initially. This subject has been reviewed [71].

A number of clinical tests are available to assess the state of the pulp; none is totally reliable because they may be ineffective, or may elicit only a response from a normal part of the damaged pulp. After all the tests, the practitioner must use judgement to decide the probable state of the pulp and the most appropriate treatment.

Clinical tests

The following clinical tests are used:

1. Application of electric current.
2. Application of cold.
3. Application of heat.
4. Examination of radiograph.
5. Assessment of blood flow.
6. Cavity preparation without anaesthesia.

Application of electric current

Electric current is usually applied from a battery-operated 'electric pulp tester'. The pulp tester is usually monopolar with an electrode being placed on the tooth under investigation; the circuit is completed by the patient contacting a ground electrode or the handle of the pulp tester. The teeth being investigated should be isolated and dried before the electrode, coated with a conducting medium, e.g. fluoride gel, is applied to the tooth. The current is variable, either under the operator's control or increased automatically over a period of time. The output characteristics of four types of pulp tester have been investigated [30]. They all produced negative pulses of electricity of the order of several hundred volts with a maximum current of a few milliamps; however, the waveform of each type investigated was distinctly different. When the patient feels a sensation, he or she lets go of the handle of the pulp tester so breaking the circuit; the reading of this lowest current to elicit a response is recorded.

In a clinical study of sound teeth it was found that teeth responded over a range of values, with posterior teeth requiring higher settings than anterior teeth [29]. Teeth with acutely inflamed pulps tend to respond at lower levels than sound control teeth, while teeth with partially necrotic pulps tend to respond at higher levels. The position of the electrode on the tooth has varied in different investigations; although the middle of the labial surface has been widely used [29], the lowest readings in adults are obtained from the incisal edge [3].

A response at a high setting may occur with a damaged pulp, by leakage through the periodontal tissues, or through a receded normal pulp. A lack of response may occur because a tooth is root filled, a pulp is necrotic, a vital pulp has receded, the pulp is in a state of shock (e.g. in traumatized teeth), or if the circuit is incomplete.

Application of cold

Cold is usually applied to a dried tooth by touching it intermittently with a pledget of cotton wool covered in ice crystals as a result of evaporation of ethyl chloride. It may also be applied by a stick of ice; this may be conveniently made by filling a sterilized discarded needle cover with water and placing it in a freezer. The application of cold usually elicits a painful response in a healthy anterior tooth as the small amount of tooth substance is cooled very rapidly; the test may work less well on posterior teeth because of their greater mass. A response indicates that the nerve fibres in the pulp are alive; an exaggerated response may indicate an inflamed pulp while no response may occur when the coronal pulp is necrotic, the pulp has receded, insufficient cooling occurred or, in traumatized teeth, the pulp is in a state of shock. A prolonged and lingering response to the application of cold usually indicates an irreversibly damaged pulp [28].

Application of heat

Heat is usually applied by a heated stick of gutta-percha temporary filling material being placed intermittently on the dried tooth surface, with a small amount of petroleum jelly being used as a lubricant. A response indicates that the pulpal nerve fibres are active. A lack of response may occur if the pulp is necrotic, the pulp has receded or insufficient heating occurred. Heat is generally considered particularly effective in diagnosing a pulp with irreversible pulpitis, for pain that lingers after the application of heat is often as a result of C-fibre stimulation; however, in one clinical study, heat was not found to be more effective than cold for diagnosis [28].

Examination of radiographs

Two radiographic views may be examined – the bitewing film and the periapical film. The bitewing film provides information about the crown of the tooth and the superficial part of the root. It gives a two-dimensional view of the extent of restorations, the extent of caries, the presence of recurrent caries, the amount of irritation dentine, the size of the pulp chamber and evidence of internal resorption. The periapical film additionally provides evidence of periradicular radiolucencies. Where teeth have large restorations, the distance between the base of the cavity and the pulp is small, and irritants could therefore affect the pulp more readily than in a tooth with a small restoration. The closer the caries is to the pulp and the larger the lesion, the greater is the threat to the pulp. The formation of irritation dentine in response to caries indicates that the pulp has most probably responded successfully to the irritant, as does a diminutive-sized pulp chamber. On the other hand the lack of irritation dentine formation to caries and an abnormally large-sized pulp chamber compared with the other teeth in the mouth could indicate that the coronal pulp became necrotic at an earlier age. Internal resorption, which should not be confused with external resorption, indicates irreversible pulpitis. Periradicular radiolucencies which may not always be at the apex indicate pulpal necrosis, which may be partial or total.

Assessment of blood flow

Laser Doppler flowmeters may be used to assess blood flow in teeth, but as yet no flowmeter has been developed specifically for dental use. The technique involves directing a low-energy laser beam along a fibreoptic cable to the tooth surface, where the light passes along the direction of enamel prisms and dentinal tubules to the pulp [60]. Some light is reflected off moving red blood cells in the pulpal capillaries. The reflected light is passed back to the flowmeter where the frequency-shifted light is detected for strength of signal and pulsatility. Currently available flowmeters display the signal on a screen, from which the clinician must interpret whether the pulp is alive and healthy, or dead. The accuracy of assessing pulp vitality is dependent on machine variables, and can be improved by mathematical analysis of the signal [59]. Laser Doppler flowmetry has been used to detect pulpal vitality in traumatized teeth at a stage when other tests are inconclusive [61]. Currently available flowmeters require careful setting-up to record useful signals from teeth, but it is hoped that a flowmeter which is simple to operate will be developed for dental use.

Cavity preparation without anaesthesia

This procedure is only performed when all other tests have failed to give a diagnosis. If the dentine is sensitive to drilling, it indicates that the pulp is alive but not necessarily healthy, for the pulp could be inflamed. A lack of sensitivity occurs if the pulp is necrotic. In a tooth with a healthy pulp which has receded a long way, there may be no sensitivity because the tubules being drilled do not connect with odontoblast processes as a result of tubular sclerosis or formation of irritation dentine.

Diagnosis

After performing as many tests as appropriate, the clinician hopes to be able to arrive at a diagnosis. If the diagnosis is uncertain in a symptomless tooth, it is usual to assume that the pulp is normal in the absence of definite contrary evidence. However, if the tooth has caused symptoms but is now quiet, the pulp must be regarded as suspect. While a policy of observation may be appropriate in some cases, root canal treatment should be carried out if advanced restorative procedures are planned on a tooth with a questionable pulp.

Pulpal irritants

The dental pulp may be irritated by dental caries, cavity preparation, dental materials, bacterial leakage around restorations, traumatic injuries or exposure of dentine. These will now be considered in detail.

Dental caries

This is the main cause of pulpal injury. When dental caries first affects dentine, the odontoblasts respond by tubular sclerosis and irritation dentine formation [82]. Tubular sclerosis is an accelerated form of peritubular dentine but the process continues further than normal with complete occlusion of the affected tubules by apatite crystals. It is a protective mechanism and occurs at the distal extremities of the odontoblast processes. This sclerotic dentine is more highly mineralized than the original dentine and, if examined in a ground section by transmitted light, would appear transparent [76]. Irritation dentine is an accelerated form of regular secondary dentine; because it has been formed more quickly its tubular pattern is less regular, and the degree of irregularity indicates its rate of formation. It is confined to the tubules affected by the carious lesion.

If the carious lesion progresses, the enamel surface breaks down and bacteria enter the dentine; the rate of decay usually accelerates. The lesion may be divided into zones: an outer zone of destruction, a middle zone of bacterial penetration and an inner zone of demineralization. The pulp responds by continued irritation dentine formation. The zone of destruction contains dentine partially destroyed by proteolytic enzymes from the mixed flora of microorganisms. The tubules are filled with microorganisms and they can be found particularly in shrinkage clefts in the rotten dentine. This dentine can be readily removed by hand excavators in active lesions and often has a light colour. In slowly progressing or arrested lesions this dentine is darker and has a leathery consistency.

The next zone, the zone of penetration, contains microorganisms within the dentinal tubules. The structure of the dentine when examined in a demineralized histological section is otherwise normal; some tubules are deeply infected while others contain no microorganisms. A variety of microorganisms have been recovered from this zone; many lactobacilli have been found but fewer streptococci [31]. More recently deep carious dentine has been shown to contain predominantly anaerobic bacteria (*Propionibacterium, Eubacterium, Arachnia* and lactobacilli) [43]. Ahead of the zone of microorganism penetration is a zone of demineralization, frequently considered to be devoid of bacteria because the conditions for bacterial survival are too unfavourable; however, small numbers of anaerobic bacteria have recently been demonstrated in this zone [44].

In the early dentine lesion the pulp is protected by the zone of tubular sclerosis and by irritation dentine, and is likely to be of normal histological appearance. No inflammatory cells can be observed in the pulp until caries has penetrated to within 1.1 mm, and inflammation is mild until the microorganisms are within 0.5 mm [70]. As the early dentine carious lesion progresses, the sclerotic zone of dentine becomes demineralized and the lesion subsequently advances into the irritation dentine. When bacteria invade this dentine, severe pulpal changes such as abscess formation often occur. Therefore until the caries is very deep, the pulp is likely to be no more than reversibly damaged. Treatment should normally consist of removal of carious dentine and insertion of a restoration. This has been shown to result in pulpal recovery [56].

The pulp is not infected until late in the carious process, typically when the irritation dentine is invaded. Infection of the inflamed pulp is localized to necrotic tissue in a pulp abscess [52]. Wider infection of the pulp only occurs after necrosis.

Cavity preparation

The preparation of dentine with rotary instruments can have a damaging effect on the pulp unless measures are taken to minimize injury. Cavity preparation without waterspray causes significantly more pulpal damage than when waterspray is used [57,78]. The waterspray must be continuously directed at the revolving bur; if the spray is obstructed by tooth structure or the bur allowed to stall or to cut when the operator has removed the foot from the activating switch, pulpal damage may occur. Various studies into the pulpal effects of high-speed instrumentation have been reviewed [74], and it was found to be acceptable provided adequate water coolant spray was used; the use of air coolant alone was considered unsatisfactory.

The area of dentine prepared can have a profound effect on the pulpal response. The more tubules that are exposed, the more routes to the pulp. Small cavities are likely to be less damaging to the pulp than large ones; in addition, in a small cavity prepared to treat a carious lesion, most of the exposed dentinal tubules will be blocked by tubular sclerosis as a result of the carious lesion. The deeper the cavity, the greater is the potential for damage: the pulp is closer, odontoblast processes may have been cut, more tubules will have been exposed, and the tubules have a larger diameter. However, there is no correlation between thickness of remaining dentine and pulpal damage [57,67]. Only when cavities are very deep, with the remaining dentine less than 0.3 mm thick, does some pulpal damage occur [78]. Prolonged drying of cavities causes odontoblast aspiration – their cell bodies move into the dentinal tubules, but there is no permanent damage to the pulp [6].

Veneer crown preparations are potentially the most damaging to the pulp, and on occasions irreversible pulpal damage has been caused by preparation with insufficient water-spray. When local anaesthetics containing adrenaline are used for crown preparation, the pulp is at particular risk of damage because of its reduced blood flow [47].

There are few reports on the pulpal response to the use of lasers for cavity preparation; two studies [54,85] have reported no long-term adverse effects from the Nd:YAG laser, however some short-term pulpal damage may occur at high energy levels (S. Kim, personal communication).

Dental materials

There is a very considerable volume of literature on the irritant effects of dental filling materials [35,68,69]. However during the last 20 years, much of the earlier work on the irritancy of various materials has been brought into question [4,8,14,18,24,84].

Silicate cement has long been regarded as the most irritating restorative material due to its acidity [77,88]; however, the cement *per se* is bland but it is the manner in which it is used that causes the pulpal reaction [15]. The cement contracts on setting, causing a gap to occur between it and the tooth, into which bacteria grow [13]; the teeth containing bacteria in the gap have inflamed pulps [4]. When bacteria are deliberately excluded, there is an excellent pulpal response to the material itself [15,24]. Elimination of bacteria may be achieved experimentally by surface-sealing the restoration with zinc oxide–eugenol cement, but it is not a clinically applicable procedure. The important point is that such a restoration must be lined by a suitable base material to prevent bacterial leakage.

Composite resin has also been regarded as irritant to the pulp, but the blandness of this class of material has now been demonstrated together with the important contribution of bacterial contamination to pulpal reaction [12,80]. It is important to acid-etch the cavity margins to allow the composite resin to seal the margins of the restoration and thereby eliminate bacteria from the cavity [12]. From a clinical standpoint, etching enamel margins and the use of a cavity liner have been considered necessary not only to prevent a pulpal inflammatory reaction, but also to reduce a reaction should the seal be imperfect.

The use of dentine bonding agents to prevent marginal leakage around composite resin restorations has been investigated for many years, but their long-term stability has often been a matter of concern. In recent years considerable development of these agents has been undertaken, and a favourable pulpal response has been reported to some [25,33,86].

Pulpal damage may occur from temporary crown materials, not because of their inherent toxicity but as a result of marginal leakage and bacterial invasion of dentinal tubules. It is recommended that temporary crowns should not be used for long periods and they must always be adequately cemented [10].

Although there is now considerable evidence to show the blandness of dental filling materials placed in teeth, many materials, particularly when freshly mixed, have been shown to be toxic to cell cultures [16]; however, dentine has a moderating effect [53].

Bacterial leakage

Bacterial leakage around restorations is not solely confined to composite resin and silicate cement materials, as a similar pattern occurs with amalgam restorations [4]. The bacteria from the oral cavity leak around the restoration after its placement, rather than surviving from the time of its placement. The lack of importance of bacterial contamination at the time of cavity preparation has been shown in a study of pulpal exposures [22]. There is a good correlation between bacterial leakage around restorations and pulpal inflammation [17,18].

Pulps respond to irritation from bacterial leakage by inflammation, tubular sclerosis and formation of irritation dentine so that after some months the bacteria cease to irritate [79]. However, measures should be taken to prevent pulpal damage during the period before the pulp has walled itself off; these consist of cavity lining, use of cavity varnish in appropriate instances, use of a dentine-bonding agent and etching of enamel for resin-based materials, or use of an adhesive cement.

In operative dentistry the main reason for placing a cavity lining (in some parts of the world referred to as a base) is to prevent damage to the pulp from bacterial leakage around restorations. Former reasons such as material irritancy or thermal protection have been severely criticized [10,15].

The choice of lining material in cavities without pulpal exposures would appear to be a matter of operator preference in many instances. Cements based on calcium hydroxide, glass ionomer, zinc phosphate, zinc polycarboxylate or zinc oxide–eugenol all appear to be satisfactory under amalgam, and have been widely used. Zinc oxide–eugenol cement has the benefit of prolonged antibacterial activity. Under resin-based restorative materials, zinc oxide–eugenol cement is inappropriate, unless separated by a covering layer of alternative cement (e.g. glass ionomer), as otherwise the eugenol may plasticize the resin. The durability of some calcium hydroxide cements has been questioned, particularly if the overlying restoration is imperfect [10,25].

Exposure of dentine

This may occur by fracture of part of the tooth, by a restoration failing to cover the entire area of prepared dentine, or by abrasion and erosion of the overlying cementum or enamel. In the early period after exposure of dentine by trauma or cavity preparation, the pulp is sensitive to stimuli and may become inflamed, particularly if bacteria colonize the surface of exposed dentine and enter the tubules. The pulp responds to the low-grade irritation by tubular sclerosis and irritation dentine formation, thereby protecting itself and making it less sensitive to stimuli [62].

Some patients complain of dentine sensitivity in undamaged or non-restored teeth, usually at their necks where there is exposed dentine. The affected tubules are open and communicate with the pulp. Sensitivity may be reduced by application of potassium oxalate which not only occludes the tubules but also reduces nerve activity [62]. The good work of repair can be undone by assault with acidic solutions, particularly in patients who continue to erode their teeth either with acidic drinks and foods, or by regurgitation [10].

Management of deep caries

With the treatment of any carious cavity in dentine, it is accepted that the margins, and the amelodentinal junction in particular, must be caries-free as detected by an absence of softening with a probe and a lack of discoloration. However, there has been less agreement over whether all carious dentine overlying the pulp should be removed [34]. In a tooth which is considered to have a healthy pulp, the prognosis for the pulp is better if exposure during caries removal is avoided [21].

A view prevails that if carious dentine remains, it will allow the carious process to continue. There is an opposite view that clinical evidence supports the leaving of a small amount of caries under a well-executed restoration; in this circumstance the caries becomes arrested [32]. Since very few restorations form a hermetic seal [4,13], a high incidence of recurrent caries would be expected if the former view were entirely correct. The latter view is full of clinical imprecision; how much is a little caries, and when does a little become an unacceptably large amount? What is meant by carious dentine? Clinical opinions conflict with scientific evidence. In one study only 64% of clinically hard dentine floors were bacteria-free [73]; therefore, in a third of teeth where the clinician thought he had a clean floor, he was wrong. The problem may be rationalized by use of an indicator dye placed in the prepared cavity; the dye stains the superficial infected dentine but not the deeper demineralized non-infected dentine [36]. This deeper non-staining layer has been shown to remineralize, thereby justifying its retention. The use of acid red dye offers the clinician the most logical approach to the removal of carious dentine, in that it conserves remineralizable dentine.

The basis for what tissue to remove must rest on an understanding of the carious lesion. The zone nearest the pulp is one of demineralization with minimal bacterial contamination, the next zone is one of infection, while the outermost zone is one of destruction of dentine. In treating a carious lesion, the destroyed zone should be removed. Most operators would feel comfortable removing the zone of infection; the use of acid red dye should achieve this, although it may not be absolute at a microscopic level because of the variability of bacterial penetration in dentinal tubules [73].

Many operators rely on the natural colour of affected dentine for deciding when a cavity is caries-free. Carious dentine is frequently discoloured yellow or brown but it can on occasions be the same colour as normal dentine; the lighter colour is usually indicative of more active caries. On the other hand a deep lesion may extend into dentine modified by tubular sclerosis or dead tracts, or into irritation dentine; these are darker than normal dentine, but must not be regarded as carious simply because of their colour. Hardness of carious dentine is a better indicator of disease activity.

If carious dentine is left, the clinician is unaware whether it has extended to involve the pulp. If the pulp is already involved, it becomes an expensive error to crown such a tooth when the crown later needs to be modified or destroyed to carry out root canal treatment. If removal of all the cariously infected dentine leads to the pulp, then root canal treatment is appropriate and should be carried out, except in the case of an immature tooth where pulpotomy may be indicated (Chapter 10). There is no justification for leaving the deeper part of the carious lesion simply because the operator is frightened of exposing the pulp [58]. Some operators, when treating symptomless teeth with deep carious lesions, prefer to remove most of the carious dentine, place a fortified zinc oxide–eugenol temporary filling for several months and then return to remove the remaining carious dentine several months later; this is known as indirect pulp capping. The procedure allows the pulp to lay down defences prior to complete caries removal.

Following removal of the carious dentine stained by acid red dye, a protective lining should be placed in a very deep cavity; a calcium hydroxide material, which stimulates pulpal repair, is commonly used. Over this an antibacterial base should be placed; zinc oxide–eugenol cement is very effective because it slowly leaches eugenol which will kill any remaining microorganisms [45], and is a more effective bactericide than calcium hydroxide materials [48]. The durability of calcium hydroxide cement as the sole base under amalgam has been questioned by the finding of softened material on removal of the overlying restoration 1–2 years later [10,23,25].

Pulp exposure

Exposure of the pulp may arise as a result of traumatic injury to the tooth, or accidentally by instruments during cavity preparation. In both instances the pulp is regarded as being normal prior to the injury. Treatment is usually by pulp capping or pulpotomy; provided that treatment is not unnecessarily delayed, which would allow infection, a good rate of success can be achieved.

Pulp capping

The pulpal wound should be cleaned of debris and the haemorrhage arrested by careful swabbing with sterile cotton buds or paper points laid across the wound. When the wound is dry, the pulp-capping material should be placed over the exposure. This should be followed by a zinc oxide–eugenol base and a permanent restoration [39].

The most widely used materials for pulp capping have contained calcium hydroxide [75,87]. The use of a proprietary calcium hydroxide cement has achieved a high success rate [66] although a similar, now discontinued, material was unsuccessful [65]. Under favourable circumstances, the pulp responds by laying down irritation dentine under the exposure site to form a dentine bridge. With most proprietary materials this bridge forms close to the capping material, but with calcium hydroxide itself the barrier is formed further away from the material [81]. The dentine bridge is not formed by calcium from the pulp-capping material [2].

The importance of preventing bacterial contamination at the time of exposure has previously been stressed [63]: however it is now known that contamination for periods up to 24 h does not adversely affect pulpal survival [22]. In an experiment where the cavities were left open to salivary contamination for 24 h, prior to being washed, dried and the pulp-capping material placed, the success rate was equivalent to that in those teeth capped immediately [22]. In contrast, the success rate in teeth exposed to saliva for 7 days is considerably lower [22]. The size of the exposure has also been considered to affect the outcome, although there is no evidence to support it.

The long-term success of pulp capping clinically is good [39,51]; however, a lower rate has been found at the histological level. This is attributed to bacterial penetration around the overlying restoration, and through the imperfect dentine bridge [25]. The pulp-capping material should be covered by a base; zinc oxide-eugenol cement would seem the most appropriate and has been found to improve the quality of dentine bridges [49].

Zinc oxide–eugenol cement has been an unsuccessful pulp-capping material [38], and this is because of its irritancy at concentrations greater than 10^{-3} mol/l [45]. However, when this material is separated from the pulp by a layer of intact dentine, the concentration of eugenol at the odontoblast level is sufficiently low to prevent permanent pulpal damage. Former explanations about impurities in the cement causing pulpal damage cannot now be accepted.

Preparations containing an antibiotic and a steroid, e.g. Ledermix, have been advocated for pulp capping on the grounds that the antibiotic would kill the microorganisms, and the steroid would reduce any pulpal inflammation, thereby alleviating pain. In one study such a material did not cause dentine bridge formation but the pulp underwent extending necrosis [64]. Better success rates have been achieved with calcium hydroxide-based materials. Steroid–antibiotic preparations have found use as a palliative dressing prior to undertaking root canal treatment in cariously exposed teeth.

Pulpotomy

For treatment of traumatized anterior teeth, an alternative technique of pulpotomy has been used. The traditional method has been to remove the coronal pulp and place calcium hydroxide on the radicular pulp. However, partial pulpotomy has been more widely practised in recent years with a high rate of success [26]. It involves cutting, with a turbine bur under waterspray, a small 2 mm deep cavity into the pulp surrounded by a shelf of dentine, placing calcium hydroxide and covering it with a base and restoration.

Traumatic injuries

These may be caused by direct blows to the anterior teeth or indirectly by a blow to the mandible, resulting in fracture of cusps, particularly of molars. The extent of damage may range from infraction of enamel through lost cusps to a split tooth which cannot be restored. Direct trauma to the anterior teeth often results in fractures which are horizontal or oblique [1], while with indirect trauma, fractures are generally vertical.

Trauma to anterior teeth most commonly affects sound teeth in children. These teeth frequently have large pulps and wide dentinal tubules so any injury which exposes dentine can potentially damage the pulp, therefore early treatment is necessary. Traumatic injuries may damage the blood supply to the pulp, which as a result may calcify or die. The endodontic aspects of traumatic injuries are further considered in Chapter 11.

Cracked cusps

A patient may complain of poorly localized pain from an unidentified posterior tooth on biting or the application of cold drinks [19,20]. Clinically and radiographically there is often no evidence of caries, and the offending tooth, although it contains a restoration, may not be heavily restored. The affected pulp responds normally to electrical stimulation. Careful examination of the teeth in that quadrant, particularly with an intraoral light, may reveal one with vertical hairline cracks; mandibular molars are the most frequently affected [20]. The pain may be reproduced if the patient is asked to close with an object, e.g. a cotton-wool roll, placed between that and the opposing teeth. When this fails to produce a response, cold in the form of ice may be applied to the teeth; a hypersensitive response will indicate the offending tooth. The mechanism of this pain on biting may be explained [7,10]: the crack contains bacteria whose toxins pass down the dentinal tubules to cause pulpal inflammation. As the cusp is wedged by chewing there is fluid movement in the crack and the communicating tubules; this elicits pain in an already sensitive tooth.

If there is sufficient evidence to identify the cracked cusp, treatment should be carried out. The form of treatment will depend on whether there have been symptoms of reversible or irreversible pulpitis. In the case of reversible pulpitis and if there is a loose cusp, any restoration should be removed together with the loose cusp; the tooth is restored as appropriate for the shape and size of cavity. If no loose cusp is detected, the tooth may be restored with composite resin attached to etched enamel in an attempt to hold it together, or alternatively an onlay or crown restoration may be constructed. When there is inadequate evidence as to which cusp on what tooth is cracked, it is wise to wait: the cusp which some months later breaks off may not be the one that was considered most likely. There are occasions in patients who grind and clench their teeth, when it is not just a small piece of cusp that fractures but the whole tooth that splits vertically; at this stage the treatment is usually extraction.

In patients who exhibit very worn teeth, it is inadvisable to wait for an observable cracked cusp to fracture; the tooth should be prepared for a crown restoration; following placement of the temporary crown, relief from pain is normally achieved. Where there have been symptoms of irreversible pulpitis, pulpal extirpation and root canal filling will be required. During root canal treatment it is advisable to place a band (e.g. stainless-steel orthodontic band) around the tooth to stop it splitting, and to reduce the tooth out of occlusion.

Pulpal response to periodontal disease and treatment

Periodontal disease does not cause pathological change in the pulp until major lateral canals become contaminated by plaque [27]. The normality of the pulp is maintained because of the intact layer of cementum on the root surface. If this layer is resorbed then pulpal inflammation under the affected tubules occurs [5]. The pulp responds to the stimuli by formation of tubular sclerosis and irritation dentine [40].

It has been shown that scaling or root-planing procedures which remove cementum may cause pulpal inflammation, and frequently the formation of irritation dentine [5,40]. However, the response to scaling was not severe and did not adversely affect pulp vitality. Following scaling, dentinal tubules become opened and the teeth are hypersensitive; after several weeks the sensitivity decreases, presumably as the tubules become blocked by mineral deposits [10].

Pulpal response to intra-alveolar surgery

It has usually been considered that pulpal necrosis and abscess formation will follow surgical cutting or severance of a root near its apex. However, orthognathic surgery has led to the roots of some teeth being cut without undesirable sequelae. The effect on the remaining pulp of severing roots in the apical region has been investigated [42]. It was found that if all the roots of a tooth were severed, the coronal pulp underwent necrosis but inflammation did not occur. After 1 year there was no evidence of inflammatory cells and cementum had formed on the cut root surface and on the root canal walls near the cut surface. Where several roots of a multi-rooted tooth were cut through but one root remained intact, the entire coronal pulp maintained its vitality. The cut surface of the apical fragment became covered by cementum, while its pulp remained normal. It appears from this study that accidental surgical damage to the roots of healthy teeth causes far less injury than was previously considered. The situation might not be so favourable if the teeth lack a complete covering of enamel which is necessary to exclude infection, or if at a later date enamel or cementum is breached.

References

1. ANDREASEN JO, ANDREASEN FM (1994) *Textbook and Color Atlas of Traumatic Injuries to the Teeth*, 3rd edn. Copenhagen, Denmark: Munksgaard.
2. ATTALLA MN, NOUJAIM AA (1969) Role of calcium hydroxide in the formation of reparative dentine. *Journal of the Canadian Dental Association* **35**, 267–269.
3. BENDER IB, LANDAU MA, FONSECCA S, TROWBRIDGE HO (1989) The optimum placement-site of the electrode in electric pulp testing of the 12 anterior teeth. *Journal of the American Dental Association* **118**, 305–310.
4. BERGENHOLTZ G, COX CF, LOESCHE WJ, SYED SA (1982) Bacterial leakage around dental restorations: its effect on the pulp. *Journal of Oral Pathology* **11**, 439–450.
5. BERGENHOLTZ G, LINDHE J (1978) Effect of experimentally induced marginal periodontitis and periodontal scaling on the dental pulp. *Journal of Clinical Periodontology* **5**, 59–73.
6. BRÄNNSTRÖM M (1968) The effect of dentin desiccation and aspirated odontoblasts on the pulp. *Journal of Prosthetic Dentistry* **20**, 165–171.
7. BRÄNNSTRÖM M (1982) *Dentin and Pulp in Restorative Dentistry*. London, UK: Wolfe Medical Publications.
8. BRÄNNSTRÖM M (1984) Communication between the oral cavity and the dental pulp associated with restorative treatment. *Operative Dentistry* **9**, 57–68.
9. BRÄNNSTRÖM M (1986) The hydrodynamic theory of dentinal pain: sensation in preparations, caries and the dentinal crack syndrome. *Journal of Endodontics* **12**, 453–457.
10. BRÄNNSTRÖM M (1986) The cause of postrestorative sensitivity and its prevention. *Journal of Endodontics* **12**, 475–481.
11. BRÄNNSTRÖM M, GARBEROGLIO R (1972) The dentinal tubules and the odontoblast processes. A scanning electron microscopic study. *Acta Odontologica Scandinavica* **30**, 291–311.
12. BRÄNNSTRÖM M, NORDENVALL KJ (1978) Bacterial penetration, pulpal reaction and the inner surface of Concise Enamel Bond. Composite fillings in etched and unetched cavities. *Journal of Dental Research* **57**, 3–10.
13. BRÄNNSTRÖM M, NYBORG H (1971) The presence of bacteria in cavities filled with silicate cement and composite resin materials. *Swedish Dental Journal* **64**, 149–155.
14. BRÄNNSTRÖM M, VOJINOVIC O (1976) Response of the dental pulp to invasion of bacteria around three filling materials. *Journal of Dentistry for Children* **43**, 83–89.
15. BRÄNNSTRÖM M, VOJINOVIC O, NORDENVALL KJ (1979) Bacteria and pulpal reactions under silicate cement restorations. *Journal of Prosthetic Dentistry* **41**, 290–295.
16. BROWNE RM (1988) The *in vitro* assessment of the cytotoxicity of dental materials – does it have a role? *International Endodontic Journal* **21**, 50–58.
17. BROWNE RM, TOBIAS RS (1986) Microbial microleakage and pulpal inflammation: a review. *Endodontics and Dental Traumatology* **2**, 177–183.
18. BROWNE RM, TOBIAS RS, CROMBIE IK, PLANT CG (1983) Bacterial microleakage and pulpal inflammation in experimental cavities. *International Endodontic Journal* **16**, 147–155.
19. CAMERON CE (1964) Cracked–tooth syndrome. *Journal of the American Dental Association* **68**, 405–411.
20. CAMERON CE (1976) The cracked tooth syndrome: additional findings. *Journal of the American Dental Association* **93**, 971–975.
21. COTTON WR (1974) Bacterial contamination as a factor in healing of pulp exposures. *Oral Surgery, Oral Medicine, Oral Pathology* **38**, 441–450.
22. COX CF, BERGENHOLTZ G, FITZGERALD M ET AL. (1982) Capping of the dental pulp mechanically exposed to the oral microflora – a 5 week observation of wound healing in the monkey. *Journal of Oral Pathology* **11**, 327–339.

23. COX CF, BERGENHOLTZ G, HEYS DR, SYED SA, FITZ-GERALD M, HEYS RJ (1985) Pulp capping of the dental pulp mechanically exposed to the oral microflora: a 1–2 year observation of wound healing in the monkey. *Journal of Oral Pathology* **14**, 156–168.

24. COX CF, KEALL CL, KEALL HJ, OSTRO E, BERGEN-HOLTZ G (1987) Biocompatibility of surface-sealed dental materials against exposed pulps. *Journal of Prosthetic Dentistry* **57**, 1–8.

25. COX CF, SUZUKI S (1994) Re-evaluating pulp protection: calcium hydroxide liners vs. cohesive hybridization. *Journal of the American Dental Association* **125**, 823–831.

26. CVEK M (1978) A clinical report on partial pulpotomy and capping with calcium hydroxide in permanent incisors with complicated crown fracture. *Journal of Endodontics* **4**, 232–237.

27. CZARNECKI RT, SCHILDER H (1979) A histological evaluation of the human pulp in teeth with varying degrees of periodontal disease. *Journal of Endodontics* **5**, 242–253.

28. DUMMER PMH, HICKS R, HUWS D (1980) Clinical signs and symptoms in pulp disease. *International Endodontic Journal* **13**, 27–35.

29. DUMMER PMH, TANNER M (1986) The response of caries-free, unfilled teeth to electrical excitation: a comparison of two new pulp testers. *International Endodontic Journal* **19**, 172–177.

30. DUMMER PMH, TANNER M, MCCARTHY JP (1986) A laboratory study of four electric pulp testers. *International Endodontic Journal* **19**, 161–171.

31. EDWARDSSON S (1974) Bacteriological studies on deep areas of carious dentine. *Odontologisk Revy* **25** (suppl 32), 1–143.

32. FAIRBOURN DR, CHARBENEAU GT, LOESCHE WJ (1980) Effect of Improved Dycal and IRM on bacteria in deep carious lesions. *Journal of the American Dental Association* **100**, 547–552.

33. FELTON D, BERGENHOLTZ G, COX CF (1989) Inhibition of bacterial growth under composite restorations following GLUMA pretreatment. *Journal of Dental Research* **68**, 491–495.

34. FISHER FJ (1981) The treatment of carious dentine. *British Dental Journal* **150**, 159–162.

35. FRANK RM (1975) Reactions of dentin and pulp to drugs and restorative materials. *Journal of Dental Research* **54**, B176–187.

36. FUSAYAMA T (1979) Two layers of carious dentin: diagnosis and treatment. *Operative Dentistry* **4**, 63–70.

37. GAZELIUS B, OLGART L, EDWALL B, EDWALL L (1986) Non-invasive recording of blood flow in human dental pulp. *Endodontics and Dental Traumatology* **2**, 219–221.

38. GLASS RL, ZANDER HA (1949) Pulp healing. *Journal of Dental Research* **28**, 97–107.

39. HASKELL EW, STANLEY HR, CHELLIMI J, STRING-FELLOW H (1978) Direct pulp capping treatment: a long-term follow-up. *Journal of the American Dental Association* **97**, 607–612.

40. HATTLER AB, LISTGARTEN MA (1984) Pulpal response to root planing in a rat model. *Journal of Endodontics* **10**, 471–476.

41. HEYERAAS KJ (1984) Pulpal, microvascular, and tissue pressure. *Journal of Dental Research* **64**, 585–589.

42. HITCHCOCK R, ELLIS E, COX CF (1985) Intentional vital root transection: a 52-week histopathologic study in *Macaca mulatta*. *Oral Surgery, Oral Medicine, Oral Pathology* **60**, 2–14.

43. HOSHINO E (1985) Predominant obligate anaerobes in human carious dentin. *Journal of Dental Research* **64**, 1195–1198.

44. HOSHINO E, ANDO N, SATO M, KOTA K (1992) Bacterial invasion of non-exposed dental pulp. *International Endodontic Journal* **25**, 2–5.

45. HUME WR (1988) *In vitro* studies on the local pharmacodynamics, pharmacology and toxicology of eugenol and zinc oxide-eugenol. *International Endodontic Journal* **21**, 130–134.

46. KIM S (1984) Regulation of pulpal blood flow. *Journal of Dental Research* **64**, 590–596.

47. KIM S (1986) Ligamental injection: a physiological explanation of its efficacy. *Journal of Endodontics* **12**, 486–491.

48. KING JB, CRAWFORD JJ, LINDAHL RL (1965) Indirect pulp capping: a bacteriologic study of deep carious dentine in human teeth. *Oral Surgery, Oral Medicine, Oral Pathology* **20**, 663–671.

49. LANGER M, ULMANSKY M, SELA J (1970) Behaviour of human dental pulp to Calxyl with or without zinc oxide eugenol. *Archives of Oral Biology* **15**, 189–194.

50. LUNDY T, STANLEY HR (1969) Correlation of pulpal histopathology and clinical symptoms in human teeth subjected to experimental irritation. *Oral Surgery, Oral Medicine, Oral Pathology* **27**, 187–201.

51. MCWALTER GM, EL-KAFRAWY AH, MITCHELL DF (1976) Long-term study of pulp capping in monkeys with three agents. *Journal of the American Dental Association* **93**, 105–110.

52. MASSLER M, PAWLAK J (1977) The affected and infected pulp. *Oral Surgery, Oral Medicine, Oral Pathology* **43**, 929–947.

53. MERYON SD (1988) The model cavity method incorporating dentine. *International Endodontic Journal* **21**, 79–84.

54. MISERENDINO LJ, LEVY GC, ABT E, RIZOIU IM (1994) Histologic effects of a thermally cooled Nd:YAG laser on the dental pulp and supporting structures of rabbit teeth. *Oral Surgery, Oral Medicine, Oral Pathology* **78**, 93–100.

55. MJÖR IA, TRONSTAD L (1972) Experimentally induced pulpitis. *Oral Surgery, Oral Medicine, Oral Pathology* **34**, 102–108.

56. MJÖR IA, TRONSTAD L (1974) The healing of experimentally induced pulpitis. *Oral Surgery, Oral Medicine, Oral Pathology* **38**, 115–121.

57. MORRANT GA (1977) Dental instrumentation and pulpal injury. Part II clinical considerations. *Journal of the British Endodontic Society* **10**, 55–63.

58. NYGARD-OSTBY B (1972) Caries profunda and 'indirect pulp capping'. *Oral Surgery, Oral Medicine, Oral Pathology* **33**, 788–790.

59. ODOR TM, PITT FORD TR, MCDONALD F (1996) Effect of wavelength and bandwidth on the clinical reliability of laser Doppler recordings. *Endodontics and Dental Traumatology* **12**, 9–15.

60. ODOR TM, WATSON TF, PITT FORD TR, MCDONALD F (1996) Pattern of transmission of laser light in teeth. *International Endodontic Journal* **29**, 228–234.

61. OLGART L, GAZELIUS B, LINDH-STRÖMBERG U (1988) Laser Doppler flowmetry in assessing vitality in luxated permanent teeth. *International Endodontic Journal* **21**, 300–306.

62. PASHLEY DH (1986) Dentin permeability, dentin sensitivity and treatment through tubule occlusion. *Journal of Endodontics* **12**, 465–474.

63. PATERSON RC (1974) Management of the deep cavity. *British Dental Journal* **137**, 250–252.

64. PATERSON RC (1976) Corticosteroids and the exposed pulp. *British Dental Journal* **140**, 174–177.

65. PITT FORD TR (1980) Pulpal response to MPC for capping exposures. *Oral Surgery, Oral Medicine, Oral Pathology* **50**, 81–88.

66. PITT FORD TR, ROBERTS GJ (1991) Immediate and delayed direct pulp capping with the use of a new visible light-cured calcium hydroxide preparation. *Oral Surgery, Oral Medicine, Oral Pathology* **71**, 338–342.

67. PLANT CG, ANDERSON RJ (1978) The effect of cavity depth on the pulpal response to restorative materials. *British Dental Journal* **144**, 10–13.

68. PLANT CG, JONES DW (1976) The damaging effects of restorative materials. Part 1 – Physical and chemical properties. *British Dental Journal* **140**, 373–377.

69. PLANT CG, JONES DW (1976) The damaging effects of restorative materials. Part 2 – Pulpal effects related to physical and chemical properties. *British Dental Journal* **140**, 406–412.

70. REEVES R, STANLEY HR (1966) The relationship of bacterial penetration and pulpal pathosis in carious teeth. *Oral Surgery, Oral Medicine, Oral Pathology* **22**, 59–65.

71. ROWE AHR, PITT FORD TR (1990) The assessment of pulpal vitality. *International Endodontic Journal* **23**, 77–83.

72. SELTZER S, BENDER IB, ZIONTZ M (1963) The dynamics of pulp inflammation: correlations between diagnostic data and actual histologic findings in the pulp. *Oral Surgery, Oral Medicine, Oral Pathology* **16**, 846–871, 969–977.

73. SHOVELTON DS (1968) A study of deep carious dentine. *International Dental Journal* **18**, 392–405.

74. STANLEY HR (1961) Traumatic capacity of high-speed and ultrasonic dental instrumentation. *Journal of the American Dental Association* **63**, 749–766.

75. STANLEY HR, LUNDY T (1972) Dycal therapy for pulp exposures. *Oral Surgery, Oral Medicine, Oral Pathology* **34**, 818–827.

76. STANLEY HR, PEREIRA JC, SPIEGAL E, BROOM C, SCHULTZ M (1983) The detection and prevalence of reactive and physiologic sclerotic dentin, reparative dentin and dead tracts beneath various types of dental lesions according to tooth surface and age. *Journal of Oral Pathology* **12**, 257–289.

77. STANLEY HR, SWERDLOW H, BUONOCORE MG (1967) Pulp reactions to anterior restorative materials. *Journal of the American Dental Association* **75**, 132–141.

78. SWERDLOW H, STANLEY HR (1959) Reaction of the human dental pulp to cavity preparation. Part II at 150,000 rpm with an air-water spray. *Journal of Prosthetic Dentistry* **9**, 121–131.

79. TOBIAS RS, PLANT CG, BROWNE RM (1982) Reduction in pulpal inflammation beneath surface-sealed silicates. *International Endodontic Journal* **15**, 173–180.

80. TORSTENSON B, NORDENVALL KJ, BRÄNNSTRÖM M (1982) Pulpal reaction and microorganisms under Clearfil composite resin in deep cavities with acid etched dentin. *Swedish Dental Journal* **6**, 167–176.

81. TRONSTAD L (1974) Reaction of the exposed pulp to Dycal treatment. *Oral Surgery, Oral Medicine, Oral Pathology* **38**, 945–953.

82. TROWBRIDGE HO (1981) Pathogenesis of pulpitis resulting from dental caries. *Journal of Endodontics* **7**, 52–60.

83. VAN HASSEL HJ (1971) Physiology of the human dental pulp. *Oral Surgery, Oral Medicine, Oral Pathology* **32**, 126–134.

84. WATTS A (1979) Bacterial contamination and the toxicity of silicate and zinc phosphate cements. *British Dental Journal* **146**, 7–13.

85. WHITE JM, GOODIS HE, SETCOS JC, EAKLE WS, HULSCHER BE, ROSE CL (1993) Effects of pulsed Nd:YAG laser energy on human teeth: a three-year follow-up study. *Journal of the American Dental Association* **124(7)**, 45–51.

86. WHITE KC, COX CF, KANKA J, DIXON DL, FARMER JB, SNUGS HM (1994) Pulpal response to adhesive resin systems applied to acid–etched vital dentin: damp versus dry primer application. *Quintessence International* **25**, 259–268.

87. ZANDER HA (1939) Reaction of the pulp to calcium hydroxide. *Journal of Dental Research* **18**, 373–379.

88. ZANDER HA (1946) The reaction of dental pulps to silicate cements. *Journal of the American Dental Association* **33**, 1233–1243.

5

Basic instrumentation in endodontics

J. Webber

Introduction	instruments and posts
Instruments for access cavity preparation	**Instruments for filling root canals**
Basic instrument pack	Lateral condensation
Burs	Vertical condensation
Rubber dam	Hybrid techniques
Instruments for root canal preparation	Thermoplasticized injectable gutta-percha
Hand instruments	Gutta-percha carrier devices
Power-assisted root canal instruments	**Equipment for storing instruments**
Electronic canal-measuring devices	**Sterilization of endodontic instruments**
Measuring instruments, gauges and stands	**Equipment for improving visibility**
Instruments for retrieving broken	**References**

Introduction

It is now widely accepted that success in root canal treatment depends upon the thorough cleaning and shaping of the root canal system and the placement of a three-dimensional root canal filling of gutta-percha and inert sealer [59]. To fulfil these objectives, many different instruments, each with a specific purpose, must be available. Some of these instruments have been used for many years, whilst others are newer and highly technical. This increase in technology has led to a situation where it is essential to evaluate the functions and limitations of the many available products which are grouped according to their use.

Instruments for access cavity preparation

Basic instrument pack

A typical set-up (Figure 5.1) includes some instruments familiar in restorative dentistry and others which have been specially adapted for endodontics.

The endodontic explorer is a double-ended, extra-long (approximately 15 mm), sharp instrument designed to help in the location of canal orifices and probing for fractures on the pulp chamber floor. A long spoon excavator is required to scoop out pulp chamber contents and flick away pulp stones during access cavity preparation. A front-surfaced mouth mirror is best suited for visibility deep within the pulp chamber. Endodontic locking tweezers are ideally suited to the handling of paper points, gutta-percha points and root canal instruments. Both Briault and periodontal probes are necessary for the initial assessment of the tooth for caries and the localized periodontal condition. Flat plastic instruments and amalgam pluggers are needed to place interappointment restorations. An endodontic millimetre ruler should be available to assess root canal length.

The irrigating syringe (Figure 5.2) is important to deposit endodontic irrigants in the pulp chamber. Many designs of syringe have

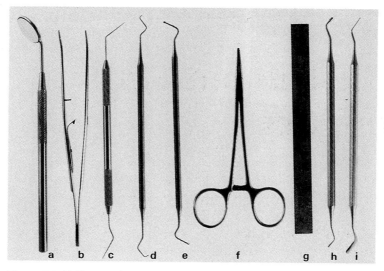

Figure 5.1 (a) Front surface mirror; (b) endodontic locking tweezers; (c) DG16 endodontic explorer; (d) Briault probe; (e) long-shank excavator; (f) surgical haemostat; (g) millimetre ruler; (h) amalgam plugger; (i) flat plastic.

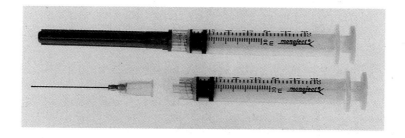

Figure 5.2 Monoject endodontic irrigating syringe, which is of Luer-Lok design and has a notched needle.

been marketed, but the Luer-Lok type remains the syringe of choice. The barrel tip prevents needle dislodgement occurring during irrigation, whilst the tip itself is notched to prevent accidental forcing of irrigant into the periapical tissues.

Burs

Several types of bur will be required to accomplish good access preparation (Figure 5.3).

Friction grip

Friction grip tapered fissure burs 557 (ISO 010) or 701 (ISO 012) are used in the initial stages of access preparation to establish the correct outline form.

Round

Round burs, normal and extra-long, size 2 (ISO 010), size 4 (ISO 014) and size 6 (ISO 018), are used to lift the roof off the pulp chamber and eliminate overhanging dentine. The longer and smaller sizes can be used to find calcified canals.

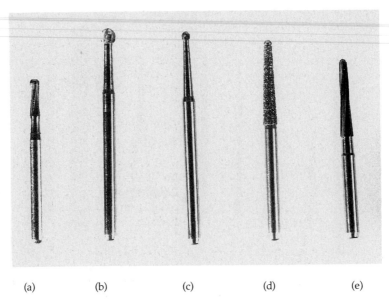

Figure 5.3 Access cavity burs: (a) FG 557 ISO 010 (TC); (b) FG ISO round 018 (long); (c) FG ISO round 010 (long); (d) FG safe-ended diamond 332 ISO 018; (e) FG safe-ended TC, Endo Z (Maillefer).

Safe-ended burs

A safe-ended diamond or tungsten-carbide bur, the Endo Z bur (Figure 5.3), both with a non-cutting tip, is used to taper and smooth the access cavity preparation. The non-cutting tip prevents gouging on the floor of the pulp chamber, where important landmarks could be lost in pinpointing the location of root canals.

Gates-Glidden burs

The Gates-Glidden bur (Figure 5.4) is a one-piece rotary cutting instrument, now widely used in all root canal preparation techniques. This bur has a bud-shaped cutting point mounted on a fine shaft attached to a latch-type shank. The bud is further modified by having a fine blunt tip which acts as a path-finder within the root canal, without damaging the walls or creating false pathways. It should be used slowly in a handpiece and only where a pathway is present for the tip to follow. If the bud jams against the canal walls, fracture should occur at the junction of

the shaft with the shank and not at the tip of the instrument. Thus, removal of the fractured instrument from the canal is easy. Gates-Glidden burs are made in stainless steel and bur diameter ranges from 0.5 to 1.5 mm. The basic properties of Gates-Glidden drills have been extensively studied [37,41,42].

The Gates-Glidden bur has three main uses:

1. The coronal two-thirds of molar canals are generally wider and less curved than the apical third, therefore these parts can be quickly and safely prepared with Gates-Glidden burs. The importance of early flaring of the root canal during preparation has been demonstrated [39].
2. The Gates-Glidden bur is useful for removing gutta-percha from a canal during post-space preparation or during retreatment.
3. The bur may be used to widen the canal when an instrument has fractured within it, to aid retrieval of the broken instrument. If the tip of the Gates-Glidden drill is flattened off (Gates-Glidden belly bur; Figure 5.4), visibility is improved.

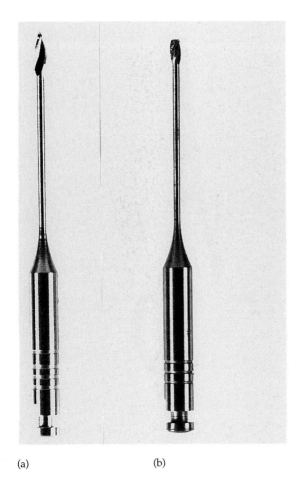

(a)   (b)

Figure 5.4 Gates-Glidden drills: (a) size 3 (ISO 090);
(b) size 3 belly bur.

Rubber dam

The rubber dam is used to:

1. Protect the patient from inhalation or ingestion of instruments, medicaments and debris. There are various safety devices available, but these are not a substitute for rubber dam as they do not fully protect the patient.
2. Provide a clean, dry field of operation free from salivary contamination.
3. Prevent the tongue and cheeks from obstructing the operating field.
4. Prevent the patient from rinsing the mouth and interfering with the efficiency of the treatment.

Rubber dam is purchased in 150 mm squares, and comes in various thicknesses.

The thicker material has the advantage of a tight fit around the neck of the tooth, thus providing a hermetic seal, without the use of floss ligatures. The thicker material does not tear easily and better protects the underlying soft tissues.

Instruments for applying rubber dam

Rubber dam punch. Several types of punch are available and most are able to punch five or six holes ranging in diameter from 0.5 to 2.5 mm (Figure 5.5). The important consideration in a punch is that it cuts a clean hole in the rubber. If a cut is incomplete, it is likely that the rubber will tear on being stretched. The size of hole that is punched is important: the ease of application with a large hole must be balanced by seal at the cervical margin.

Forceps. Several types are available and choice is a matter of personal preference (Figure 5.5). The forceps are used to place, adjust and remove the rubber dam clamp. Some makes of forceps require adjustment to their working ends prior to first use; if the ends are too large, it is difficult to disengage the clamp on the tooth, therefore reshaping is required.

Lubricants, floss and tape. If more than one tooth is to be isolated, it is sometimes difficult to pass the rubber between the teeth. If the contact point is tight but smooth, the use of a lubricant on the undersurface of the dam is very helpful. Brushless shaving cream or a water-soluble tasteless lubricant jelly are available.

The trick of getting rubber through tight contacts is to knife a single layer of rubber through the contact point. The rubber is stretched and positioned vertically above the contact point. It is then gently forced through the point as a single layer of rubber. It is important that the rubber remains as a single layer and does not fold over on contact with the teeth.

Sometimes knifing is insufficient and the rubber must be forced through the contacts by dental floss or tape. This technique has been described fully [14–16, 56].

Rubber dam frame. The rubber dam must be stretched over the patient's mouth, so as not

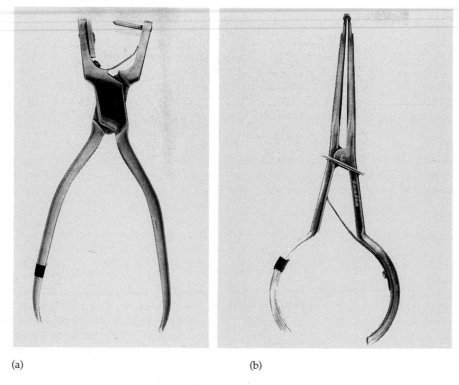

(a)   (b)

Figure 5.5 (a) Rubber dam punch and (b) clamp forceps.

to obscure the operator's vision and to provide patient comfort. Rubber dam frames (Figure 5.6) are available in a variety of shapes and sizes, and are predominantly made from plastic, which has the advantage of being radiolucent, so it is unnecessary to remove it for radiographs. Frames are shaped so that they do not impinge on the patient's face.

Rubber dam clamps. Clamp selection need not be large, but to choose from the dozens available, the function of the clamp and the effect of design must be understood. Clamps have

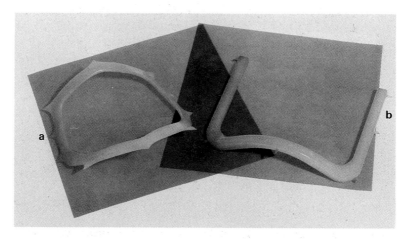

Figure 5.6 Rubber dam frames: (a) Nygard-Ostby frame; (b) Starlite Visiframe.

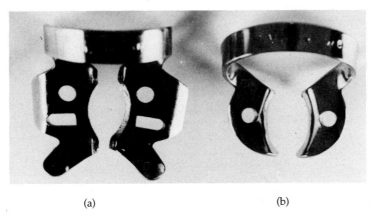

(a)   (b)

Figure 5.7 Rubber dam clamps: (a) winged clamp with bland jaws (Ash 7A); (b) wingless clamp with retentive jaws (Ivory W8).

two uses: first, they anchor the dam to the tooth, and second, they retract the gingivae. In endodontics, only anchorage is of concern. Most modern clamps are made from stainless steel; older ones were made from plated steel, which is corroded by sodium hypochlorite.

Clamps consist of a pair of jaws joined by a spring bow. They may be wingless or winged (Figure 5.7). The latter have a protrusion attached to each jaw. The wings are used to attach the rubber dam to the clamp so that both clamp and rubber may be applied to the tooth together. Clamps may be retentive or bland (Figure 5.7). Retentive clamps are designed to make a four-point contact with the tooth and have narrow, curved and slightly inverted jaws, which may displace gingival tissue to grip the tooth below the level of greatest circumference; they are very useful on partly erupted teeth. Bland clamps have flat jaws which grip the tooth around its entire circumference and because of their flatness, they are less likely to impinge on the gingivae. However, they can only be used where a tooth is fully erupted and has a cervical constriction that prevents the clamp from slipping off the tooth.

A basic assortment of clamps may consist of the following (Figure 5.8): Ivory pattern 00,

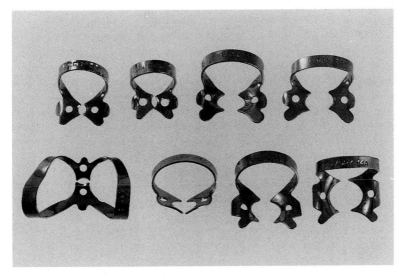

Figure 5.8 Basic assortment of clamps. Top row, left to right: patterns 00, 0, 1, 2A. Bottom row: patterns 9, W8A, 14, 14A.

0, 1, 2A, 9, W8A, 14 and 14A. The winged 14A and the wingless W8A are for molars, the 2A and 1 for premolars, and the 9 for incisors. A range of lettered Ash clamps, which are generally smaller, may also be used.

Method of application. In root canal treatment, it is sufficient to isolate only one tooth and this makes rubber dam application extremely simple. Essentially, there are two methods of application. In the first, the rubber dam is attached to the clamp and frame before it is placed on to the tooth. In the second, the clamp is attached to the tooth before the dam is placed over the clamp. The method used is a matter of preference. Although the rubber dam can be placed single-handed, the assistance of a trained dental nurse facilitates the procedure. While it may be possible to place a clamp on a tooth without encroaching on the gingivae, this cannot be guaranteed, and therefore the use of local anaesthesia is a wise precaution.

Applying rubber dam and clamp as a single unit. As a safety measure against clamp fracture during insertion, a 450 mm piece of floss is passed through one of the holes in the jaw of the clamp and knotted. This is wound around the bow of the clamp, threaded through the hole in the opposite jaw and tied again. A winged clamp is chosen, e.g. a 14A on a molar; the clamp is tried on the tooth to check for fit and stability. If satisfactory, the clamp is removed and put to one side. The rubber dam is then placed on the frame before an appropriately sized hole is punched. The clamp is then inserted into the rubber so that the wings engage the edges of the hole. The clamp forceps then engage the clamp and the combination is carried to the mouth where the clamp is positioned on the tooth. Once the clamp is firmly seated, the forceps are removed and a plastic instrument used to lift the rubber from the wings on to the side of the tooth (Figure 5.9). If more than one tooth is to be isolated, the rubber is knifed through each succeeding contact point, as described above.

Applying rubber dam to a clamped tooth. A wingless clamp is selected and tried on the

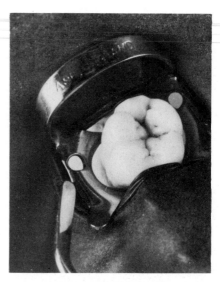

Figure 5.9 After the clamp is positioned on the tooth, the rubber is lifted off the wings with a flat plastic instrument.

tooth to check the fit and stability. The rubber dam is punched with the correct-size hole and lubricated. The success of this operation depends on dry fingers and stretching the dam so that the punched hole is made large enough to be passed over the bow of the clamp. Once the bow has been negotiated, the dam is re-stretched in a mesial direction so that it may now be passed over one jaw and then the other.

Oraseal. At times, regardless of how well the tooth is isolated, seepage of saliva may occur. To prevent this Oraseal putty (Ultradent Products, Salt Lake City, UT, USA) can be applied around the margins of the tooth to provide a totally impervious barrier (Figure 5.10).

Removal of rubber dam. If a single tooth has been isolated, the dam falls free as soon as the clamp is removed. In multiple isolation, the dam may be pulled through each contact, although it is much easier if the dam is stretched sideways and cut with scissors. Care must be taken to protect the patient's lips as this is done. After removal of the dam, it must be checked to ensure that the dam has not been torn and that a piece does not remain interdentally, as this would cause considerable postoperative discomfort.

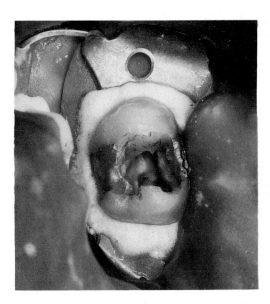

Figure 5.10 Oraseal putty applied around the edge of the rubber dam to achieve a seal (courtesy of Dr E. Saunders).

Bridgework. Generally, this is not a problem because the tooth to be treated is managed like a single tooth and the rubber allowed to cover the pontic. However, a problem may arise when the abutment has a ceramic retainer, and inspection shows that the ceramic is delicate and may fracture if clamped. If a natural tooth is present distal to the bridge, it may be used as the anchor tooth, and the dam is also attached to the tooth mesial to the bridge. The rubber above the bridge is then slit with scissors and allowed to lie alongside the bridge.

Broken-down teeth. Where insufficient tooth remains for clamp placement, it may be possible to remove enough soft tissue surgically, or by electrosurgery, to allow a clamp to be placed. It may be better not to clamp the broken-down tooth because of poor clamp stability and trauma to the gingivae, but to clamp the teeth mesial and distal to it. The dam is punched in three positions corresponding to the two anchor teeth and the broken-down tooth, and these holes are joined by cutting through with scissors. The dam can now be stretched over the mesial and distal clamps and this facilitates access to

the broken-down tooth. Protection against contamination from saliva is obtained by the use of cotton-wool rolls placed beneath the dam on the buccal side, and by the use of an aspirator on the lingual side, as well as the use of Oraseal.

Instruments for root canal preparation

Hand instruments

Hand instruments are grouped according to usage by the International Organization for Standardization (ISO), working alongside the American National Standards Institute (ANSI). These organizations have defined terminology, dimensions, physical properties, measuring systems and quality control of endodontic instruments and materials [3,31].

Standardization

The development of worldwide standards for endodontic instruments and materials has occurred since the 1950s, when it was realized that a considerable amount of variation existed between root canal instruments of different manufacturers. At that time proposals for standardizing instruments were produced [30] and covered the following:

1. The diameter and taper of each instrument and filling point.
2. The graduated increase in size from one instrument to the next.
3. An instrument-numbering system based on the diameter of the instrument.

These proposals have been widely accepted, and endodontic hand instruments, i.e. files, reamers and barbed broaches, are standardized in relation to size, colour coding and physical properties [31]. Table 5.1 lists the relevant information on sizing and colour coding for files and reamers; d_1 represents the diameter of the projection of the working part at the tip end, and is its nominal size; d_3 represents a point at 16 mm from d_1 where the cutting part of the instrument ends and is 0.32 mm larger. The taper is a constant

Table 5.1 Nominal sizes, diameters d_1 and colour of root canal files and reamers

Size	d_1 (mm)	Colour
008	0.08	Grey
010	0.10	Purple
015	0.15	White
020	0.20	Yellow
025	0.25	Red
030	0.30	Blue
035	0.35	Green
040	0.40	Black
045	0.45	White
050	0.50	Yellow
055	0.55	Red
060	0.60	Blue
070	0.70	Green
080	0.80	Black
090	0.90	White
100	1.00	Yellow
110	1.10	Red
120	1.20	Blue
130	1.30	Green
140	1.40	Black

0.02 mm per 1 mm of cutting flute. The length of instruments ranges from 21 to 31 mm, with 25 mm being the most commonly used.

Barbed broaches

These are made from soft steel wire (Figure 5.11). The barbs are formed by cutting into the metal and forcing the cut portion away from the shaft, so that the tip of the barb points towards the handle. The cuts are made eccentrically around the shaft so that it is not weakened excessively at any one point. Barbed broaches are mainly used for the removal of pulp tissue from root canals, but also for removal of cotton-wool dressings.

Provided the instrument is loose within the canal and the barb is used to engage soft tissue only, the risk of fracture is minimal. However, as soon as the barbed broach is wedged against the wall of the canal, the barbs are flattened against the shaft. When an attempt is made to remove the instrument from the canal, the sharp barb tips dig into the canal wall and resist its withdrawal. Considerable force may be necessary to free the jammed instrument and there is a risk of either fracturing the shaft of the instrument or at least some of the individual delicate barbs. For this reason, the instrument should never be used to shape canal walls.

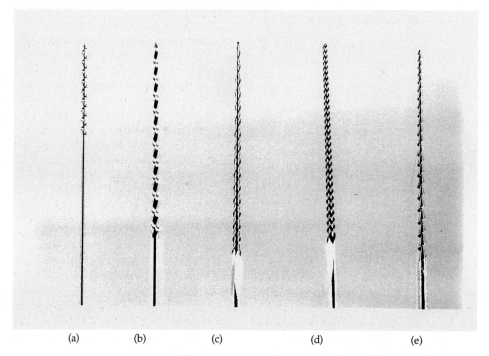

| (a) | (b) | (c) | (d) | (e) |

Figure 5.11 Hand instruments: (a) barbed broach; (b) reamer; (c) K-flex file; (d) Flexofile; (e) Hedstrom file.

Reamers

Reamers (Figure 5.11) are usually made from stainless steel by twisting tapered lengths of wire which have a triangular or square cross-section, to form an instrument with sharp cutting edges along the spiral. Although cross-section is a manufacturer's prerogative, the smaller sizes (15–50) are usually manufactured from a square blank, while the larger sizes are manufactured from a triangular blank.

Reamers are used to enlarge and shape an irregularly shaped root canal into a cavity of round cross-section. The basic action is a half-turn twist and pull which shaves the canal wall, removing dentine chips from the root canal. However, anatomically, no root canal is round in cross-section and none can be prepared so [21,25,66]. Reamers are widely used in cleaning and shaping procedures, and during the Schilder method of canal preparation [59].

Files

There are various types of root canal file, and they are usually made from stainless steel. The following are the main types:

1. K-file.
2. K-flex.
3. Flexofile.
4. Flex-R.
5. Hedstrom and Safety Hedstrom.
6. S-file.

Files are predominantly used with a filing or rasping action, in which there is little or no rotation of the instrument in the root canal, except for the Flex-R instrument. Some preparation filing techniques, e.g. stepback, create a large amount of canal debris, which may be extruded apically or block canals [2].

K-file. This instrument is manufactured from stainless-steel wire which is ground into square or triangular cross-sections (Figure 5.11). The blank is twisted into a tighter series of spirals than a reamer to produce from 0.9 to 1.9 cutting edges per millimetre length [50]; some K-files are ground. When a K-file is manufactured from a triangular cross-section it demonstrates superior cutting efficiency [55,68], and as a result of its increased flexibility is more likely to follow canal curvature than a file with a square cross-section.

K-flex file. The K-flex file (Figure 5.11) has a cross-section that is rhomboid-shaped and the twisted instrument has a series of cutting flutes with alternate sharp (<60°) cutting edges and obtuse non-cutting edges. The cutting efficiency of the K-flex file is greater than many brands of K-file, due to its increased flexibility [13,36] and ability to remove debris as its alternating blades provide a reservoir for debris [51,55]. A disadvantage of this file is its quicker loss of cutting efficiency.

Flexofile. This instrument (Figure 5.11) is manufactured by Maillefer in the same manner as the K-file but it has a triangular cross-section that gives sharper cutting blades and more room for debris than the conventional K-file. The stainless steel is extremely flexible and the instrument resists fracture. The file tip is non-cutting (Batt).

Flex-R file. Most root canal instruments have a sharp tip [43]. Removal of the sharp cutting edges from the tip of the instrument helps to prevent undesirable ledge formation [53]. The notion that the tip of the instrument demonstrates potentially active cutting surfaces led to the theory of balanced force and the eventual design of the Flex-R file [58]. The Flex-R design eliminates the possibility of ledge formation by removing the cutting surfaces at the tip's leading edge (Figure 5.12). This enables the tip to ride along the canal rather than gouge into it. At the same time, the triangular cross-sectional area of the Flex-R file provides flexibility to negotiate severely curved canals.

The balanced-force technique of clockwise rotation with anti-clockwise rotation and apical pressure has been shown to create less canal blockage and less extruded apical debris than the stepback technique [47]. The technique has been advocated for curved canals as larger non-precurved files can be used without canal transportation or ledging [61].

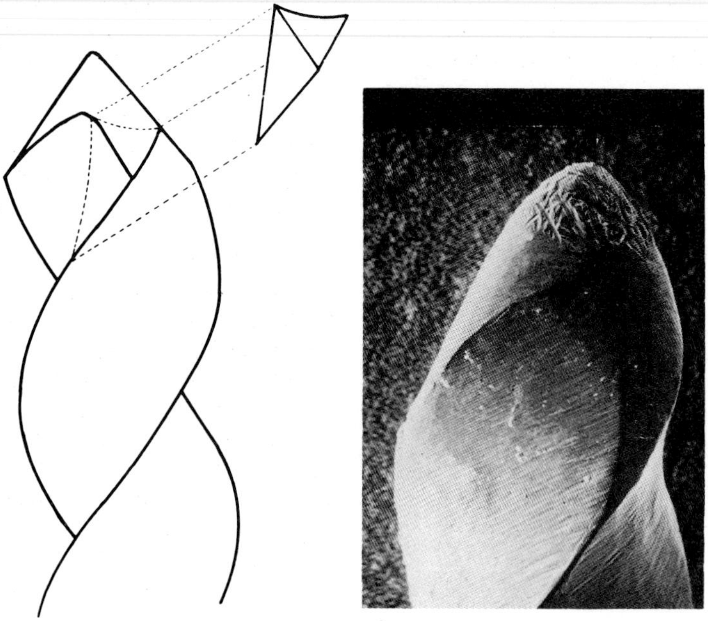

Figure 5.12 Flex-R file design: (a) outlined part indicates material removed to eliminate sharp cutting edge close to the tip; (b) scanning electron micrograph shows tip of instrument with modified blades (courtesy of Dr J.B. Roane).

Hedstrom and Safety Hedstrom. The Hedstrom file (Figures 5.11 and 5.13) is made by machining a steel blank of round cross-section to produce elevated cutting edges. The tapering effect appears to form a series of intersecting cones. Although the design leads to a flexible instrument [27,28], the instrument is inherently weak due to the small shaft diameter and is therefore prone to breakage. The Hedstrom file has been reported to have a low cutting efficiency compared with other files as it only cuts on the withdrawal stroke [68]; nevertheless it can be used to flare canal orifices and remove broken instruments, gutta-percha and silver points.

The Safety Hedstrom file (Kerr) features a non-cutting safety side along the length of the blade (Figure 5.13), which reduces the potential for strip perforations. The non-cutting side is oriented to the side of the canal where cutting is not desired, and is indicated by a flattened side on the handle. The file is used with a traditional vertical filing technique.

S-file. Originally developed in Sweden, this instrument has an S-shaped cross-section which has been produced by grinding. This

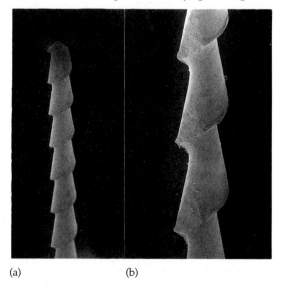

(a)   (b)

Figure 5.13 Scanning electron micrographs of (a) Hedstrom file and (b) higher magnification Safety Hedstrom file with non-cutting side.

results in a stiffer instrument than the conventional Hedstrom file. A millimetre scale is etched on to the shaft of the instrument to facilitate length control. The instrument has good cutting efficiency in either a filing or reaming action [51]; the instrument therefore could be classified as a hybrid design.

New instrument design and technology

Nickel–titanium file. In 1988, the properties of a file manufactured from nickel–titanium (Ni–Ti) alloy were reported [67]. This file demonstrates greater elastic flexibility in bending, and greater resistance to torsional fracture than stainless steel. There are now several commercial versions. Ni–Ti files have a non-cutting tip, cannot be precurved, and tend to straighten curved root canals less than stainless-steel files [19].

Profile-Series 29

In the present ISO system of hand instrument sizes, the tip diameter at d_1 increases by 0.02 mm for sizes 06–10, 0.05 mm for sizes 10–60 and 0.1 mm for larger sizes. The percentage difference between tip diameters of sizes 10–15 is 50%, whilst between sizes 55 and 60 the difference is only 9%. The variable percentage changes appear illogical and support the clinical impression that between ISO sizes 10 and 35, there are insufficient instruments. This is blamed for problems such as ledging that occur during apical preparation of root canals.

Profile-Series 29 instruments (Tulsa Dental), manufactured in stainless steel, address this problem with new instrument sizes that have a constant increase of 29% in d_1 tip diameter. Therefore in the critical smaller sizes, the range of maximal use, there are more instruments than in the ISO range, and in the less critical larger sizes there are fewer instruments. In the Profile-Series 29, 13 instruments replace 20 in the ISO series. The new size 1 Profile 29 corresponds to ISO size 10 and the first five instruments in the new series are all narrower at d_1 than their counterparts in the ISO series.

Golden-Mediums. Maillefer have produced a series of intermediate-size instruments to complement ISO standard-size instruments.

The new instruments roughly correspond in size to halfway between standard ISO sizes and are numbered 12, 17, 22, 27, 32 and 37. Whilst this system addresses the problem of too few instruments in the smaller sizes, it does not achieve linear dimensional change at d_1. Golden-Mediums are part of the Flexofile range.

MAC Files and Double MAC Files. The MAC file is a new instrument manufactured from Ni–Ti, and has a working surface demonstrating dissimilar helical angles with blades that spiral round the shaft at different rates. According to the manufacturer this allows the instrument to stay relatively loose within the canal and balances the forces of the file against the canal wall during rotation to prevent canal transportation. The Double MAC has a series of increasing tapers from 0.03 to 0.55 mm/mm length (Figure 5.14).

Canal Master U. The Canal Master U (CMU) hand instrument (Figure 5.15) was developed in the late 1980s [69]. The instrument is used to prepare the apical third of the canal, and has a non-cutting pilot tip, a 1 mm length cutting blade, and a parallel-sided shaft with a smaller diameter than the cutting blade. It is designed to improve debris removal and reduce apically extruded debris [54]; further, it has been reported to create a well-centred canal preparation without ledging and transportation [5,18].

Recently, a Ni–Ti CMU hand instrument has been developed, and it produces a better canal preparation than other files [19].

Flexogate. Similar in design and use to the CMU hand instrument, the Flexogate (Figure 5.15) is a logical development of the Gates-Glidden drill. Whereas the latter is used during conventional coronal preparation of the canal, the Flexogate's task is enlarging the apical region of the canal. The Flexogate demonstrates a non-cutting guiding tip and debris evacuation zone which helps to maintain root canal configuration during instrumentation [8].

Whilst the Flexogate can fracture more easily during torsion than the CMU, it has a breakage point approximately 16 mm from the tip, which ensures its retrieval in the event of separation [9]. The bending moment

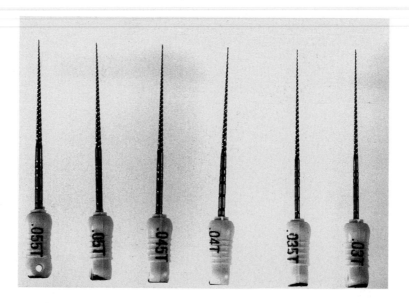

Figure 5.14 Double MAC files are produced in a series of tapers from 0.03 to 0.055; tip size is 0.2 mm.

of the Flexogate and the CMU are well below standards' specifications for files, leading to considerable flexibility in curved canals [9].

Power-assisted root canal instruments

Reciprocating handpieces

Specifically designed handpieces providing a mechanical action to a root canal cutting instrument have been available for 30 years. They are all designed to reduce the time spent in canal preparation.

Giromatic. The first of the mechanized handpieces, and now little used by endodontists, accepts barbed-broach-type files (Rispi) and three-sided files (Heli files). The continuous rotation of the driveshaft in the handpiece is transformed into an alternating quarter-turn movement of the file.

M4 Safety Handpiece. This handpiece, manufactured by Kerr, has a simplified chuck mechanism activated by thumb pressure to accommodate a plastic-handled root canal instrument (Figure 5.16). The handpiece lets

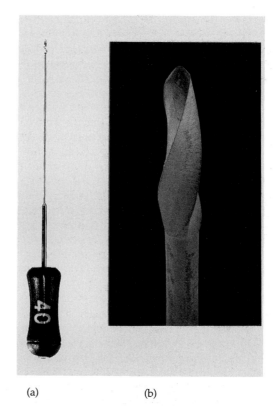

(a)   (b)

Figure 5.15 (a) Canal Master U size 40; (b) scanning electron micrograph of head of Maillefer Flexogate.

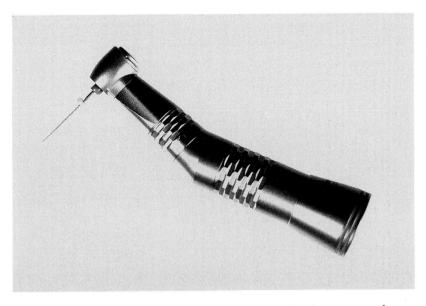

Figure 5.16 Kerr M4 Safety handpiece, which accepts most hand instruments, shown with a Safety Hedstrom.

the instrument glide along the walls of the canal by mimicking commonly used hand movements. The M4 has a 4:1 gear ratio, which even at full speed demonstrates minimal torquing.

Canal Finder System. The Canal Finder System consists of a contra-angle handpiece powered by a micromotor that runs at speeds <3000 rpm, producing a reciprocal screwing action which enables the file to cleave, rather than abrade the canal wall, and advance along the path of least resistance, maintaining the original pathway. Specially designed files rotate the file slightly when resistance from the canal is met. The system is of benefit in initial penetration of extremely curved and narrow canals [38]; it has a tendency to straighten canals with over-instrumentation and widening of the apical foramen, but does not clean better than hand preparation [26].

Canal Master System. The rotary version of the Canal Master System is principally used for coronal flaring of the body of the canal as far as its curvature. These instruments have a 2 mm non-cutting tip and a 2 mm cutting

head. The latch-type instruments for use in a contra-angle handpiece are sized ISO 50–100. Recently, a totally engine-driven version in Ni–Ti has been developed.

Ultrasonic instrumentation

The use of ultrasonic energy to prepare root canals was first described in the 1950s [45,57], although commercial production took another 20 years.

Cavi-Endo. This was the first ultrasonic unit (Figure 5.17) specifically designed for endodontic use. The machine is a modified Cavitron which contains an irrigant reservoir that supplies a continuous flow of sodium hypochlorite through a specially designed handpiece on to the energized file. The files are available in two types (Figure 5.18): a stainless-steel K-file with a colour-coded shaft, and a safe-ended file coated with diamond particles. As the file vibrates within the root canal (at 25 kHz) an acoustic streaming effect is set up within the irrigant. Endosonic files, sizes 15, 20 and 25, are used to prepare the apical part of the canal, while the safe-ended diamond files flare the coronal

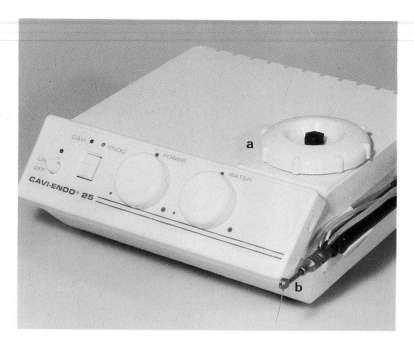

Figure 5.17 Cavi-Endo unit which can be used as a scaler or for endosonic use. The reservoir (a) supplies a constant flow of irrigant through the special handpiece (b).

part of the canal. Evidence suggests that canal preparation using the Cavi-Endo system results in superior canal debridement over hand preparation [12,20]. However, caution is advisable as over-preparation could result in straightening of the canal and even strip perforation [10].

Piezoelectric. These units are supplied with a multifunctional handpiece, into which different tips are fitted. This unit is additionally used for the location of calcified canals, removal of broken instruments, removal of cemented posts, and for root-end cavity preparation during periradicular surgery (see Chapter 9).

Atraumatic post removal can be achieved with the use of a tip similar to an ultrasonic scaler tip. After removing the core material, the tip of the ultrasonic instrument is activated against the luting cement and against the metal post. A high power setting is used to break up the cement lute; within a short time the post becomes loose and can easily be retrieved. Unlike other more aggressive methods of post removal there is little loss

of tooth structure and root damage is minimized.

Sonic instrumentation

The Endo MM1500 (Figure 5.19) was developed as a sonic vibratory handpiece to be attached to the turbine line of a dental unit. The handpiece operates at a frequency of 1500 Hz and accepts specially designed Micro-Mega files: the Helisonic file, Rispisonic file and Shaper file (Figure 5.20). The Shaper file adequately cleans the apical third of the root canal, while the Rispisonic file is more suitable for the coronal two-thirds [6], and has superior cutting efficiency [52].

The root canal instrument vibrates in a simpler pattern than ultrasonic files. A continuous flow of water is delivered through the handpiece on to the instrument. An adjustable depth stop controls instrument length. The sonic method improves the ease and extent of instrumentation, thus reducing operator fatigue [4,65]; it also produces less apical extrusion of debris [17]. Sonic instrumentation avoids transportation of curved canals in the smaller sizes [70].

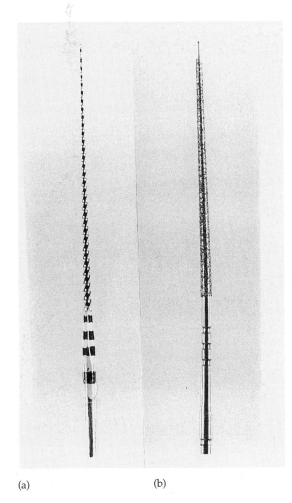

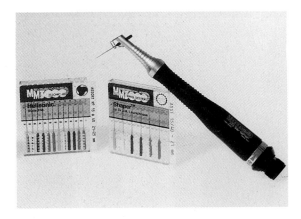

Figure 5.19 Sonic vibratory handpiece, Micro-Mega 1500, shown with special files.

Nitimatic system

The Nitimatic system has a handpiece run by an electric motor which provides load-torque compensation and constant speed, even at very low speed. The handpiece has a 16:1 gear reduction contra-angle for use at extremely low speed (300 rpm) with Ni–Ti files (sensor files) and a 1:1 contra-angle for obturation with Ni–Ti condensers. Small files, sizes 15–30, have flat cutting spirals rather than blades, which plane the canal wall to produce an extremely smooth finish. In addition, the file has an eccentric tip which enables it to negotiate around curves and natural ledges. Larger files have two or more spiralled blades which intersect at intervals

(a)   (b)

Figure 5.18 Cavi-Endo ultrasonic files: (a) size 15 stainless-steel K-file; (b) diamond-coated safe-ended file.

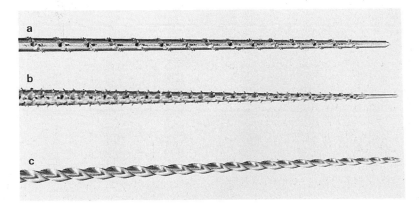

Figure 5.20 Specially designed files for Micro-Mega sonic handpiece: (a) Shaper file; (b) Rispi file; (c) Heli file.

along the shaft of the instrument; at the intersection, there are twice as many cutting edges. There has been little evaluation of Ni–Ti sensor files; however, recently [19], these files created a better-centred canal preparation than hand files.

The Nitimatic system has recently incorporated a new file (McXim; Figure 5.21), which prepares the canal in a crown-down action similar to the Double MAC file. The files have a constant size 25 tip, but are available in five different tapers, from 0.03 to 0.055.

ProFile 0.04 Taper Series 29

Manufactured by Tulsa Dental Products, these Ni–Ti engine files are similar to Series 29 hand instruments, but with a 0.04 mm/mm tapered shaft. The instruments are used in a high-torque rotary handpiece at a speed of 300 rpm, which provides a reaming action, producing a centred and tapered preparation. The flat outer edges of the file (U-file design) prevent threading of the instrument into the canal wall, help to keep the instrument well centred, and plane rather than cut the canal wall.

Electronic canal-measuring devices

The concept of measuring canal length electrically goes back many years [63]. Recent electronic apex locator devices rely on the impedance between an electrode placed on the oral mucosa and an electrode passed through a root canal in contact with the periodontal ligament being constant [62]. Modern equipment is reliable and may give a visual display, or emit an audible sound [11]; an example is shown in Figure 5.22. Root canal length should be measured by an apex locator and confirmed radiographically, thus reducing the number of X-ray exposures [11].

While these devices are useful in determining root canal length, they must be used carefully to avoid errors. The presence of fluid (pus, exudate or sodium hypochlorite irrigant)

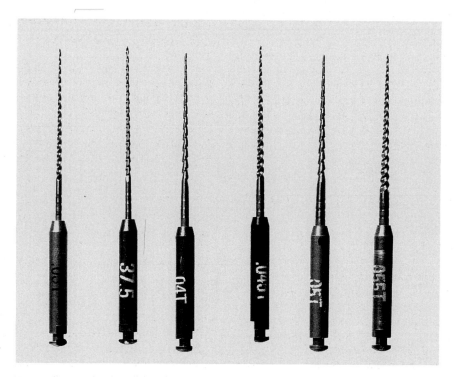

Figure 5.21 McXim engine files for use in the Nitimatic handpiece; taper increases from 0.03 to 0.055, but tip size is constant at 0.25 mm.

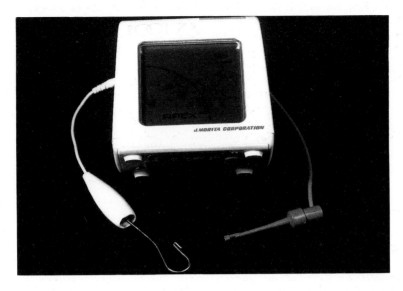

Figure 5.22 Root ZX apex locator with a visual display is shown with its electrical leads.

may hinder correct estimation of working length. A major influencing factor is the size of the apical foramen [29]; when this is large, the apex locator may give a reading short of the apex. However, when the apex is small, an accurate reading within 0.5 mm of the apical foramen is likely. One apex locator has been developed in which the canal probe is covered by an insulating sleeve to overcome the problem of canal contents. Another apex locator (Root ZX, Morita, Kyoto, Japan) may be used in a wet canal and even in the presence of electrolytes.

Measuring instruments, gauges and stands

The importance of instrumentation to a known canal length cannot be overstressed. A rubber stop provides the simplest and most positive stop to instrumentation. A ruler is necessary to set the stop, or alternative measuring devices have been developed to make the procedure easier. Rubber stops are already placed on some makes of file; alternatively they can be placed using a dispenser. A stand is useful as the instruments can be placed in order, and are easily accessible at

the chairside. A number of these are commercially available (Figure 5.23).

Instruments for retrieving broken instruments and posts

As prevention is much easier than the removal of a fractured instrument from the root canal, all root canal instruments should be used carefully. When an instrument fractures, it may be possible to remove it with one of a number of different instruments; techniques are covered in Chapter 13.

Forceps

Fine-beaked forceps can be used to remove a broken instrument only if the end of the fractured instrument is visible and not jammed firmly within the canal (Figure 5.24).

Cancellier kit

If the obstruction is loose but not free, Cancellier extractors (Excellence in Endodontics), which are simply hollow pluggers, can be used to fit over the obstruction. A single drop of cyanoacrylate glue deposited into the Cancellier sticks the instrument into the

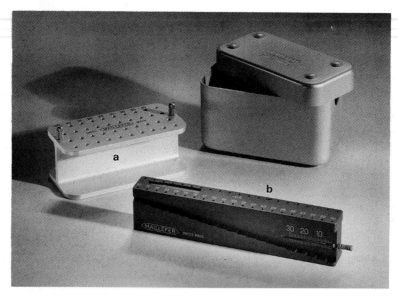

Figure 5.23 (a) Storage box with its stand that will hold up to 40 files; (b) measuring block for precise and quick setting of file working length.

extractor, and it is retrieved. A common solvent, e.g. xylene, will dissolve the cyanoacrylate so that the Cancellier can be cleaned and reused.

Masserann kit

The Masserann kit (Figure 5.25) can be used to free an obstruction which is jammed in the canal. The principle of this method consists of freeing around the periphery of a broken post or instrument using hollow trepan burs, whose inner diameter corresponds to the diameter of the broken post or instrument. The trench created around the broken instrument reduces the resistance of the fragment to removal and also creates space for the insertion of a second instrument in the kit,

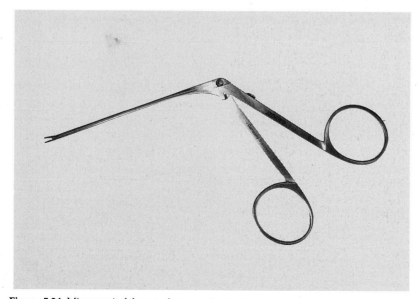

Figure 5.24 Microsurgical forceps for removing broken instruments.

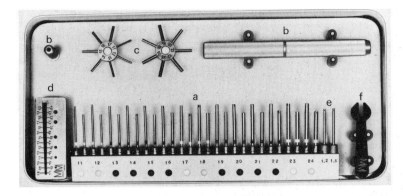

Figure 5.25 Masserann kit (Micro-Mega) containing (a) a range of trepans, (b) handle, (c, d) gauges, (e) extractors and (f) a spanner for removing the trepans from handles.

which grips and extracts the broken instrument [46].

Post remover

Many techniques have been devised to remove cemented posts, from simple drilling with burs to sophisticated post pullers such as the Eggler or Thomas extractor [44]. These devices (Figure 5.26) exert a strong pull on

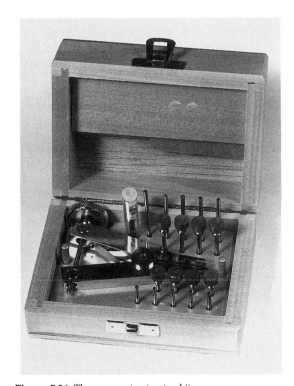

Figure 5.26 Thomas post extractor kit.

the post and there is a risk of tooth fracture. Atraumatic post removal can be achieved with an ultrasonic scaler tip.

Instruments for filling root canals

The final stage of root canal treatment is three-dimensional filling of the root canal system. The instruments used depend on the technique employed to obturate the canal.

Lateral condensation

Hand spreaders

Manufactured from stainless steel, hand spreaders are designed to facilitate the placement of accessory gutta-percha points around a well-fitting master gutta-percha point during the lateral condensation method (Figure 5.27). Their diameter and shape are not standardized, making it difficult to match spreaders with accessory gutta-percha points. There is also variation amongst manufacturers in sizing [32].

Finger spreaders

These instruments are colour-coded to match either standardized or accessory gutta-percha points. Their short length affords a high degree of tactile sense and allows them to rotate freely around their axis, thus freeing

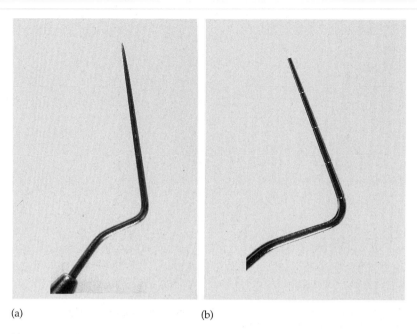

(a)   (b)

Figure 5.27 (a) Long-handled spreader for lateral condensation. (b) Schilder plugger for vertical condensation of gutta-percha.

the instrument for easy removal (Figure 5.28). The depth of spreader penetration is important for the quality of the final apical seal [1]; spreaders should be capable of reaching to within 1–2 mm of the apical stop alongside the master gutta-percha point. A variety of spreaders of different lengths and widths is required.

Vertical condensation

Schilder pluggers

Schilder pluggers (Figure 5.27), manufactured by Caulk, consist of long-handled instruments which are of larger diameter than spreaders and have a blunt end; they are used to pack thermally softened gutta-percha into the root canal. The different-diameter pluggers have reference lines on the tips to allow the assessment of plugger depth. It is very important to realize when the plugger is engaging a cushion of softened gutta-percha, rather than the resistance of the canal wall. These pluggers may also be used to pack calcium hydroxide into root canals.

Heat carrier – Touch 'n Heat

In the vertical condensation technique, segments of gutta-percha are removed by a heat source so that the remaining gutta-percha point left in the canal can be vertically condensed with pre-fitted Schilder pluggers in waves. The application of a heat source in this technique has been facilitated by the introduction of the Analytic Technology Touch 'n Heat unit (5004 model; Figure 5.29). The tips of the Touch 'n Heat unit are heated rapidly and internally to concentrate the heat at the tip at a controlled temperature. A contact spring on the front of the handpiece activates the heater at the slightest touch. It can also be used as a heat source for warm lateral condensation. Electrically-heated pluggers have been further developed with the introduction of System B (Analytic Technology).

Hybrid techniques

Thermomechanical compaction

This technique utilizes the principle of a reverse turning screw which softens gutta-

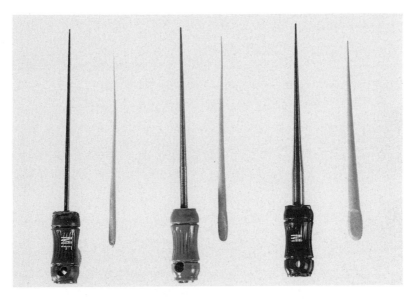

Figure 5.28 Finger spreaders with corresponding accessory gutta-percha points (Kerr medium fine, fine and medium).

percha and forces and compacts it ahead of and lateral to the rotating compactor shaft [64]. Compacting instruments are engine-operated and have a screw-type thread. The Maillefer gutta-condensor (Figure 5.30) is rotated in a forward direction at 8000 rpm alongside a well-fitting standardized gutta-percha point. The instrument heats and softens by friction the gutta-percha, which is forced ahead of the instrument approximately

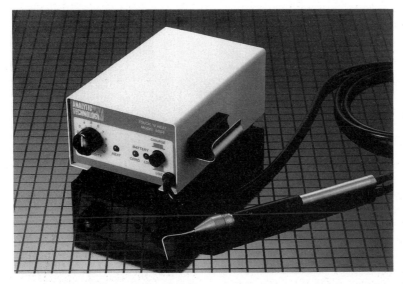

Figure 5.29 Analytic Technology Touch 'n Heat. The tip of the handpiece heats up rapidly and is used to remove gutta-percha in vertical condensation (courtesy of Analytic Technology).

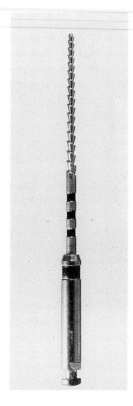

Figure 5.30 Maillefer gutta-condensor for thermomechanical compaction of gutta-percha.

2–3 mm. As the bulk of gutta-percha in the canal builds up, the compactor is forced out of the canal. The result is a well-condensed three-dimensional root canal filling which, when used in conjunction with sealer, produces a comparable apical seal to lateral condensation [34]. If the compactor is used in reverse, it screws into the root and breaks. Without the presence of a good apical stop, it is possible to overfill the root canal using this technique. Overfilling can be prevented by laterally condensing three or four accessory gutta-percha points, prior to thermomechanical compaction [35,64].

Warm lateral condensation

The Endotec condenser (Figure 5.31) consists of a battery-operated heated root canal spreader. The handpiece is a rechargeable battery to which is attached a fine metal tube shaped as a condenser, that contains a heating element, controlled by a push-button.

The heat softens the gutta-percha in the root canal so that it can be better condensed. If the operator is heavy-handed, the fine condenser may be damaged.

Thermoplasticized injectable gutta-percha

Injecting softened gutta-percha into the root canal was first introduced about 20 years ago [71]. Subsequent developments have led to the production of two commercial systems, which differ in the temperature at which the gutta-percha is extruded.

Obtura II heated gutta-percha system

This second-generation high-temperature delivery system is capable of taking the temperature of gutta-percha in the heating chamber to 200°C. The gutta-percha is introduced at a much lower temperature into the root canal from a delivery unit that resembles a glue gun. The gutta-percha is delivered through a 20- or 23-gauge needle. The delivery unit (Figure 5.32) is connected by an electric cord to a control box that adjusts the temperature of the heating element. Precise temperature control (the manufacturer recommends 185°C) and uniform viscosity of the extruded gutta-percha, which has a working time of 3–5 min in the root canal, provide good results [7]. Thermal protectors are available to insulate the heating unit and prevent burning of the patient's lip. Applicator tips, made from silver, are reusable, bendable and sterilizable.

There are advantages in a device that reduces obturation time [60], although it is necessary to master the technique [23]. Concern has been expressed about the heat generated by the Obtura system; however, due to the short injection time and rapid cooling, the heat has not been shown to cause damage [22, 24].

Ultrafil system

This system of injectable thermoplasticized gutta-percha (Hygenic) differs from the Obtura II system in that the material is extruded at a lower temperature, 70°C. The system consists of:

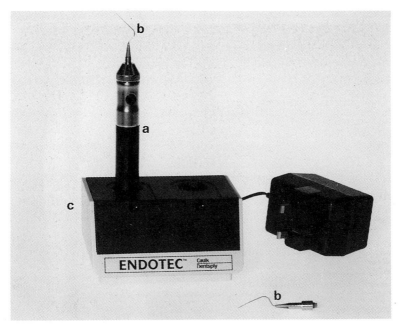

Figure 5.31 Endotec heated lateral spreader. The handpiece (a) contains a rechargeable battery and has a replaceable tip (b) which is heated internally. The main unit (c) is a battery charger.

1. Pre-filled disposable cannulae containing gutta-percha with 22-gauge stainless-steel needles. The cannulae can be obtained with gutta-percha in three different viscosities.

2. An autoclavable syringe.
3. A portable heating unit.

The preloaded disposable cannulae are heated in the portable heating unit (Figure

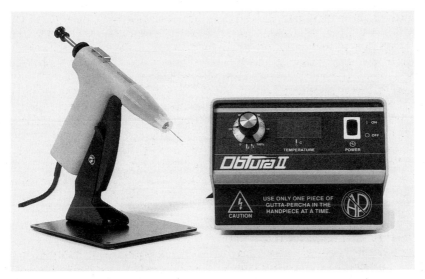

Figure 5.32 Obtura II heated gutta-percha system. The heated delivery gun (a) extrudes gutta-percha through the fine needle; the temperature is controlled by the main unit (b).

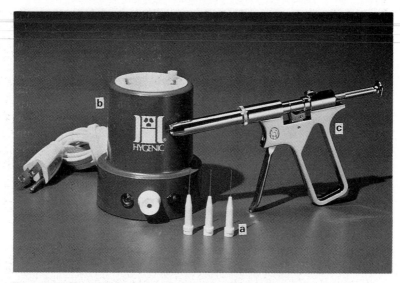

Figure 5.33 Hygenic Ultrafil system. Cannulae filled with gutta-percha (a) are heated in the main unit (b); when the gutta-percha has softened, the cannula is loaded into the delivery syringe (c) (courtesy of Hygenic).

5.33), and once the correct temperature is reached, obturation is performed by inserting the cannula into the syringe and squeezing the trigger to express the softened gutta-percha, which should be used in conjunction with a suitable root canal sealer. The success of this technique has been reported [48,49]; the root canal filling shows very close adaptation to the root canal wall, and as the gutta-percha has been shown to penetrate dentinal tubules, the use of sealer has been questioned.

Gutta-percha carrier devices

Thermafil

In 1978, a technique was described of moulding heated gutta-percha to a root canal file, which could then be carried to the prepared canal. The coronal section was sectioned with a bur and the apical part left in the canal [33]. The technique is now commercially available as the Thermafil endodontic obturator (Tulsa Dental Products).

Stainless steel, titanium or plastic carriers, which have been coated with a particular type of gutta-percha (Figure 5.34), are placed into a special heating unit to soften the

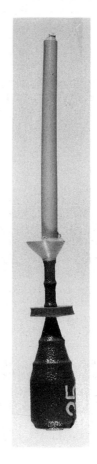

Figure 5.34 Thermafil obturator. The plastic carrier is coated with gutta-percha.

gutta-percha. The heated gutta-percha has excellent flow properties and when the carrier is placed in the root canal it forces the softened gutta-percha to the apex. The carriers are pre-notched, sized and colour-coded (ISO sizes 20–140). The flexible metal carriers, especially in the smaller sizes, are suitable for insertion into very curved canals. Whilst high clinical success has been achieved, good canal preparation is a prerequisite. The leaving of a solid core filling material in the root canal has been questioned when possible retreatment may be required in the future.

Trifecta technique

This technique (Hygenic) uses thermoplasticized gutta-percha (SuccessFil), injected on to the tip of either a titanium or plastic core carrier and available in ISO sizes 20–40. The carriers, with their gutta-percha coating, are carried into the apical part of the canal and, when turned anti-clockwise and withdrawn, leave a softened segment of gutta-percha which can then be condensed with a pre-fitted plugger. The remainder of the canal is filled with injectable gutta-percha from an Ultrafil syringe. SuccessFil gutta-percha is preheated in a syringe in the Ultrafil heating unit. The sealing ability of the Trifecta technique has been reported [40].

Inject-R-Fill

Inject-R-Fill (Moyco/Union Broach) is a thermal gutta-percha injection device, designed for back-filling the canal after the apical part of the canal has been plugged by gutta-percha during warm vertical condensation. It consists of a stainless-steel carrier prefilled with conventional gutta-percha (Figure 5.35) which is warmed over an open flame. When the carrier is inserted into the canal orifice, the handle is pushed towards the canal to drive the heat-softened gutta-percha into the canal. The gutta-percha contents flow into the canal, whilst the excess flows into the access cavity. Rotation of the handle withdraws the empty device from the canal. The gutta-percha is then condensed with a plugger until the filling is flush with the chamber floor.

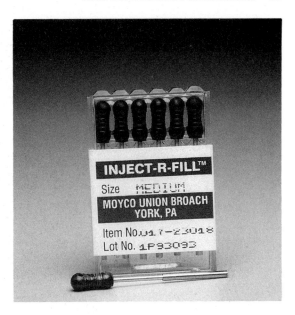

Figure 5.35 Inject-R-Fill. A stainless-steel tube contains gutta-percha, which after heating is forced out of the tube by pressure from the handle.

J S Quick-Fill

This relatively new technique (J S Dental) uses thermomechanical compaction, with a compacting instrument pre-coated with gutta-percha (Figure 5.36). The compacting instrument is a reverse-turning screw which softens the gutta-percha by frictional heat, and compacts it ahead of and lateral to the rotating shaft.

Multiphase gutta-percha

An engine-driven Ni–Ti condenser has been developed. Gutta-percha in syringes is heated to 79°C in a heater. Multiphase I gutta-percha has the composition and properties of gutta-percha used for filling points, and after heating is extruded from the syringe on to an appropriately sized condenser. This is then covered with Multiphase II gutta-percha, which has a lower melting range. The double-coated condenser is inserted into the canal and the handpiece run at 3000–4000 rpm. The reverse-screw action of the condenser forces the gutta-percha into the canal. The single-sized PAC MAC condenser, which has a size 0.25 mm tip with 0.90 mm at its handle, has enough flexibility to condense around curves.

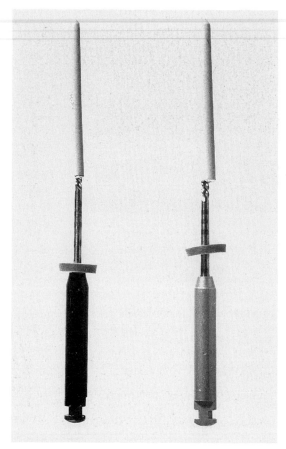

Figure 5.36 J S Quick-Fill. A thermocompactor instrument precoated with gutta-percha.

Equipment for storing instruments

Prearranged sets of instruments can be sterilized and stored in boxes, which are available in a variety of sizes with or without compartments (Figure 5.23). Some have been specially designed to take a full complement of endodontic instruments and one such box is the RAF model (Figure 5.37), which has a stand for files and a grip for cleaning hand instruments, medicament trays and pellet containers. Alternatively, instruments can be autoclaved and stored in transparent paper bags and laid out on an open plastic tray (Figure 5.37). Root canal hand instruments can be stored in sets, e.g. of sizes 15–40, in sterilizable Pyrex glass test tubes (Figure 5.37); different-coloured test tube covers can be used to identify various lengths and types of instruments.

Sterilization of endodontic instruments

While it is generally recognized that the aim of root canal preparation is to eliminate infection from a canal, it is very important that all instruments used in the root canal should be sterile, or at least have been sterilized between patients.

Various methods have been advocated.

Pressure steam (autoclaving) sterilization

Dental hand instruments and root canal files are normally sterilized by autoclaving. This is effective and has the advantage of a reasonably short cycle – 3 min at 134°C. However, heating up and cooling down extend the clinical cycle to about 15 min. As autoclaves are pressure vessels, they need to be checked for safety on a regular basis. A disadvantage is that cotton wool and paper points must be dried after sterilization and non-stainless steel instruments may corrode.

Dry-heat sterilization

Hand instruments and other materials such as cotton wool and paper points can be placed in metal boxes, sterilized and sealed afterwards until used. Recommended dry-heat sterilization is performed at 160°C for 60 min. When the preheating and cooling-down period after sterilization are included, a complete cycle of 90 min may be excessive in a busy dental surgery.

Sterile packs

Increasingly, disposable items are produced in sterile blister packs; these were initially confined to syringes, needles, scalpel blades and sutures but now include some files and paper points.

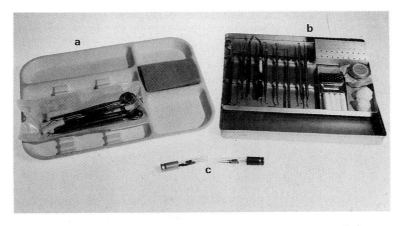

Figure 5.37 (a) Plastic tray containing instruments in a transparent sterile bag; (b) metal RAF tray containing instruments which can be sterilized together; (c) files can be stored and sterilized in Pyrex test tubes.

Gas sterilization

Sterilizers using ethylene oxide, alcohol and other chemicals are available, and these operate at similar temperatures to steam autoclaves. Because water is absent from the system, cotton wool and paper points do not get wet and so do not need to be dried; also metal instruments do not corrode.

Bead or salt sterilization

This method is effective, provided the instrument to be sterilized is held in the heat-conducting material for a minimum of 10 s. Temperature variations within the well may occur and this may lead to imperfect sterilization. It is normally only used to reduce contamination during treatment, as files are

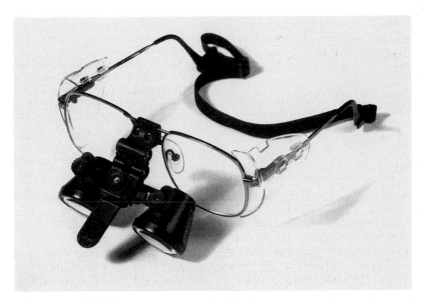

Figure 5.38 Orascoptic telescopes attached to spectacles for enhanced vision.

autoclaved between patients. Bead sterilizers have also been criticized because it is relatively easy to carry beads into the root canal and cause an obstruction.

Chemical disinfectant

Chemical disinfection is useful for those items which would be damaged by methods of sterilization. Disinfectants such as sodium hypochlorite and glutaraldehyde may be used to wipe over working surfaces and glass slabs. Gutta-percha points may be effectively disinfected by immersion in sodium hypochlorite or 70% alcohol.

Equipment for improving visibility

Endodontic treatment, both conventional and surgical, involves procedures often performed in areas of reduced visibility. A dental operating light may be insufficient to enhance operator vision. Under these circumstances, there is a need for improved illumination and magnification, either separately or combined.

Dental telescopes

These are now available in many designs, but are more practical when attached to spectacles which contain the clinician's correct prescription. Different levels of magnification can be obtained with varying depth of field to enhance the operator's vision in searching for canal orifices. Orascoptic telescopes (Advanced Dental Concepts, Madison, WI, USA) can be attached to the frame and can be pushed up when not required (Figure 5.38).

References

1. ALLISON DA, WEBER CR, WALTON RE (1979) The influence of the method of canal preparation on the quality of apical and coronal obturation. *Journal of Endodontics* **5,** 298–304.
2. AL-OMARI MAO, DUMMER PMH (1995) Canal blockage and debris extrusion with eight preparation techniques. *Journal of Endodontics* **21,** 154–158.
3. AMERICAN NATIONAL STANDARDS INSTITUTE (1988) *Revised American National Standards Institute/American Dental Association Specification no. 28 for Root Canal Files and Reamers, Type K.* New York, NY, USA: American National Standards Institute.
4. BARNETT F, GODICK B, TRONSTAD L (1985) Clinical suitability of a sonic vibratory endodontic instrument. *Endodontics and Dental Traumatology* **1,** 77–81.
5. BAUMGARTNER JC, MARTIN H, SABALA CL, STRITTMATER EJ, WILDEY WL, QUIGLEY NC (1992) Histomorphometric comparison of canals prepared by four techniques. *Journal of Endodontics* **18,** 530–534.
6. BOLANOS OR, SINAI IH, GONSKY MR, SRINVASAN R (1988) A comparison of engine and air-driven instrumentation methods with hand instrumentation. *Journal of Endodontics* **8,** 392–396.
7. BUDD CS, WELLER RN, KULILD JC (1991) A comparison of thermoplasticized injectable gutta-percha obturation techniques. *Journal of Endodontics* **17,** 260–264.
8. CAMPS J, MACOUIN G, PERTOT WJ (1994) Effects of the Flexogates and Canal Master U on root canal configuration in simulated curved canals. *International Endodontic Journal* **27,** 21–25.
9. CAMPS JJ, PERTOT WJ (1994) Torsional properties of stainless steel Canal Master U and Flexogates. *International Endodontic Journal* **27,** 334–338.
10. CHENAIL BL, TEPLITSKY PE (1988) Endosonics in curved root canals. Part II. *Journal of Endodontics* **14,** 214–217.
11. CHONG BS, PITT FORD TR (1994) Apex locators in endodontics: which, when and how? *Dental Update* **21,** 328–330.
12. CUNNINGHAM WT, MARTIN H, FORREST W (1982) Evaluation of root canal debridement by the endosonic ultrasonic synergistic system. *Oral Surgery, Oral Medicine, Oral Pathology* **53,** 401–404.
13. DOLAN DW, CRAIG RG (1982) Bending and torsion of endodontic files with rhombus cross sections. *Journal of Endodontics* **8,** 260–264.
14. ELDERTON RJ (1971) A modern approach to the use of rubber dam. Part 1. *Dental Practitioner and Dental Record* **21,** 187–193.
15. ELDERTON RJ (1971) A modern approach to the use of rubber dam. Part 2. *Dental Practitioner and Dental Record* **21,** 226–232.
16. ELDERTON RJ (1971) A modern approach to the use of rubber dam. Part 3. *Dental Practitioner and Dental Record* **21,** 267–273.
17. FAIRBOURN DR, MCWALTER GM, MONTGOMERY S (1987) The effect of four preparation techniques on the amount of apically extruded debris. *Journal of Endodontics* **13,** 102–108.
18. GILLES JA, DEL RIO CE (1990) Comparison of the Canal Master endodontic instrument and K-type files for enlargement of curved root canals. *Journal of Endodontics* **16,** 561–565.
19. GLOSSON CR, HALLER RH, DOVE SB, DEL RIO CE (1995) A comparison of root canal preparations using Ni–Ti hand, Ni–Ti engine-driven, and K-flex endodontic instruments. *Journal of Endodontics* **21,** 146–151.

20. GOODMAN A, READER A, BECK M, MELFI R, MEYERS W (1985) An *in vitro* comparison of the efficacy of the step-back technique versus a step-back/ultrasonic technique in human mandibular molars. *Journal of Endodontics* **11**, 249–256.

21. GUTIERREZ JH, GARCIA J (1968) Microscopic and macroscopic investigation on results of mechanical preparation of root canals. *Oral Surgery, Oral Medicine, Oral Pathology* **25**, 108–116.

22. GUTMANN JL, CREEL DC, BOWLES WH (1987) Evaluation of heat transfer during root canal obturation with thermoplasticized gutta-percha. Part I. *In vitro* heat level during extrusion. *Journal of Endodontics* **13**, 378–383.

23. GUTMANN JL, RAKUSIN H (1987) Perspectives on root canal obturation with thermoplasticized injectable gutta-percha. *International Endodontic Journal* **20**, 261–270.

24. GUTMANN JL, RAKUSIN H, POWE R, BOWLES WH (1987) Evaluation of heat transfer during root canal obturation with thermoplasticized gutta-percha. Part II. *In vivo* response to heat levels generated. *Journal of Endodontics* **13**, 441–448.

25. HAGA CS (1968) Microscopic measurements of root canal preparations following instrumentation. *Journal of the British Endodontic Society* **2**, 41–46.

26. HAIKEL Y, ALLEMANN C (1988) Effectiveness of four methods for preparing root canals. A scanning electron microscopic evaluation. *Journal of Endodontics* **14**, 340–345.

27. HARTY FJ, STOCK CJR (1974) A comparison of the flexibility of Giromatic and hand operated instruments in endodontics. *Journal of the British Endodontic Society* **7**, 64–71.

28. HARTY FJ, STOCK CJR (1974) The Giromatic system compared with hand instrumentation in endodontics. *British Dental Journal* **137**, 239–244.

29. HUANG L (1987) An experimental study of the principle of electronic root canal measurement. *Journal of Endodontics* **13**, 60–64.

30. INGLE JI, LEVINE M (1958) The need for uniformity of endodontic instruments, equipment and filling materials. In: Grossman LI (ed.) *Transactions of the Second International Conference on Endodontics*, pp. 123–143. Philadelphia, PA, USA: University of Pennsylvania.

31. INTERNATIONAL ORGANIZATION FOR STANDARDIZATION (ISO) (1992) *Dental Root Canal Instruments – Part 1: Specification for Files, Reamers, Barbed Broaches, Rasps, Paste Carriers, Explorers and Cotton Broaches.* ISO 3630–1: 1992. London, UK: British Standards Institution.

32. JEROME CE, HICKS ML, PELLEU GB (1988) Compatibility of accessory gutta-percha cones used with two types of spreaders. *Journal of Endodontics* **14**, 428–434.

33. JOHNSON WB (1978) A new gutta-percha technique. *Journal of Endodontics* **4**, 184–188.

34. KEREKES K, ROWE AHR (1982) Thermo-mechanical compaction of gutta-percha root filling. *International Endodontic Journal* **15**, 27–35.

35. KERSTEN HW, FRANSMAN R, THODEN VAN VELZEN SK (1986) Thermomechanical compaction of gutta-percha. I. A comparison of several compaction procedures. *International Endodontic Journal* **19**, 125–133.

36. KRUPP JD, BRANTLEY WA, GERSTEIN H (1984) An investigation of the torsional and bending properties of seven brands of endodontic files. *Journal of Endodontics* **10**, 372–380.

37. LAUSTEN LL, LUEBKE NH, BRANTLEY WA (1993) Bending and metallurgical properties of rotary endodontic instruments. IV. Gates Glidden and Peeso drills. *Journal of Endodontics* **19**, 440–447.

38. LEVY G, ABOU-RASS M (1990) Endodontic file design and dynamics in automated root canal preparation. *Alpha Omegan* **83**, 68–72.

39. LIM KC, WEBBER J (1985) The effect of root canal preparation on the shape of the curved root canal. *International Endodontic Journal* **18**, 233–239.

40. LLOYD A, THOMPSON J, GUTMANN JL, DUMMER PMH (1995) Sealability of the Trifecta technique in the presence or absence of a smear layer. *International Endodontic Journal* **28**, 35–40.

41. LUEBKE NH, BRANTLEY WA (1990) Physical dimensions and torsional properties of rotary endodontic instruments 1. Gates Glidden drills. *Journal of Endodontics* **16**, 438–441.

42. LUEBKE NH, BRANTLEY WA (1991) Torsional and metallurgical properties of rotary endodontic instruments 2. Stainless steel Gates Glidden drills. *Journal of Endodontics* **17**, 319–323.

43. LUKS S (1959) An analysis of root canal instruments. *Journal of the American Dental Association* **58(3)**, 85–92.

44. MACHTOU P, SARFATI P, COHEN AG (1989) Post removal prior to retreatment. *Journal of Endodontics* **15**, 552–554.

45. MARTIN H (1976) Ultrasonic disinfection of the root canal. *Oral Surgery, Oral Medicine, Oral Pathology* **42**, 92–99.

46. MASSERANN J (1971) Entfernen metallischer Fragmente aus Wurzelkanälen. *Journal of the British Endodontic Society* **5**, 55–59.

47. MCKENDRY DJ (1990) Comparison of balanced forces, endosonic and step-back filing instrumentation techniques: quantification of extruded apical debris. *Journal of Endodontics* **16**, 24–27.

48. MICHANOWICZ A, CZONSTKOWSKY M (1984) Sealing properties of an injection-thermoplasticized low-temperature (70°C) gutta-percha: a preliminary study. *Journal of Endodontics* **10**, 563–566.

49. MICHANOWICZ AE, CZONSTKOWSKY M, PIESCO NP (1986) Low-temperature (70°C) injection gutta-percha: a scanning electron microscopic investigation. *Journal of Endodontics* **12**, 64–67.

50. MISERENDINO LJ (1991) Instruments, materials and devices. In: Cohen S, Burns RC (eds) *Pathways of the*

Pulp, 5th edn, pp. 388–432. St Louis, MO, USA: Mosby–Year Book.

51. MISERENDINO LJ, BRANTLEY WA, WALIA HD, GERSTEIN H (1988) Cutting efficiency of endodontic hand instruments. Part 4. Comparison of hybrid and traditional instrument designs. *Journal of Endodontics* **14**, 451–454.

52. MISERENDINO LJ, MISERENDINO CA, MOSER JB, HEUER MA, OSETEK EM (1988) Cutting efficiency of endodontic instruments. Part III. Comparison of sonic and ultrasonic instrument systems. *Journal of Endodontics* **14**, 24–30.

53. MISERENDINO LJ, MOSER JB, HEUER MA, OSETEK EM (1986) Cutting efficiency of endodontic instruments. Part II. Analysis of tip design. *Journal of Endodontics* **12**, 8–12.

54. MYERS GL, MONTGOMERY S (1991) A comparison of weights of debris extruded apically by conventional filing and Canal Master techniques. *Journal of Endodontics* **17**, 275–279.

55. NEWMAN JG, BRANTLEY WA, GERSTEIN H (1983) A study of the cutting efficiency of seven brands of endodontic files in linear motion. *Journal of Endodontics* **9**, 316–322.

56. REUTER JE (1983) The isolation of teeth and the protection of the patient during endodontic treatment. *International Endodontic Journal* **16**, 173–181.

57. RICHMAN MJ (1957) Use of ultrasonics in root canal therapy and root resection. *Journal of Dental Medicine* **12**, 12–18.

58. ROANE JB, SABALA C, DUNCANSON MG (1985) The 'balanced force' concept for instrumentation of curved canals. *Journal of Endodontics* **11**, 203–211.

59. SCHILDER H (1974) Cleaning and shaping the root canal. *Dental Clinics of North America* **18**, 269–296.

60. SOBARZO-NAVARRO V (1991) Clinical experience in root canal obturation by an injection thermoplasticized gutta-percha technique. *Journal of Endodontics* **17**, 389–391.

61. SOUTHARD DW, OSWALD RJ, NATKIN E (1987) Instrumentation of curved molar root canals with the Roane technique. *Journal of Endodontics* **13**, 479–489.

62. SUNADA I (1962) New method of measuring the length of the root canal. *Journal of Dental Research* **41**, 375–387.

63. SUZUKI K (1942) Experimental study on iontophoresis. *Japanese Journal of Stomatology* **16**, 411–417.

64. TAGGER M, TAMSE A, KATZ A, KORZEN BH (1984) Evaluation of the apical seal produced by a hybrid root canal filling method, combining lateral condensation and thermatic compaction. *Journal of Endodontics* **10**, 299–303.

65. TRONSTAD L, BARNETT F, SCHWARTZBEN L, FRASCA P (1985) Effectiveness and safety of a sonic vibratory endodontic instrument. *Endodontics and Dental Traumatology* **1**, 69–76.

66. VESSEY RA (1969) The effect of filing versus reaming on the shape of the prepared root canal. *Oral Surgery, Oral Medicine, Oral Pathology* **27**, 543–547.

67. WALIA HM, BRANTLEY WA, GERSTEIN H (1988) An initial investigation of the bending and torsional properties of Nitinol root canal files. *Journal of Endodontics* **14**, 346–351.

68. WEBBER J, MOSER JB, HEUER MA (1980) A method of determining the cutting efficiency of root canal instruments in linear motion. *Journal of Endodontics* **6**, 829–834.

69. WILDEY WL, SENIA ES (1989) A new root canal instrument and instrumentation technique: a preliminary report. *Oral Surgery, Oral Medicine, Oral Pathology* **67**, 198–207.

70. YAHYA AS, ELDEEB ME (1989) Effect of sonic ultrasonic instrumentation on canal preparation. *Journal of Endodontics* **15**, 235–239.

71. YEE FS, MARLIN J, KRAKOW AA, GRON P (1977) Three-dimensional obturation of the root canal using injection molded thermoplasticized dental gutta-percha. *Journal of Endodontics* **3**, 168–174.

6

Preparation of the root canal system

E.M. Saunders and W.P. Saunders

Introduction

Root canal therapy may be defined as the complete removal of the irreversibly damaged pulp followed by thorough cleaning, shaping and obturation of the root canal system so that the tooth may remain as a functional unit within the dental arch. Elective extirpation of a vital, symptomless pulp may be necessary where a treatment plan involves the provision of overdentures [24] or where realignment of the angulation of crown to root by means of a post and core is required.

The object of treatment is to clean the root canal system of infected and toxic debris and to shape the root canal to receive a filling material which will seal the entire canal system from the periodontal tissues and from the oral cavity. This creates an environment which is aimed at preserving normal periradicular tissues or restoring these tissues to health.

The rationale of treatment lies in the fact that the non-vital pulp, being avascular, has no defence mechanisms. The damaged tissue within the root canal undergoes autolysis and the resulting breakdown products will diffuse into the surrounding tissues and cause periradicular irritation associated with the portals of.exit. Although bacterial contamination of the root canal system is considered to be the most common cause of periradicular inflammation [10], the latter can occur in the absence of detectable microorganisms and may be associated with endotoxins [63]. The complex anatomy of the root canal system, especially the apical delta, makes its complete debridement virtually impossible. It is essential, therefore, that root canal treatment must include sealing of the entire root canal system. This:

1. Prevents tissue fluid percolating into the root canal and providing a culture medium for any residual microorganisms.
2. Prevents microorganisms, which may subsequently contaminate the root canal by leakage coronally, from exiting into the periradicular tissues [61].
3. Prevents toxic byproducts from both necrotic tissue and microorganisms egressing into the periradicular tissues.

Treatment of the root canal may be carried out in two ways, either conventionally through an access cavity cut in the crown of the tooth or by surgical means. However, non-surgical conventional root canal filling or retreatment should always be considered as the primary method of case management as success rates with surgical endodontics are less predictable and the procedure tends to be more unpleasant for the patient. Surgical endodontics may be necessary, however, when it is not possible to negotiate and prepare the full length of the canal and seal the canal system adequately. Difficulties which may occur are:

1. A sharp bend in the apical portion of the root canal. Improved quality and flexibility of instruments used in canal preparation has meant that curved canals are not the problem that they used to be. However, curves >60° may be difficult to prepare adequately.
2. An obstruction in the root canal which cannot be removed or bypassed, such as

an old root canal filling, a fractured instrument or post.
3. Calcification within the pulp chamber and the root canal. Reparative dentine forms initially in the coronal portion of the root canal system and this may make location of the canal entrance extremely difficult.
4. Failure of conventional root canal treatment, e.g. continued pain after root canal filling, or in cases where there is no evidence of reduction in the size of a periradicular radiolucency following root canal retreatment and repetition of root canal retreatment is considered inappropriate.

The presence, on radiographic examination, of a large periapical radiolucency is not a contraindication to conventional root canal treatment, provided that the source of irritation, namely the necrotic pulp, can be removed and the canal system cleaned and subsequently obturated (Figure 6.1). However, it should be appreciated that large lesions could be cystic.

Method and rationale for conventional root canal treatment

Preoperative radiographic examination

It is essential that at least one undistorted preoperative periapical radiograph is taken prior to the commencement of treatment. This radiograph should project the tooth to as near its actual size as possible and show the full root(s) and approximately 2–3 mm of periradicular tissues (Figure 6.2). On many occasions a second radiograph from a slightly different horizontal angle, parallax shift, may be helpful in interpreting canal anatomy. The radiograph should be taken, ideally using a paralleling technique and a film-holder, to ensure minimal distortion of the processed image [27]. This will allow standardization of images and make possible meaningful comparisons of the state of the periradicular tissues over time. The use of a film-holder ensures that when a radiograph of a maxillary molar is taken, the zygoma is not super-

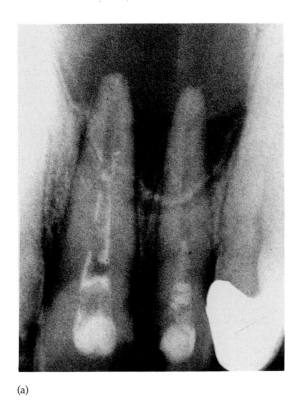

(a)

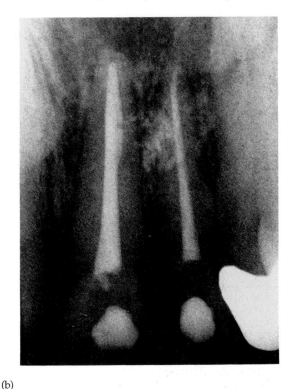

(b)

Figure 6.1 (a) A very large periradicular radiolucency associated with inadequately root filled ⁄12 ; (b) after repreparation and several changes of calcium hydroxide intracanal dressings over 18 months, bony healing was well advanced: the canals were dried and obturated. Recourse to surgery was not required.

imposed on the root apices of the relevant tooth. Processing of the film must be done in such a way that allows a permanent and

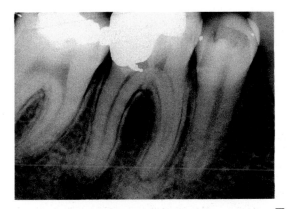

Figure 6.2 A preoperative periapical radiograph of 6̄7̄ showing condensing osteitis around the apex of the mesial root. Mesial horizontal angulation of the X-ray beam separates the two mesial canals: the mesiobuccal canal appearing the more distal (MBD rule), the parallax shift.

stable record to be kept. If a direct digital imaging system is available, this may be used to produce an image of the tooth. The main advantages of digital imaging are the speed of image production and the reduction in radiation per image [51].

The processed radiograph should be carefully examined to establish the basic anatomy of the pulp chamber and the root canals. This will allow anticipation of possible problems together with any features of note that may influence the treatment. These include the type of coronal restoration, numbers of roots, extra or branching canals, the presence of curves, presence of calcification within the pulp chamber and root canals and any iatrogenic damage that may have occurred. The size and location of any periradicular radiolucency should also be noted. It must be appreciated, however, that a radiograph is only a two-dimensional representation of a three-dimensional object and interpretation should always be carried out with this in

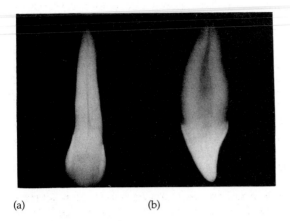

(a)   (b)

Figure 6.3 Two views of the same maxillary canine: (a) the normal clinical radiographic view showing the narrow mesiodistal dimension of the canal; (b) the mesiodistal view gives a better indication of the wide irregular shape of the coronal two-thirds of the canal.

mind. For example, a root canal that looks quite narrow mesiodistally on a normal clinical buccolingual view may be much wider in a buccolingual dimension (Figure 6.3). In addition, a high proportion of roots have some degree of curvature which may not be evident on the radiograph. If the curve of the

root is directly towards or away from the direction of the X-ray beam, as with the palatal root of a maxillary molar, for example, it will appear straight (Figure 6.4). It may be necessary to take more than one radiograph to confirm suspicions as to the number and position of roots and canals or presence of fractures of the root.

Preparation of the tooth prior to root canal treatment

It is essential that contamination of the root canal system by microorganisms is reduced to a minimum during root canal treatment. To achieve this, the steps involved are:

1. Preparation and isolation of the clinical crown.
2. Disinfection of the crown and its immediate environment.
3. Adherence to a surgically clean technique.

Preparation of the crown

It is essential that all caries and defective restorations are removed and a sound coronal

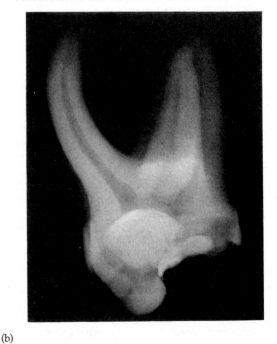

(a)   (b)

Figure 6.4 (a) In the normal clinical radiographic view of a maxillary molar the palatal root and its canal can appear virtually straight; (b) the same tooth viewed mesiodistally shows the true buccal curvature of the palatal root.

restoration placed. The tooth should be restored in such a way that contamination and coronal leakage cannot take place during treatment or between visits. A permanent type of restorative material such as amalgam, resin composite, glass ionomer, glass cermet or resin-modified glass ionomer are suitable for this purpose. The use of these materials to restore the crown will also make placement of rubber dam easier. Temporary restorative materials are less satisfactory as they tend to be weak. Their use should therefore be confined to sealing of the access cavity only.

Isolation of the crown

The use of rubber dam must be considered mandatory during root canal treatment as it:

1. Prevents the inhalation and ingestion of debris, instruments, irrigants and restorative materials.
2. Eliminates salivary contamination and therefore microorganisms and moisture from the operating field.
3. Improves access to the operating area by retracting and thus also protecting adjacent soft tissues; this improves visibility of the working area for the operator.
4. Relaxes the patient, reduces conversation and eliminates rinsing of the mouth.

It can therefore be appreciated that not only will operator stress be greatly reduced by the use of rubber dam but also the potential for better-quality treatment is considerably enhanced. When rubber dam placement becomes a team effort between dental nurse and clinician, it will be streamlined and cost-effective. Its use will then be seen as a positive advantage and will become integrated into normal practice.

If rubber dam cannot be used to isolate the tooth, then serious consideration should be given to abandoning root canal treatment, particularly if a posterior tooth is involved. Other methods have been employed to avoid salivary contamination of the root canal and possible ingestion or inhalation of instruments, irrigant and medicaments, but it must be emphasized that these are not foolproof and are no longer recommended.

The inhalation or swallowing of hand-held endodontic instruments by a patient in the absence of rubber dam is a serious but preventable accident and, as such, is indefensible. If an instrument is lost in this way, arrangements must be made for immediate radiographs of the chest and abdomen to be taken so that the precise location of the instrument can be ascertained. The practitioner must inform his or her defence organization immediately should such an unfortunate occurrence take place. When an instrument has been ingested, its passage through the alimentary tract must be monitored by radiography. Thankfully, in most instances, the instrument is passed uneventfully. If it is not passed or it is inhaled, then major surgery will be required to remove it (Figure 6.5).

The only reliable way of preventing such accidents is to use rubber dam. There is no one recommended or correct way to place rubber dam. The method selected will depend on the tooth to be treated and also, to a large extent, on personal preference. The

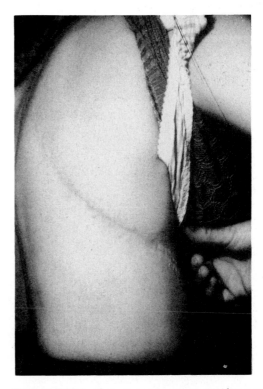

Figure 6.5 Major thoracic surgery was required to remove an inhaled endodontic file. Such serious consequences could have been avoided with rubber dam isolation.

clinician should have a flexible approach, choosing the most effective and easiest technique for each case (Chapter 5). With practice and some ingenuity it is almost always possible to place rubber dam quickly and effectively.

Disinfection of the crown

Rubber dam is placed on the appropriate tooth or teeth, and checked to ensure that there is no leakage. If leakage is suspected then the area may be caulked using a proprietary seal (Oraseal, Ultradent, Salt Lake City, UT, USA; see Figure 5.10). The crowns and surrounding dam should then be disinfected by swabbing with an antiseptic solution.

Surgical cleanliness

The number of microorganisms entering the root canal must be minimized. It is essential that all instruments are sterilized prior to the commencement of root canal treatment and must not be contaminated thereafter, except by the contents of the canals.

Access to the root canal

Local anaesthesia is essential when vital tissue is present in the tooth. It is also recommended in most other cases. Patients tend to be more relaxed when the tooth is anaesthetized and therefore both patient and clinician are less tense. If local anaesthesia is not used it is advisable to apply topical anaesthetic to the gingival tissues of any tooth which is to receive a rubber dam clamp.

It is now necessary to gain access to the pulp chamber and root canal(s) of the tooth. The outline of the access cavity should be carried out according to the principles described in Chapter 3. The temptation to enter the pulp chamber through an existing cavity or restoration in the crown of the tooth must be resisted. To attempt root canal preparation through an approximal cavity may lead to instrument fracture or perforation of the root canal. Properly designed and prepared access cavities will eliminate many potential problems during canal preparation and obturation.

Design principles for the access cavity

These are as follows:

1. The access cavity should enable root canal instruments to be introduced into the canals to their apical constriction without undue bending and binding coronally.
2. The access cavity must be large enough to allow complete debridement of the pulp chamber. The roof of the pulp chamber must be removed completely; if this is not achieved, access to the canals becomes difficult, if not impossible. Also, infected and necrotic materials will be retained within the pulp chamber which may then be transferred to the root canals during instrumentation. Breakdown products from such remnants may be responsible for subsequent discoloration of the crown. Overhangs on the wall of the pulp chamber must be removed (Figure 6.6).
3. In multirooted teeth great care must be taken not to damage the floor of the pulp chamber. Not only is there a possibility of perforation, but the contour of the floor is such that the openings to the root canal

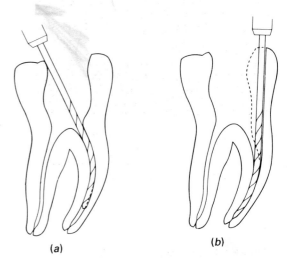

(a)   (b)

Figure 6.6 (a) The instrument needs to be bent excessively because of the curvature of the mesial root; instrumentation is difficult and may lead to ledge formation; (b) removal of dentine from the mesial wall of the access cavity and canal allows instrumentation without undue bending.

tend to be funnel-shaped (Figure 6.7). If this natural anatomy is destroyed, subsequent instrumentation is more difficult.

4. The access cavity should funnel into the canal orifices. In multirooted teeth the orifices of the root canals should be at the periphery of the base of the access cavity so that instruments may be slipped down the walls of the cavity and into the root canals. The occlusal projection of the access cavity should be larger than the base, to allow better visualization of the floor of the pulp chamber, especially if an operating microscope is used.

A sound knowledge of pulpal anatomy is essential in order to carry out these principles of access cavity preparation (Chapter 3).

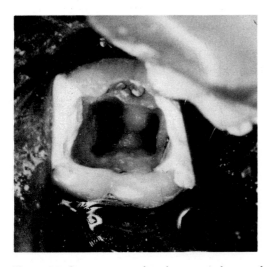

Figure 6.7 Great care must be taken not to damage the natural shape of the floor of the pulp chamber during access cavity preparation. In the case of a mandibular first molar the central dome-shaped floor falls naturally towards the canal orifices.

Access cavity preparation

Method

Before access to the pulp chamber is undertaken the preoperative radiograph should be examined carefully (Figure 6.2). Much information can be gleaned which will be of considerable help during preparation of the access cavity. This can include some indication of the size of the pulp chamber in the vertical axis, evidence of the crown-root angulation in one plane and the inclination of the roots compared with that of the adjacent teeth. In the case of root canal treatment to an anterior tooth, placement of rubber dam may include a number of adjacent teeth. This can make X-ray film placement easier, and avoids inappropriate superimposition of the clamp on the root on the radiographic image.

Access should be a two-stage procedure. The initial penetration of the crown of the tooth is done using a bur in a high-speed handpiece. The correct outline of the cavity is cut into dentine. In tilted or crowned posterior teeth, it may be advisable to do the initial access preparation prior to placement of the rubber dam in order to avoid obscuring the orientation of the tooth relative to the adjacent ones. If this relationship is lost, the access cavity may deviate off course and even result in perforation.

The second stage of access preparation is best done with burs in a low-speed handpiece. These may be fissure or tapered fissure burs with a non-cutting tip (Batt, Maillefer, Ballaigues, Switzerland) or round burs. They should have long shanks so that the head of the handpiece does not interfere with coronal tooth tissue or with vision. Angle of penetration and depth may be gauged from the preoperative radiograph. In molars the initial penetration of the pulp chamber should be directed towards the axis of the largest canal, that is, the palatal canal of a maxillary molar and the distal canal of a mandibular molar. This canal should be the easiest to find and will set the correct depth (Figure 6.8). The roof of the pulp chamber is then removed completely using the cutting action of the bur only on the withdrawal stroke. This avoids the possibility of damage to the floor of the pulp chamber. A hand-held endodontic explorer (DG16, Hu Friedy, Chicago, IL, USA) is very useful to probe the floor of the pulp chamber to detect the openings of the canals and to ascertain if additional canals are present (Figure 6.9).

If difficulty in locating canals in molars is encountered then an ultrasonic probe (CT4 or UT4: Excellence in Endodontics, San Diego,

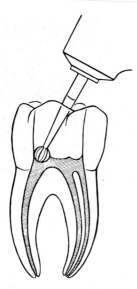

Figure 6.8 Initial penetration of the pulp chamber should be directed towards the axis of the largest canal. The pulp chamber will be at its widest in this area, is easiest to find and will set the correct depth and position for location of the remaining orifices.

CA, USA) may be used to remove more hard tissue over the area where the orifice is expected.

In cases where great difficulty is experienced in locating the canal it may be necessary to use a long-shanked or goose-necked round bur in a low-speed handpiece to remove coronal calcified material. It is essential that this procedure is done slowly with

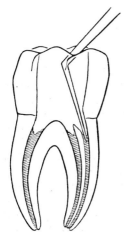

Figure 6.9 A fine endodontic explorer is used to probe the overlying dentine to expose the calcified canal entrance.

extreme caution and that radiographic confirmation of the angulation of the burr relative to the root canal is made to avoid perforation [34].

Removal of pulpal tissue

Vital teeth

In teeth with a relatively wide, single, straight canal, the contents of the pulp chamber and radicular pulp are removed together using a barbed broach. These instruments should only be used in the straight part of the canal and should never bind against the wall as the barbs are fragile. The largest barbed broach which will fit loosely in the canal is selected. It is inserted into the pulp tissue, rotated through 90° so that the barbs engage, and then removed. If the pulp is not detached in one piece, a second attempt with a new broach will be necessary. In fine canals, or where tissue fragmentation has occurred, vital tissue should be removed with files [34]. Haemorrhage from a hyperaemic pulp must be washed immediately from the pulp chamber, otherwise discoloration of the crown may result.

Barbed broaches are not easy to use in multirooted teeth. Contents of the pulp chamber can be removed with sharp, long-shafted spoon excavators and each radicular pulp then extirpated by using short-handled fine barbed broaches (Maillefer) or, in the case of narrow curved canals, with K-files or Hedstrom files. Broaches are difficult to clean at the chairside and should therefore be discarded after single use.

Non-vital teeth

The removal of necrotic pulp remnants from non-vital teeth is carried out during the preparation of the root canal system using a combination of cleaning and shaping with files and irrigation. This is universally called biomechanical preparation.

Preparation of the canal

Removal of agents which initiate or perpetuate periapical inflammation, such as necrotic pulp debris and microorganisms, will minimize exacerbations and promote uneventful healing. Complete cleaning and shaping should therefore be completed, if possible, at the first visit.

In order to minimize patient discomfort and increase the success rate, all instrumentation should be kept within the confines of the root canal and efforts made to avoid extrusion of contaminated debris into the periradicular tissues [65].

Correct instrumentation, debridement and obturation of the root canal system, without the use of any intermediate intracanal sterilizing agent, often leads to a successful result. However, the converse is not true. No amount of chemotherapy, unless preceded by correct and adequate instrumentation, will lead to a satisfactory outcome. It must also be borne in mind that the ability of the final root canal filling to seal the canal can be no better than the preparatory cleaning and shaping of the canal system will allow.

Root canal irrigation

The goals of root canal irrigation are to flush pulpal debris and dentine slurry from the root canal and to help lubricate endodontic instruments, thereby facilitating their cutting action. The ideal irrigant solution should:

1. Dissolve organic debris.
2. Flush out inorganic and organic debris.
3. Lubricate endodontic instruments.
4. Eliminate microorganisms.
5. Be relatively non-toxic.
6. Be inexpensive.

Sodium hypochlorite with its antiseptic and tissue-dissolving properties is considered the irrigant of choice (Chapter 7). However, regardless of which irrigant is selected, an adequate volume must be used and irrigant must be kept within the confines of the root canal system. Care must be taken to ensure that the irrigant is allowed to escape freely into the pulp chamber and that it is never delivered with undue force, as this could cause extrusion through the apex with resulting inflammation and afterpain.

The solution should be delivered in copious amounts and this can be achieved most

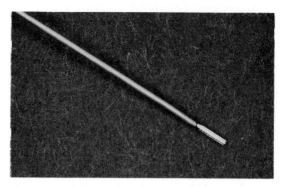

Figure 6.10 A 27-gauge endodontic needle allows maximum penetration for effective irrigation with less likelihood of extrusion of irrigant into the periradicular tissues.

simply by means of a Luer-Lok syringe and a 27-gauge endodontic-tipped needle (Figure 6.10). The special tip has one side cut away and allows some backflow of liquid, thereby reducing the possibility of forcing irrigant into the periradicular tissues. Little fluid exchange takes place below the opening of the needle [2,20,69].

Irrigant solution can also be delivered very effectively in large amounts by ultrasonic, sonic and mechanical reciprocating instruments equipped with an irrigating system which will accept sodium hypochlorite (Figure 6.11). The efficacy of irrigation with ultrasonics is time-dependent [23] and is superior to syringe irrigation alone in narrow canals.

Other materials for lubrication

Instruments work more efficiently if the cutting flutes are lubricated during use. Various materials and chemicals can be used in paste or liquid form to lubricate. These include a chlorhexidine soap (Hibiscrub: ICI, Macclesfield, UK), glycerine, File-eze (Ultradent), a 17% ethylenediaminetetraacetic acid (EDTA) water-soluble paste and RC Prep (15% EDTA, 10% urea peroxide: Premier Dental Products, Philadelphia, PA, USA). However, RC Prep contains carbowax which is not water-soluble, making its complete removal from the root canal system difficult using conventional irrigation techniques after preparation is complete [78].

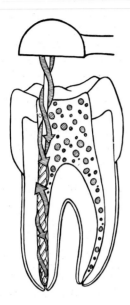

Figure 6.11 A continuous flow of irrigant solution is delivered very effectively using ultrasonics.

Influence of root canal morphology on endodontic preparation

Some teeth may have simple straight roots but the majority have some degree of curvature, especially in the apical third. The internal diameter of the canal may also vary from fine to large depending on the particular tooth and the amount of reparative dentine that has been laid down. The latter is related to the age of the patient and the previous history of the tooth, including physical trauma, caries experience and coronal restoration. The canal may be roughly circular in cross-section along most of its length, or only the apical part of the root canal may be round, the remainder being oval or irregular in cross-section. A particular example of the problems likely to be encountered during bio-mechanical preparation can be seen in the two radiographic views of a maxillary canine (Figure 6.3). This lack of uniformity of shape makes preparation more difficult than it might at first appear. Reamers, when used with a reaming action in a straight canal, produce a round cross-section [38,70] but a reaming technique cannot be used in irregularly shaped and curved canals. When an instrument is used with a complete rotating action in a canal with apical curvature, instead of a round shape, a gouged cavity will be created (Figure 6.12). If reaming is continued iatrogenic root perforation is likely. The result is not only afterpain, but a canal shape which is very difficult to obturate three-dimensionally. As the majority of canals have some degree of curvature along their length, it is wise to assume this and select a preparation technique which takes curvature into consideration. To overcome some of the problems experienced with preparation of the curved root canal, files which are very flexible have been produced.

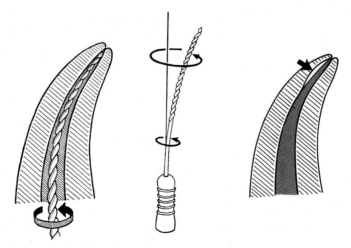

Figure 6.12 An endodontic instrument used in a rotary movement in a curved canal will create a gouged cavity at the apical extent of preparation.

Root canal preparation can be achieved with either hand-held or mechanically driven instruments, or a combination of both. A multiplicity of methods have been applied to root canal preparation. The simplicity or sophistication of the approach will depend to a certain extent on the anatomy of the canal itself, on the technique selected for obturation, and on the clinician's preference. The basic objectives of removal of tissue debris and bacteria and of canal shaping prior to final obturation remain the same however, regardless of the technique used to achieve them.

The objectives of root canal preparation are to:

1. Eliminate microorganisms.
2. Remove remaining pulp tissue.
3. Remove debris.
4. Shape the root canal system so that it may be obturated.

The requirements are that:

1. The prepared canal should include the original canal (i.e. not be straightened or transposed).
2. The canal should end in an apical narrowing.
3. The canal preparation should taper smoothly from crown to apex.

Canal preparation should be considered as having two important components:

1. The manner in which the files are moved.
2. The sequence of the preparation technique selected. In addition, the design of the file will influence its efficiency and the resulting canal shape.

Movement of files

Files can be used in a number of ways.

1. *Stem winding, watch winding or twiddling.* The file is used with a 45° rotational movement clockwise and anticlockwise with gentle apical force. The canal becomes enlarged and the file can be moved apically into the root canal. This movement is useful when penetrating fine canals and in retreatment cases. Files are usually precurved prior to use in this way.
2. *Quarter turn and pull.* This causes more aggressive cutting than stem winding and tends to remove more material from the wall.
3. *Apical–coronal filing.* The file is applied to the wall of the root canal and moved in and out of the canal at an amplitude of 1–2 mm. This movement is especially efficient with Hedstrom files.

To ensure that all the walls of the root canal are cut, circumferential filing is done. The need for this can be clearly appreciated from Figure 6.3.

4. *Balanced-force technique.* This technique was first described by Roane et al. [55]. Files are not precurved with this technique. The movement of the file is clockwise and anticlockwise and its action is based upon Newton's third law. The file is placed into the canal until it first binds and then advanced further by clockwise rotation, usually through approximately 60°. The file cuts into the root canal wall and creates threads in the dentine as it moves apically. This is the power phase. The anticlockwise rotation, through approximately 120°, is carried out with some apical pressure so that the file does not unscrew out of the canal. During this movement the threads of dentine formed during the power phase are cut from the wall. This is the so-called control phase. Often an audible click can be heard which resembles an instrument fracturing, but is merely the dentine being cut from the wall. The file is then removed and the flutes cleaned of debris. If difficulty is encountered in removing the file then a small rotation clockwise, of about 30°, allows the file to be freed. In nearly all studies where this manipulation of the file has been compared with other methods, the balanced-force technique has been shown to be superior in shaping the canal [9,60,67], with less likelihood of iatrogenic damage. The reason for this is that the files tend to remain more centrally placed within the root canal which means that the canal can be prepared to a larger size without compromising the structure of the root (Figure 6.13). This combination of a larger size and smooth, even flare which

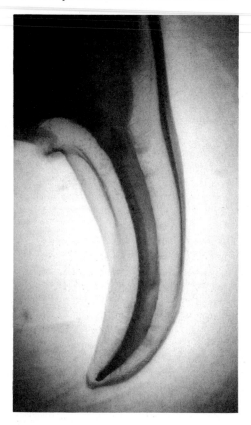

Figure 6.13 Preparation of the curved root canal, using the modified double-flared technique with balanced force movement of files, results in a canal which is large enough to allow three-dimensional obturation but still remains centred within the root. Cleared tooth specimen.

follows the natural curvature of the canal probably results in a cleaner canal and certainly one that is easier to obturate with gutta-percha.

Whatever the technique employed, files must not be misused or overused. Liberal use of small-sized flexible files is advocated and damaged instruments must be discarded. All preparation techniques must be accompanied by copious irrigation.

Factors influencing efficiency of hand instruments

Size

Conventional files are produced in various diameters but the taper is the same. As the file increases in diameter, so the flexibility is reduced and this means that a curved canal will tend to be straightened during preparation. This may create a ledge at the curve (Figure 6.14). The International Organization for Standardization (ISO) sizing for files means that the diameter of the narrower files tends to increase disproportionately quicker than those that are wider, and this may affect the preparation of fine root canals. To overcome this problem some manufacturers have introduced files which increase in diameter in smaller increments (Chapter 5). In addition, the taper of some of the newer files is greater than usual, making coronal cutting easier to achieve during apical movement of the file.

Cross-sectional shape

As has already been described in Chapter 5, the cross-sectional shape varies between files. Files with a triangular cross-sectional shape are more flexible than those with a square cross-section.

Type of file

Preparation is usually carried out with a flexible K-file, although filing in the long axis of the canal is more efficiently achieved with a Hedstrom file. More recently, nickel–titanium files have been introduced. These are extremely flexible, but smaller sizes may not be very efficient when used with a filing action, as insufficient lateral force can be applied [17,72]. However, a more recent study has found that nickel–titanium files used with linear movement shape the canal effectively with minimal iatrogenic damage [77].

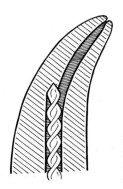

Figure 6.14 Large inflexible instruments have a tendency to straighten curved canals by creating a ledge in the outer wall of the apical part.

Shape of the file tip

It has been shown that if the cutting blades at the tip of the file are removed, the incidence of straightening the root canal during preparation is reduced [58]. A more parabolic shape is produced by eliminating the cutting blades of the tip and first flute of the instrument. A number of manufacturers have introduced these modified-tipped instruments.

Method of instrumentation

Measurement of the working length of the root canal

The working length of the root canal establishes the apical extent of instrumentation and the ultimate level of the root canal filling. The stage at which this length is determined will vary depending on which preparation technique is employed. It is generally accepted that the apical extent of instrumentation will be at the apical constriction, which, as a general guideline, and depending on the patient's age and the history of the tooth, is 0.5–2 mm from the anatomical or radiographic apex (Figure 3.6). If instrumentation is confined to the root canal with neither apical perforation nor incomplete instrumentation, there will be not only a reduced incidence of postoperative pain but also a better long-term prognosis [36]. The working length must therefore be verified accurately prior to instrumentation in the apical third of the root canal.

A sound point of reference must be identified on the occlusal surface of the tooth. In the case of an anterior tooth this is usually the incisal edge and, on a posterior tooth, a cusp or marginal ridge (Figure 6.15). It is important that the reference point remains sound and reproducible throughout the treatment and should be noted in the patient's records. In some instances, it will be necessary to reduce weak cusps or to smooth traumatized incisal edges to avoid fracture during the course of treatment or to create a flatter and more accurate reference. Reference points should not be on temporary restorations which could wear or fracture between appointments.

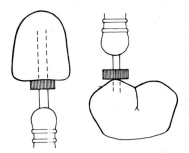

Figure 6.15 A silicone stop set at right angles to the shaft of the instrument must mark a sound and reproducible point of occlusal reference.

With knowledge of the average lengths of teeth and an undistorted preoperative radiograph, not only can a rough estimate of the working length be made, but the correct size of the initial path-finding file can be selected. With very fine canals this may be size 06, 08 or 10. The instrument must be fine enough to negotiate the full length of the canal but not so loose that it moves during taking of the radiograph. Very fine instruments can be difficult to see in their entirety on the film. In the case of most single-rooted teeth and larger molar canals, a size 15, 20 or 25 file can be used.

A rubber stop must be placed perpendicular to the shaft of the instrument. By setting this stop 1 mm short of the estimated working length, penetration of the file past the apical constriction can usually be avoided and subsequent postoperative discomfort eliminated. The file should be precurved unless the balanced force method of instrumentation is being used. Precurving can be done by using a proprietary bending instrument (Maillefer) or by inserting the file tip into a sterile cotton-wool roll and bending the shank to produce a gradual curve. The curve on the instrument should be appropriate to that of the canal. The file is then gently passed up the root canal until it has reached the estimated working length or its progress has been impeded by the apical constriction. The stop is then adjusted to the reference point and a radiograph taken. It is essential that the radiograph should be of high quality and this may be achieved using a film holder (Endo Ray, Rinn, Chicago, IL, USA) [26] (Figure 6.16). The instrument is withdrawn

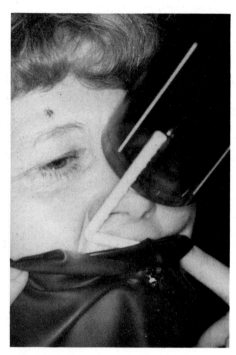

Figure 6.16 By using a paralleling technique with a film-holder which allows the rubber dam to remain in place, working length can be ascertained from an undistorted radiograph. The angulation of the radiograph can then be accurately reproduced in future films.

and the length from its tip to the mark is measured and recorded. If the length is incorrect by 3 mm or more, the stop should be adjusted, the instrument replaced in the canal, and a further radiograph taken. When two canals appear to be superimposed, e.g. the mesial root of mandibular molars, instead of taking individual radiographs of each canal with an instrument in place, a preferable method is to use the technique of parallax shift, and expose a single radiograph from a *mesial* horizontal angle. This will separate the two canals with the *buccal* canal always appearing the more *distally* positioned of the two (*MBD* rule) (Figure 6.2).

If the method of preparation selected involves initial coronal preparation of the root canal then calculation of the working length is delayed until the coronal part of the canal has been cleaned and shaped.

Electronic apex locators

An adjunct to radiography for determining the working length is the use of an electronic measuring device. The principle employed is based upon electrical impedance between apical tissue and oral mucosa [45]. With practice and clinical experience, these instruments are capable of accurate measurement. Although they cannot take the place of the radiographic method of working length determination, they make an excellent adjunct, and the most recently introduced models are not so easily affected by contaminated canals [59]. Apex locators have several advantages. First, they are of benefit in maxillary posterior teeth where the position of the apex may be difficult to interpret or an undistorted radiograph difficult to achieve. Second, they may prevent perforation of the apical constriction in those teeth where the apical foramen is located several millimetres from the radiographic apex. A further important advantage is the reduction in the number of radiographs required.

Root canal preparation

Currently employed methods of canal preparation can be divided into two distinct approaches: those which prepare the coronal section of the canal system first with large instruments and progress towards the apex and those which start at the apex with fine instruments and progress back towards the cervical orifice with larger instruments. Historically, after gaining access to the root canal, working length determination and apical preparation were completed first using a standardized technique which produced an almost parallel canal with a round cross-section. Difficulties encountered during preparation of the curved canal prompted a move away from this technique to one which involved less preparation of the apical third and a 'stepping back' to produce a continuous flare with its narrowest point at the apical constriction.

Although the stepback technique was an obvious improvement [53], early preparation of the apical section tended to result in over-preparation of the outer curve with transportation of the apical preparation to form an elliptically shaped defect [74]. Coronal to this apical defect, the canal had its narrowest part, which gave an hourglass shape that was difficult to obturate three-dimensionally (Figure 6.17).

In general terms cleaning and shaping of the root canal system may be begun from either the coronal or apical parts of the root canal. However, preparation of the coronal part of the canal system first is now considered to be superior as this results in a number of significant advantages.

1. Most of the microorganisms will be in the coronal third of the root canal system [66]. Early removal of these will reduce the possibility of their inoculation into the apical portion of the canal and thence into the periradicular tissues. In addition, hydrostatic pressure can occur within the root canal if working length confirmation or apical preparation is initiated at the start of preparation because the file will act like a piston in a cylinder. This pressure may force pulp debris, dentine chips, irrigant solution and microorganisms through the apical foramen [18,71]. Extrusion of material is greater when the instrument size is approximately the same as that of the apical section of the root canal [35,57].

2. Early flaring of the coronal part of the canal system prevents binding of the instruments as they are unencumbered throughout most of their length and also gives better access to the apical part of the root canal [39].

3. If removal of interferences at the base of the pulp chamber and in the coronal part of the root canal is undertaken prior to working length determination, the latter is less likely to alter during preparation (Figure 6.6).

4. Early coronal flaring allows better penetration of the irrigant solution [35].

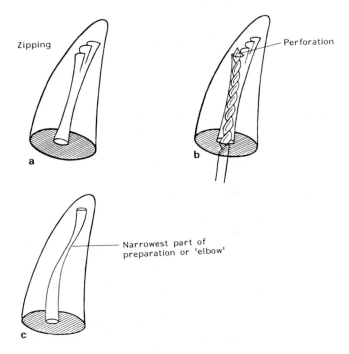

Figure 6.17 (a) Overpreparation of the outer wall of the apical curvature of the canal with inflexible instruments will cause *zipping*; (b) excessive overpreparation with non-safe-ended instruments may lead to perforation; (c) the narrowest part of the preparation is short of its apical extent and is known as the elbow.

Preparation of the root canal from the crown to the apex offers advantages which are now sufficiently compelling to warrant its routine selection.

Techniques involving initial coronal preparation

The authors' current preferred method for preparation of previously uninstrumented curved canals involves instrumentation of the coronal straight section of the root canal initially, using the balanced-force movement of files. Preparation toward the apical part of the canal is then achieved, again with balanced force, followed by sequential stepping back to meet the coronal preparation. From present research information it would appear that the combination of stepping down with a balanced-force movement will most often result in the production of a prepared canal centred within its original shape (Figure 6.13). In addition, this shape will be produced with the minimum of apical extrusion of debris and will lend itself to three-dimensional obturation with gutta-percha and sealer cement [7].

Modified double flare with balanced force

The stages of this preparation technique [62] are depicted diagrammatically in Figure 6.18.

The hand instruments used with this technique must be of good quality and must not be precurved. Conventional K-files and Hedstrom files are unsuitable. Flexible files should be used and should preferably have non-cutting tips. All instrumentation must be accompanied by copious irrigation with sodium hypochlorite and lubrication with chlorhexidine soap (Hibiscrub) or EDTA paste (File-eze).

When access to the root canal is gained and the roof of the pulp chamber has been removed, the chamber should be flooded with sodium hypochlorite. This helps to reduce the amount of necrotic debris and microorganisms in the coronal part of the root canal system. For each root canal the following stages should be carried out.

Preparation of the coronal section of the root canal

1. Check the length of the straight section of the coronal part of the root canal from the preoperative radiograph.

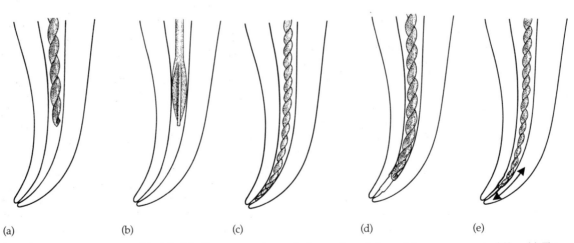

(a)　　　　　(b)　　　　　(c)　　　　　(d)　　　　　(e)

Figure 6.18 Stages in the modified double-flare preparation technique using a balanced-force movement of files. (a) The largest file which fits loosely in the straight coronal part of the canal prepares the coronal 5–7 mm using balanced force. (b) The coronal 5–7 mm is prepared with sizes 2 and 3 Gates-Gliddens. (c) A size 10 file is used initially to check canal patency and then using a size 15 or 20 file, preparation is taken apically by balanced force, checked radiographically, and the apical section enlarged to at least a size 30. (d) The apical section is stepped back using balanced force. (e) The canal is smoothed with a filing action.

2. Take a size 35 or 40 file with a stop set at that length, dip the tip in File-eze or Hibiscrub, and place it in the root canal. If the instrument feels too tight and will not seat to that length, then an instrument with smaller diameter, e.g. size 30, should be chosen. In very fine canals, this size may need to be even smaller.

3. This instrument is turned clockwise through approximately 60°. This rotation moves the file passively into the root canal.

4. Using slight apical pressure to hold the file at that length the file is turned anticlockwise approximately 120°. This is done in two finger movements of 60° each. The file is then withdrawn and the flutes cleaned with sterile gauze. The root canal is then irrigated with sodium hypochlorite.

5. This instrumentation is repeated using size 40, 45 and 50 files, or sizes which are appropriate to the width of the canal. All instrumentation must be accompanied by copious irrigation and lubrication.

6. The coronal section thus prepared is then carefully flared using Gates-Glidden burs sizes 070 and 090. These should be used at very low speed (1500 rpm) and the pulp chamber should be full of irrigant. Circumferential preparation of the root canal wall is achieved by cutting on the outward stroke of the bur. The considerable slurry generated should be washed away with irrigant. It is essential that great care is taken at this stage neither to overprepare the coronal section of the canal nor to create ledging. Overpreparation can weaken the tooth very significantly [14].

7. A size 10 file should then be passed to just short of the estimated working length to ensure that the canal remains patent.

Preparation of the apical section

1. A size 15 or 20 file is then dipped in File-eze, or Hibiscrub, and instrumented towards the apex using the balanced-force technique until just short of the estimated working length. The working length radiograph can now be taken. Such a size of file should be readily visible on the radiograph.

2. The working length is determined and the apical preparation carried out to a size 35–40 master apical file (MAF), depending on the original diameter of the root canal, using 60° clockwise – 120° anticlockwise instrumentation (balanced-force technique). Clean dentine debris should be seen in the apical few flutes of the instrument on withdrawal from the canal.

Stepping back

1. The next size of file from the MAF is then instrumented 1 mm short of the working length, using the balanced-force technique.

2. The next-sized file is then taken 2 mm short of the full working length, and the next 3 mm short of the full working length, until the prepared straight section of the canal is reached.

3. During the stepback phase of the preparation, it is essential that the patency of the canal is maintained to the full working length. This is done by introducing the master apical file to the working length after each larger instrument. This file is used to clean the canal of debris created during progressive enlargement. This is known as recapitulation. A final refining stage uses a gentle apical–coronal filing action to smooth the canal wall.

4. The root canal is finally irrigated with sodium hypochlorite. The MAF is then reintroduced and checked to ensure that the stop is correctly positioned at the working length. If the canal preparation is complete, this file can be introduced to the working length in a single movement with only gentle finger pressure on the end of the handle of the instrument and with no rotation.

5. An appropriate size of spreader should now be introduced into the root canal to ensure its penetration to within 2 mm of the working length. This final stage is important to ensure that adequate lateral condensation of gutta-percha and sealer can be achieved in the apical third of the canal [6]. The final shape of the root canal which can be accomplished with this technique is illustrated in Figure 6.13.

Stepdown technique

In the stepdown technique sequential enlargement of the root canal from pulp chamber to apex is advocated using instruments with a filing action [14,30]. Early preparation of the coronal straight section of canal is achieved with increasing sizes of Hedstrom files followed by Gates-Glidden burs; copious irrigation is essential. The working length is then established and the apical part of the preparation starts with a precurved, lubricated fine file (08, 10 or 15) used with an apical–coronal filing motion. Increasing sizes of files are used until the apical preparation has been enlarged to a minimum of size 25; the preparation is stepped back with progressively larger files to join the already enlarged coronal part.

Double-flare technique

This is a technique where files are used to enlarge the canal, starting coronally and progressing apically with decreasing file size. It is followed by a stepback enlargement of the apical third with files used with an apical–coronal filing action [25].

Crown-down pressureless technique

This preparation method involves early coronal flaring with Gates-Glidden burs. This is followed by incremental removal of canal contents using clockwise rotation of files without apical pressure; progressively smaller files are used until the working length is reached. Files are not precurved [52].

Continuous wave shaping

A more recent refinement of the stepdown method of preparation involves the creation of resistance for obturation over a few millimetres of the apical part of the root canal [15]. Initial preparation is carried out in the coronal section of the root canal with increasing diameter of files. The final coronal preparation is completed with Gates-Glidden burs. Apical preparation is then done using files with an 04 taper, i.e. twice the taper of ISO-sized files. These can be used by hand with stem-winding or balanced force, or in a low-speed handpiece. The files (Profile: Tulsa Dental Products, Tulsa, OK, USA) are not sized according to ISO standards but for each size increase of file the diameter increases by 29%. This technique for preparation is used in conjunction with continuous-wave obturation using warm gutta-percha.

Anticurvature filing

The midroot section of some curved roots may exhibit external invagination (Figure 6.19). If care is not exercised during the preparation of the canal wall associated with this invagination, perforation may occur. To avoid this danger zone, files and Gates-Glidden burs should be directed away from it towards the bulkiest portion of the root structure; this technique is termed anticurvature filing [1]. A circumferential filing technique which involves filing of the buccal, mesial and lingual or palatal walls of the root canal in a ratio of 3:1 with the furcal walls has been recommended [41]. Alternatively, with root curvatures of 10–20°, the cutting edges of the file should be removed at certain strategic sites so that less dentine will be removed from the outer curve in the apical section and from the inner curve in the midroot area [74]. This adjustment to the configuration of the instrument should reduce 'zipping' at the apex and 'elbowing' coronal to it. The problems associated with anticurvature filing have been reduced by the introduction of more flexible files but extreme care should always be taken when using engine-driven Gates-Glidden or Peeso burs (Figure 6.19).

Technique involving initial apical preparation

Current research findings indicate that all preparation techniques which prepare the coronal section first and progress towards the apex produce a prepared canal of significantly better shape and terminus than the stepback method, which is not now widely used.

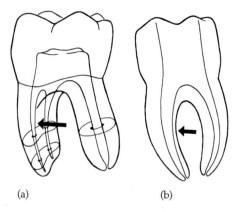

(a)   (b)

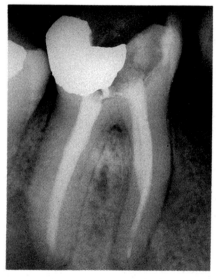

(c)

Figure 6.19 (a) Some roots exhibit external invagination in the mid-section; (b) the danger zone (arrowed) is at risk of being overprepared unless an anticurvature filing technique is used, in which instruments are deliberately kept from this wall; (c) radiograph of a root-filled mandibular molar in which anticurvature filing was not used; the danger zone in the mesial root is close to perforation.

Mechanized techniques of root canal preparation

In an attempt to speed up and facilitate root canal preparation, automated techniques have been developed. These include ultrasonic and sonic, vibratory and rotary systems.

Ultrasonic techniques

The use of ultrasonics in root canal preparation (endosonics) is not a new concept [48,49], having first been proposed in the 1950s [54]. Handpieces have been designed to transmit low-frequency ultrasonic vibration (20–42 kHz) by electromagnetic energy converted to mechanical energy (magnetostriction) to produce oscillation of files. Other instruments are powered by piezoelectric principles, where crystal deformation is converted to mechanical energy. The ultrasonic handpiece has a facility whereby a continuous flow of irrigant solution passes along the file and across its oscillating tip. A very characteristic pattern of oscillation is set up: nodes, where very little displacement of the file occurs, and antinodes where there is maximum displacement. The greatest displacement takes place at the tip of the file. The amount of tip displacement depends upon the power supplied to the instrument and also on the dimensions and design of the file used [73].

The type of irrigant used during ultrasonic endodontic preparation is important; 2.6% sodium hypochlorite produced significantly better results compared with water or a bisdequalinium acetate solution [33]. The collagen-dissolving action of sodium hypochlorite is enhanced by soft-tissue fragmentation.

The improved physical activation of the sodium hypochlorite occurs by acoustic streaming [50], which is the generation of multiple low-velocity eddy currents of liquid around the vibrating file. The rate of change of velocity from the file is large; this produces large hydrodynamic shear stresses around the file [42]. This violent agitation of irrigating solution allows cleaning of the root canal walls. Sufficiently high pressure-fields are unlikely to occur around an oscillating file within the root canal to produce cavitation [73], and no evidence of cavitation has been found [3]. However, the effect of the acoustic streaming of a large volume of irrigant will be responsible for efficient removal of bacteria and pulpal remnants during endosonic root canal preparation [4].

The movement of the file in an ultrasonic handpiece is transverse, so when the file is constrained within a fine, curved root canal, the cutting efficiency is markedly reduced. The file should be used in a gentle up-and-down motion within the root canal and can also be applied to the wall and moved circumferentially. Unconstrained in the root canal, it provides large amounts of irrigant solution for cleaning. When traditional concepts of root canal treatment are combined with ultrasonic cleaning and shaping, the results of earlier studies tended to suggest that there was greater efficiency in canal preparation than with hand filing alone [16,21,49]. The fact that only light cutting and guiding pressure are needed does help to reduce operator fatigue [50]. However, whereas both ultrasonic and hand preparation tend to result in some transportation of the canal, hand preparation appears to be superior in retaining the original canal shape [31]. With file sizes 20–35 straightening of the canal normally occurs with ultrasonic preparation [19].

There is no doubt that very efficient cleaning of the coronal and middle portions of the canal can be achieved with ultrasonics [32], but it is strongly recommended that preparation of the apical third of all canals should only be accomplished with hand instrumentation [64]. Ultrasonic cleaning is especially useful in heavily infected canals, for example, those that have been on open drainage for some time. The action of the activated irrigant helps to clean these root canals very efficiently. Because of the copious and continuous flow of irrigant delivered at the tip of the ultrasonic file, many clinicians routinely conclude their preparation of the root canal, by whatever means, with ultrasonic sodium hypochlorite irrigation (Figure 6.11).

Sonic preparation

Another group of air-driven devices operate at frequencies below 20 kHz. These sonic handpieces transmit oscillation to the tip of a file. This oscillation, when unconstrained, is elliptical in shape, with a single antinode at the tip and a node near the driver handpiece. When the file is unconstrained within the root canal, a longitudinal movement takes place which allows shaping of the root canal. Sonic preparation must be accompanied by

irrigation, and this is delivered down the file during cutting. Various special files are available for use with some sonic systems. For example, the Micro-Mega 1500 Sonic Air (Prodonta, Geneva, Switzerland) has three file types, two of which, the Rispisonic and the Shaper, are specifically made for this unit. The Rispisonic is, however, an aggressive cutter and should be used with great care.

Stepdown instrumentation is done either with Gates-Glidden drills or with the Contact Shaper file in the coronal–mid section of the canal, followed by stepback and circumferential filing. To achieve maximum benefit from sonic and ultrasonic preparation and cleaning techniques, sodium hypochlorite should be the irrigant used. It is essential that preparation of the apical few millimetres of the canal be done with hand instruments as overinstrumentation is common with all mechanical instrumentation techniques.

Power-assisted instrumentation

Power-assisted root canal instruments are currently available with claims of faster canal preparation but without iatrogenic damage. Lightspeed is an example (Lightspeed Technology, San Antonio, TX, USA); it is a nickel-titanium instrument with a flexible taperless shaft and a short cutting blade, used at 2000 rpm in a conventional high-torque handpiece.

Other methods of preparation with future clinical potential

Lasers

Lasers have been recommended for use in endodontics and specifically for root canal preparation. Root canals can be sterilized with the use of a pulsed Nd:YAG laser [56]. An *in vitro* study has shown that preparation with a laser beam is possible and results in cleaner root canal walls compared with conventional techniques [40]. Unfortunately, the use of a pulsed Nd:YAG laser in the apical part of the root canal caused damage to the periradicular tissues resulting in ankylosis [8].

However, when a KTP:YAG laser was used to prepare root canals, the temperature rises were below the safety threshold [46].

Reduced-pressure technique

A method for cleaning the root canal system using controlled cavitation within a reduced pressure system has been devised [43,44]. At a reduced pressure of 3×10^4 Pa, microscopic and macroscopic bubbles are created within the root canal. A rapid rise in pressure to 9×10^4 Pa causes these bubbles to collapse, and cavitation and hydrodynamic turbulence then occur, cleaning the wall of the root canal. The irrigant used is sodium hypochlorite. Using the same attachment to the tooth, the root canal can then be obturated with sealer. The treatment time is reported to be three times quicker than conventional instrumentation [44]. The reduced-pressure preparation technique is currently experimental with no clinical documentation.

All preparation methods, whether using hand or mechanical instrumentation, are technique sensitive. It is therefore imperative that all unfamiliar techniques be practised *in vitro* prior to clinical use.

Root canal retreatment

As the number of root canal treatment cases increases, unfortunately so too do the number of failures which require retreatment. However, clinical surveys indicate that primary root canal therapy has a considerably higher success rate than any other subsequent attempt [5,12]. Initial prevention of procedural mishaps and the need for a high standard of care are therefore critical.

Preparation of the root canal in retreatment cases varies in several respects from primary root canal treatment. The majority of retreatment cases will have obturated canals and restored coronal tooth tissue [68].

The quality of the primary root canal treatment, both that of the canal preparation and of the type and density of the root canal filling, can only be assessed radiographically. Therefore it may be difficult to predict potential problems accurately prior to commencement of retreatment. Patients tend to be more dentally aware, having experienced this type of treatment previously and may well have higher expectations. It is prudent to warn of the poorer prognosis and the time which retreatment may take.

Whether the existing coronal restoration should be removed completely, or only penetrated, in order to gain access to the root canal system, is a decision which will need to be made at the treatment-planning stage. The type of restoration, its marginal integrity, the cost of subsequent replacement and the patient's wishes are some of the factors which will influence this decision [28]. In many instances of root canal retreatment, the access cavity will need to be made larger than that required for primary treatment.

Obturating materials may be difficult to remove. Some paste fillings are relatively easy to file and irrigate from the canal, but materials such as SPAD (Quetigny, France), which sets harder than dentine, are extremely difficult to remove. It may be possible to break up hard cement using ultrasonics [29], but root perforation is always a hazard.

Gutta-percha root canal fillings can be removed from the canal system using combinations of a softening solvent and filing, or bypassing with a file which then ensnares the gutta-percha, or by using solvent and ultrasonics [29]. Old gutta-percha root canal fillings tend to be relatively hard and often need to be softened prior to attempting removal. This can be achieved with a heated instrument placed into the body of the material. Solvents used to soften gutta-percha have been evaluated [37]. Chloroform and xylene are widely used in gutta-percha removal procedures but they are toxic [13] and potentially carcinogenic [37]. Rectified white turpentine is a suitable, effective and much less toxic alternative for softening gutta-percha [22]. The present authors find oil of turpentine (BP) extremely effective, easy to procure and inexpensive.

Method for removal of gutta-percha root canal fillings

1. A heated instrument is placed into the coronal mass of gutta-percha (endodontic

plugger, or System B; Analytic Technology Redmond, WA, USA).

2. Size 070 and 090 Gates-Glidden burs may then be used to remove the gutta-percha in the coronal straight section of the canal.

3. A few drops of oil of turpentine are introduced into the coronal part of the root canal using a syringe and 27-gauge needle. Care must be taken to confine this liquid to the canal and not to allow it to contact the rubber dam, which splits almost immediately.

4. A size 25 or 30 precurved file is placed in the canal and used with a stem-winding motion. This will penetrate into the gutta-percha mass and result in removal of the material. This procedure is continued, wiping softened gutta-percha from the file at each removal. These procedures must be done carefully to avoid injection of solvent into the periradicular tissues and to avoid forcing root canal filling material beyond the root apex.

5. Continue until the estimated working length is reached. The root canal system is not irrigated during the removal of the gutta-percha to avoid dilution of the solvent.

6. A periapical radiograph is then taken to ascertain if any gutta-percha remains in the root canal.

7. Paper points, dampened in solvent, are wiped against the canal wall in an attempt to remove any remaining softened gutta-percha.

8. Preparation is completed using the balanced-force movement of the files until clean dentine is removed. Copious irrigation is essential at this stage.

However, even after achieving an apparently clean canal, root canal filling and debris may remain on the canal wall [75]. The canal should be clean enough, however, to encourage a successful outcome if failure of the primary treatment has been caused by inadequate debridement and obturation [76].

Unavoidably, during physical removal of gutta-percha and repreparation of the canal, its shape will be wider than the original preparation, resulting in a tendency for overfilling [11]. The first attempt to locate and negotiate canals, especially those which are fine and tortuous, is the most critical and failed attempts inevitably complicate future treatment. The canal anatomy may have been adversely altered during the original preparation to produce ledges and/or an hourglass shape. In order to improve the prognosis for retreatment, not only is there a requirement that canal patency be regained and all canals found and negotiated, but they must also be shaped to allow three-dimensional obturation. Ledges can sometimes be bypassed. To achieve this, the canal coronal to the ledge must be sufficiently straightened to allow a file to operate effectively. This may be achieved by anticurvature filing. The file that is then used to bypass the obstruction must be precurved quite severely at its tip and used to probe gently past the ledge [47]. If it proves impossible to bypass obstructions or ledges then cleaning, shaping and obturation of the canal coronal to the obstruction should be completed and the patient warned of the poorer prognosis.

In general, retreatment preparation is very time-consuming and often considerably more difficult than preparation of the untouched canal, with the added disadvantage of a lower success rate. The operating microscope, an excellent aid in root canal treatment, both surgical and non-surgical, will prove invaluable during retreatment cases.

Key points of root canal preparation

Irrespective of the preparation method used key points should be observed.

1. The canal should be widened whilst still retaining its preoperative shape.
2. Instruments and irrigants should be kept within the confines of the root canal system.
3. Instruments should be used sequentially.
4. Preparation should be accompanied by copious irrigation with sodium hypochlorite.

Root canal preparation is challenging, particularly in the case of fine curved canals. It requires attention to detail and is time-consuming.

References

1. ABOU-RASS M, FRANK AL, GLICK DH (1980) The anti-curvature filing method to prepare the curved root canal. *Journal of the American Dental Association* **101,** 792–794.

2. ABOU-RASS M, PICCININO MV (1982) The effectiveness of four clinical irrigation methods on the removal of root canal debris. *Oral Surgery, Oral Medicine, Oral Pathology* **54,** 323–328.

3. AHMAD M, PITT FORD TR, CRUM LA (1987) Ultrasonic debridement of root canals: an insight into the mechanisms involved. *Journal of Endodontics* **13,** 93–101.

4. AHMAD M, PITT FORD TR, CRUM LA (1987) Ultrasonic debridement of root canals: acoustic streaming and its possible role. *Journal of Endodontics* **13,** 490–499.

5. ALLEN RK, NEWTON CW, BROWN CE (1989) A statistical analysis of surgical and non-surgical endodontic retreatment cases. *Journal of Endodontics* **15,** 261–266.

6. ALLISON DA, WEBER CR, WALTON RE (1979) The influence of the method of canal preparation on the quality of apical and coronal obturation. *Journal of Endodontics* **5,** 298–304.

7. AL-OMARI MAO (1994) An ex-vivo study of root canal preparation techniques. PhD thesis. Cardiff: University of Wales.

8. BAHCALL J, HOWARD P, MISERENDINO L, WALIA H (1992) Preliminary investigation of the histological effects of laser endodontic treatment on the periradicular tissues in dogs. *Journal of Endodontics* **18,** 47–51.

9. BACKMAN CA, OSWALD RJ, PITTS DL (1992) A radiographic comparison of two root canal instrumentation techniques. *Journal of Endodontics* **18,** 19–24.

10. BAUMGARTNER JC, FALKLER WA (1991) Bacteria in the apical 5 mm of infected root canals. *Journal of Endodontics* **17,** 380–383.

11. BERGENHOLTZ G, LEKHOLM U, MILTHON R, ENGSTROM B (1979) Influence of apical overinstrumentation and overfilling on re–treated root canals. *Journal of Endodontics* **5,** 310–314.

12. BERGENHOLTZ G, LEKHOLM U, MILTHON R, HEDEN G, ODESJO B, ENGSTROM B (1979) Retreatment of endodontic fillings. *Scandinavian Journal of Dental Research* **87,** 217–224.

13. BRODIN P, ROED A, AARS H, ØRSTAVIK D (1982) Neurotoxic effects of root filling materials on rat phrenic nerve *in vitro*. *Journal of Dental Research* **61,** 1020–1023.

14. BUCHANAN LS (1991) Paradigm shifts in cleaning and shaping. *Journal of the California Dental Association* **19,** 23–33.

15. BUCHANAN LS (1994) The Buchanan continuous wave of condensation technique. A convergence of conceptual and procedural advances in obturation. *Dentistry Today* **October,** 80–85.

16. CAMERON JA (1983) The use of ultrasonics in the removal of the smear layer: a scanning electron microscopic study. *Journal of Endodontics* **9,** 289–292.

17. CAMPS J, PERTOT WJ (1995) Machining efficiency of nickel–titanium K-type files in a linear motion. *International Endodontic Journal* **28,** 279–284.

18. CHAPMAN CE (1971) The correlation between apical infection and instrumentation in endodontics. *Journal of the British Endodontic Society* **5,** 76–80.

19. CHENAIL BL, TEPLITSKY PE (1985) Endosonics in curved root canals. *Journal of Endodontics* **11,** 369–374.

20. CHOW TW (1983) Mechanical effectiveness of root canal irrigation. *Journal of Endodontics* **9,** 475–479.

21. CUNNINGHAM WT, MARTIN H, FORREST WR (1982) Evaluation of root canal debridement by the endosonic ultrasonic synergistic system. *Oral Surgery, Oral Medicine, Oral Pathology* **53,** 401–404.

22. DAMAS J, REMACLE-VOLON G, DEFLANDRE E (1986) Further studies of the mechanism of counter-irritation by turpentine. *Archives of Pharmacology* **332,** 196–202.

23. DRUTTMAN ACS, STOCK CJR (1989) An *in vitro* comparison of ultrasonic and conventional methods of irrigant replacement. *International Endodontic Journal* **22,** 174–178.

24. ETTINGER RL, KRELL K (1988) Endodontic problems in an overdenture population. *Journal of Prosthetic Dentistry* **59,** 459–462.

25. FAVA LRG (1983) The double-flared technique: an alternative for biomechanical preparation. *Journal of Endodontics* **9,** 76–80.

26. FORSBERG J (1987) Radiographic reproduction of endodontic 'working length' comparing the paralleling and the bisecting-angle techniques. *Oral Surgery, Oral Medicine, Oral Pathology* **64,** 353–360.

27. FORSBERG J, HALSE A (1994) Radiographic simulation of a periapical lesion comparing the paralleling and the bisecting-angle techniques. *International Endodontic Journal* **27,** 133–138.

28. FRIEDMAN S, STABHOLZ A (1986) Endodontic retreatment – case selection and technique. Part I. Criteria for case selection. *Journal of Endodontics* **12,** 28–33.

29. FRIEDMAN S, STABHOLZ A, TAMSE A (1990) Endodontic retreatment – case selection and technique. 3. Retreatment techniques. *Journal of Endodontics* **16,** 543–549.

30. GOERIG AC, MICHELICH RJ, SCHULTZ HH (1982) Instrumentation of root canals in molar using the step-down technique. *Journal of Endodontics* **8,** 550–554.

31. GOLDMAN M, WHITE RR, MOSER CR, TENCA JI (1988) A comparison of three methods of cleaning and shaping the root canal *in vitro*. *Journal of Endodontics* **14,** 7–12.

32. GOODMAN A, READER A, BECK M, MELFI R, MEYERS W (1985) An *in vitro* comparison of the efficacy of the step-back technique versus a step-back/ultrasonic technique in human mandibular molars. *Journal of Endodontics* **11,** 249–256.

33. GRIFFITHS BM, STOCK CJR (1986) The efficiency of irrigants in removing root canal debris when used in an ultrasonic preparation technique. *International Endodontic Journal* **19,** 277–284.

34. GUTMANN JL, DUMSHA TC, LOVDAHL PE, HOVLAND EJ (1992) *Problem Solving in Endodontics. Prevention, Identification and Management*, 2nd edn, pp. 178–180. St Louis, MO, USA: Mosby-Year Book.

35. HESSION RW (1977) Endodontic morphology. III. Canal preparation. *Oral Surgery, Oral Medicine, Oral Pathology* **44**, 775–785.

36. INGLE JI, BAKLAND LK, PETERS DL, BUCHANAN LS, MULLANEY TP (1994) Endodontic cavity preparation. In: Ingle JI, Bakland LK (eds) *Endodontics*, 4th edn, pp. 92–227. Malvern, PA, USA: Williams and Wilkins.

37. KAPLOWITZ GJ (1990) Evaluation of gutta-percha solvents. *Journal of Endodontics* **16**, 539–540.

38. KEREKES K, ROWE AHR (1982) Thermomechanical compaction of gutta-percha root filling. *International Endodontic Journal* **15**, 27–35.

39. LEEB J (1983) Canal orifice enlargement as related to biomechanical preparation. *Journal of Endodontics* **9**, 463–470.

40. LEVY G (1992) Cleaning and shaping the root canal with a Nd:YAG laser beam: a comparative study. *Journal of Endodontics* **18**, 123–127.

41. LIM SS, STOCK CJR (1987) The risk of perforation in the curved canal: anticurvature filing compared with the stepback technique. *International Endodontic Journal* **20**, 33–39.

42. LUMLEY PJ, WALMSLEY AD, LAIRD WRE (1988) Ultrasonic instruments in dentistry. 2. Endosonics. *Dental Update* **15**, 362–369.

43. LUSSI A, NUSSBACHER U, GROSREY J (1993) A novel noninstrumented technique for cleansing the root canal system. *Journal of Endodontics* **19**, 549–553.

44. LUSSI A, MESSERLI L, HOTZ P, GROSREY J (1995) A new non-instrumental technique for cleaning and filling root canals. *International Endodontic Journal* **28**, 1–6.

45. MCDONALD NJ (1992) The electronic determination of working length. *Dental Clinics of North America* **36**, 293–307.

46. MACHIDA T, WILDER-SMITH P, ARRASTIA AM, LIAW LHL, BERNS MW (1995) Root canal preparation using the second harmonic KTP:YAG laser: a thermographic and scanning electron microscopic study. *Journal of Endodontics* **21**, 88–91.

47. MANDEL E, FRIEDMAN S (1992) Endodontic retreatment: a rational approach to root canal reinstrumentation. *Journal of Endodontics* **18**, 565–569.

48. MARTIN H (1976) Ultrasonic disinfection of the root canal. *Oral Surgery, Oral Medicine, Oral Pathology* **42**, 92–99.

49. MARTIN H, CUNNINGHAM WT, NORRIS JP, COTTON WR (1980) Ultrasonic versus hand filing of dentin: a quantitative study. *Oral Surgery, Oral Medicine, Oral Pathology* **49**, 79–81.

50. MARTIN H, CUNNINGHAM W (1984) Endosonic endodontics: the ultrasonic synergistic system. *International Dental Journal* **34**, 198–203.

51. MOLTENI R (1993) Direct digital dental X-ray imaging with Visualix/VIXA. *Oral Surgery, Oral Medicine, Oral Pathology* **76**, 235–243.

52. MORGAN LF, MONTGOMERY S (1984) An evaluation of the crown-down pressureless technique. *Journal of Endodontics* **10**, 491–498.

53. MULLANEY TP (1979) Instrumentation of finely curved canals. *Dental Clinics of North America* **23**, 575–592.

54. RICHMAN MJ (1957) Use of ultrasonics in root canal therapy and root resection. *Journal of Dental Medicine* **12**, 12–18.

55. ROANE J, SABALA C, DUNCANSON MG (1985) The 'balanced force' concept for instrumentation of curved canals. *Journal of Endodontics* **11**, 203–211.

56. ROONEY J, MIDDA M, LEEMING J (1994) A laboratory investigation of the bactericidal effect of a Nd:YAG laser. *British Dental Journal* **176**, 61–64.

57. RUIZ-HUBARD EE, GUTMANN JL, WAGNER MJ (1987) A quantitative assessment of canal debris forced periapically during root canal instrumentation using two different techniques. *Journal of Endodontics* **13**, 554–558.

58. SABALA CL, ROANE JB, SOUTHARD LZ (1988) Instrumentation of curved canals using a modified tipped instrument: a comparison study. *Journal of Endodontics* **14**, 59–64.

59. SAITO T, YAMASHITA Y (1990) Electronic determination of root canal length by newly developed measuring device. Influences of the diameter of apical foramen. *Dentistry in Japan* **27**, 65–72.

60. SAUNDERS WP, SAUNDERS EM (1992) Effect of non-cutting tipped instruments on the quality of root canal preparation using a modified double-flared technique. *Journal of Endodontics* **18**, 32–36.

61. SAUNDERS WP, SAUNDERS EM (1994) Coronal leakage as a cause of failure in root-canal therapy: a review. *Endodontics and Dental Traumatology* **10**, 105–108.

62. SAUNDERS EM, SAUNDERS WP (1995) *A Manual for Root Canal Therapy*, pp. 23–26. Dundee, Scotland: University of Dundee.

63. SCHONFELD SE, GREENING AB, GLICK DH, FRANK AL, SIMON JH, HERLES SM (1982) Endotoxic activity in periapical lesions. *Oral Surgery, Oral Medicine, Oral Pathology* **53**, 82–87.

64. SCHULZ-BONGERT U, WEINE FS, SHULZ-BONGERT J (1995) Preparation of curved canals using a combined hand-filing, ultrasonic technique. *Compendium of Continuing Education in Dentistry* **16**, 272–283.

65. SELTZER S, SOLTANOFF W, SMITH J (1973) Biologic aspects of endodontics. V. Periapical tissue reactions to root canal instrumentation beyond the apex and root canal fillings short of and beyond the apex. *Oral Surgery, Oral Medicine, Oral Pathology* **36**, 725–737.

66. SHOVELTON DS (1964) The presence and distribution of micro-organisms within non-vital teeth. *British Dental Journal* **117**, 101–107.

67. SOUTHARD DW, OSWALD RJ, NATKIN E (1987) Instrumentation of curved molar root canals with the Roane technique. *Journal of Endodontics* **13**, 479–489.

68. STABHOLZ A, FRIEDMAN S (1988) Endodontic retreatment – case selection and technique. Part 2. Treatment planning for retreatment. *Journal of Endodontics* **14**, 607–614.

69. TIDMARSH BG (1982) Preparation of the root canal. *International Endodontic Journal* **15**, 53–61.

70. VESSEY RA (1969) The effect of filing versus reaming on the shape of the prepared root canal. *Oral Surgery, Oral Medicine, Oral Pathology* **27**, 543–547.

71. VANDE VISSE JE, BRILLIANT JD (1975) Effect of irrigation on the production of extruded material at the root apex during instrumentation. *Journal of Endodontics* **1**, 243–246.

72. WALIA H, COSTAS J, BRANTLEY W, GERSTEIN H (1989) Torsional ductility and cutting efficiency of the Nitinol file. *Journal of Endodontics* **15**, 174 (abstract 22).

73. WALMSLEY AD (1987) Ultrasound and root canal treatment: the need for scientific evaluation. *International Endodontic Journal* **20**, 105–111.

74. WEINE FS, KELLY RF, LIO PJ (1975) The effect of preparation procedures on original canal shape and on apical foramen shape. *Journal of Endodontics* **1**, 255–262.

75. WILCOX LR (1989) Endodontic retreatment: ultrasonics and chloroform as a final step in reinstrumentation. *Journal of Endodontics* **15**, 125–128.

76. WILCOX LR, KRELL KV, MADISON S, RITTMAN B (1987) Endodontic retreatment: evaluation of gutta-percha and sealer removal and canal reinstrumentation. *Journal of Endodontics* **13**, 453–457.

77. ZMENER O, BALBACHAN L (1995) Effectiveneess of nickel–titanium files for preparing curved root canals. *Endodontics and Dental Traumatology* **11**, 121–123.

78. ZURBRIGGEN T, DEL RIO CE, BRADY JM (1975) Post-debridement retention of endodontic reagents: a quantitative measurement with radioactive isotope. *Journal of Endodontics* **1**, 298–299.

7

Intracanal medication

D. Ørstavik

Introduction

Endodontic success or failure is related to the absence or presence of signs and symptoms of apical periodontitis [85]. Root canal treatment can therefore be considered the prevention or cure of this disease [63]. Apical periodontitis includes apical granuloma and radicular cyst as well as acute manifestations of inflammation. The aetiology of apical periodontitis is primarily a bacterial infection of the root canal system [48,55,86] (Table 7.1); consequently, the technical and pharmacological aspects of prevention and treatment are mainly aimed at controlling infection. Thus, *preventive* endodontics entails treatment of a tooth without previous signs of apical periodontitis by aseptic pulp extirpation and root canal filling. *Treatment* of a tooth

with radiographic or clinical signs of the disease is the chemomechanical elimination of infection in the pulp canal system.

The use of intracanal medicaments is an adjunct to the prevention or treatment of

Table 7.1 Association of bacteria with apical periodontitis: experimental studies in monkeys. Percentage of teeth with signs of inflammatory periapical reactions

Pulp status	Clinical	Radiographic	Histological
Lacerated, non-infected	0	0	8
Lacerated, infected	23	90	100

From Möller *et al.* (1981) [55].

apical periodontitis. Thus their primary function is to prevent canal infection where none is present, and/or to eliminate bacteria already infecting the root canal. Intracanal *medicaments* would include any agent with intended pharmacological action introduced in the root canal. Antibacterial and other active compounds currently used as irrigating solutions during instrumentation rightly belong in this category. Intracanal *dressings* more concisely describe medicaments left in the root canal to exert their effects over a longer time period.

History

The role of microorganisms in pulpless teeth was recognized more than a century ago [51], and strong caustic antiseptics were popular as intracanal medicaments at the turn of this century. Formaldehyde-containing materials, e.g. formocresol [12], and iodoform pastes [98] belong to this category and have remained popular for decades. Formulations with sulphonamides [60] and later antibiotics were tried as intracanal medicaments; Grossman's polyantibiotic paste [33] and Ledermix [75] are examples of these types of dressing.

The reduction of pain through pharmacological control of the inflammatory process has been attempted in endodontics also by the application of eugenol [50], and later corticosteroids and other anti-inflammatory drugs [59], as dressings.

Focus on the possible adverse toxic effects of medicaments [84,99] led to a more systematic selection from the list of disinfectants available for use. Phenol derivatives and iodine formulations gained popularity as medicaments in endodontics; sodium hypochlorite was confirmed as a suitable irrigant.

Calcium hydroxide, while advocated since 1930 [43], has gained popularity in endodontics in the last two decades. Calcium hydroxide has had success in a variety of clinical situations including root resorption, apexification and apexogenesis, exudation and canal infection [40]. In recent years, it has become almost a panacea endodontic medicament.

Rationale and overview of applications

The primary function of endodontic medicaments is to provide antimicrobial activity. In a few instances, other secondary functions are desirable (Table 7.2). The rationale for applying intracanal medicaments in various clinical situations has recently been reviewed [18].

Asepsis, antisepsis and disinfection

Asepsis is the assurance that no bacteria are present in the field of operation. It entails the use not only of clean, but of definitively sterile instruments and utensils, liquids, etc. In the course of treating teeth with no signs of canal infection, maintaining asepsis is the primary means of preserving a bacteria-free canal.

Antisepsis is the endeavour to eliminate infecting or contaminating microbes. In vital pulp extirpation, antiseptic measures are necessary to prevent infection if there is a breach in the chain of asepsis. Irrigating solutions and interappointment dressings need to be antibacterial in action to prevent any microorganisms which may contaminate the canal system from multiplying and establishing themselves.

Disinfection is the elimination of pathogenic microorganisms, usually by chemical or physical means. Disinfection by antiseptic agents is what is attempted in the treatment of infected teeth. Sterilization, on the other hand, implies the use of irradiation or heat to reach a state of complete freedom from microbes and cannot be applied to root canal treatment. Disinfection entails mechanical removal of tissue and debris containing

Table 7.2 Functions of intracanal medicaments

Primary function: antimicrobial activity
Antisepsis
Disinfection

Secondary functions
Hard-tissue formation
Pain control
Exudation control
Resorption control

microbes, irrigation and dressing with anti-septic agents; also, surgical removal of an infected apex serves the antiseptic efforts of treatment. The presence of radiographically discernible apical periodontitis is a sign that the root canal system is infected [86]. This state of pre-existing infection also has a negative influence on prognosis [64]. In these cases, bacterial reduction, and if possible dis-infection, of the root canal system is a pre-requisite for successful treatment.

Secondary functions of medicaments

Root canal treatment is sometimes associated with clinical features only indirectly related to infection of the canal system. Pain during and after treatment may occur, and the tissue reactions associated with affected root canals include exudation, transudation, swelling and resorption. Each of these phenomena, either singly or in conjunction with infection, have been targets for attempts at medication during, between and after treatment sessions.

Induction of hard-tissue formation

It is often considered desirable to allow hard tissue to form to continue apical root devel-opment, to close a wide foramen, or to create a mechanical barrier at a fracture line. Although the mechanism of action is largely unknown, dressings are available with claims of inducing hard-tissue formation.

Pain control

Pain is often associated with infection, and the primary means of pain control in endo-dontic treatment is infection control. Phar-macological agents which result in pain reduction through a decrease in the tissue responses in inflammation may have a role in further alleviating clinical pain from both infectious and aseptic pulpo-periodontal inflammation.

Control of exudation or bleeding

Persistent exudation in the root canal may occur, despite apparently successful clinical and technical aspects of the treatment.

Exudation reflects inflammation, however, and residual infection should be suspected. Therefore, treatment is aimed at dealing with potential infection as well as drying or coagu-lating the exudating surface.

Control of inflammatory root resorption

Trauma to the teeth may result in various forms of resorptive damage, inflammatory root resorption being the most aggressive and destructive. Inflammatory root resorption is associated with infection of the root canal combined with physical damage to the cementum; again, a primary function of treat-ment is to eliminate infection in the root canal. Secondarily, the resorption process itself may be influenced by medicaments.

Microbes of the pulp

A root canal containing an inflamed pulp is assumed to be sterile in the part apical to the inflamed area until complete or near-complete pulpal necrosis has occurred. Following pulpal necrosis, sooner or later the entire pulp canal system will become infected. A long-standing infection will have bacteria not only in the main canal but also in accessory canals and for a distance into the dentinal tubules [78]. If apical periodontitis has progressed to the point where resorption of the cementum occurs, bacteria may be found throughout the length of the tubules [95].

The source of the infecting bacteria is usually dental caries, salivary contamination through fractures, cracks or leaking fillings, or contamination of the pulp space during dental, including endodontic, treatment.

With increasing depth and time of pulp infection, the microbial flora changes from a predominantly facultative, Gram-positive flora to an almost completely anaerobic and mainly Gram-negative set of micro-organisms [28]. Strains belonging to the genera *Fusobacterium*, *Prevotella*, *Porphyro-monas*, *Peptostreptococcus*, *Veillonella* and spirochaetes are frequently isolated from teeth with apical periodontitis [87]. Faculta-tive streptococci are also common. These same types of microorganisms are found in acute exacerbations or periapical abscesses [11]. In addition, specific infections involving particular microorganisms, e.g. enterococci [54] and *Actinomyces/Arachnia* [80] may occur.

In most infected canals, several species are recovered from the root canals [87]. Many of the dominating species, e.g. *Fusobacteria, Prevotella, Porphyromonas,* may require the presence of some other, synergistic species for their survival and propagation. It may be noteworthy in this context that these same species have not been found in dentinal tubules, which when infected harbour less fastidious microorganisms, such as lactobacilli and streptococci [7].

Infected canals typically contain 2–10 different species; total numbers range from 10^3 to 10^7 [15]. Exact numbers of microorganisms are unknown as they vary from tooth to tooth, and due to a lack of established quantitative methods of collection.

Antimicrobial agents

Antibiotics

The successful use of various antibiotics, both systemically and topically, in other fields of medicine made them likely candidates for antibacterial action in the root canal. There are three main concerns about the local use of antibiotics in the root canal:

1. *Sensitization.* Topical application of an antibiotic increases the risk of the patient becoming allergic to it [96]. Life-threatening anaphylactic reactions may occur from administration of antibiotics to sensitized individuals. Induced allergy to an antibiotic may limit the options for treatment of more severe infections which would otherwise be curable with that particular drug.
2. *Development of bacterial drug resistance.* The drug kinetics of antibiotics applied in the root canal are not well known [5]. Conditions may become favourable for the development of antibiotic-resistant microbial strains, causing an infection which in turn is more difficult to treat [97]. Moreover, beyond the scope of treatment of the individual patient, the widespread use of antibiotics causes a general increase in pathogenic and indigenous microorganisms that are resistant to a variety of antibiotics [20].
3. *Limited spectrum.* No one antibiotic is efficacious against all endodontic microorganisms [6]. Given that most endodontic infections are caused by a combination of species, the chance of one antibiotic achieving effective bacterial inhibition or elimination is small.

Sulpha preparations

Sulphathiazole as part of a dressing was advocated in the 1950s and 1960s [60]. While irrefutably antibacterial, clinical studies showed variable results in comparative studies [31,77]. Moreover, although effective against many Gram-negative and Gram-positive microorganisms, sulpha drugs are ineffective against enterococci and *Pseudomonas aeruginosa.*

Penicillin

Grossman's polyantibiotic paste contained penicillin as an important ingredient. Beta-lactamase produced by several species found in the root canal makes them resistant to penicillin. This includes *P. aeruginosa* and several anaerobic Gram-negative rods.

Metronidazole

Metronidazole has good effect against several Gram-negative, anaerobic microorganisms [83]. It has been suggested for use in irrigating solutions [74], as an intracanal dressing [44] and for parenteral applications in combination with other antibiotics, particularly penicillin [91].

Tetracycline

Tetracycline shows affinity for hard tissues and may be retained on tooth surfaces [10]. It is used locally in periodontics with good clinical and bacteriological results [32], and the derivative doxycycline forms the antibiotic ingredient in Ledermix [25]. However, its antimicrobial spectrum is quite narrow, and it may be ineffective against several oral and endodontic pathogens. The fact that resistance to tetracyclines occurs through the formation of transferable R factors also suggests caution in its application.

Clindamycin

One study has reported on the use of clindamycin as an interappointment dressing, but only limited antibacterial efficacy could be demonstrated [53].

Disinfectants

While antibiotics work through biological interference with essential biochemical processes, disinfectants (Table 7.3) are a group of chemicals that act by direct toxicity to the microbes. Their action is thus quicker and more general, and they usually have a broader antibacterial spectrum than the antibiotic drugs. On the other hand, they may be more toxic to host tissues, and their action is more dose-dependent.

Aldehydes

Formaldehyde, paraformaldehyde and glutaraldehyde have been widely used in dentistry, including endodontics. They are water-soluble, protein-denaturing agents and are among the most potent disinfectants. Aldehydes have applications in the disinfection of surfaces and medical equipment that cannot be sterilized, but they are quite toxic and allergenic, and some may be carcinogenic.

Formocresol contains formaldehyde as its main ingredient and is still a widely used medicament for pulpotomy procedures, but its toxic and mutagenic properties are of concern. These same properties have caused the use of neutral buffered formalin, a popular dressing some 20 years ago, to be discontinued.

Paraformaldehyde is the polymer form of formaldehyde, best known for its inclusion in the root canal-filling materials, N2 and Endomethasone. It slowly decomposes to

Table 7.3 Root canal disinfectants

Aldehydes
Formocresol
  Dressing: 19% formaldehyde, 35% cresol, 46% water and glycerine

Halogens
Chlorine
  Irrigating solution: sodium hypochlorite 0.5% in 1% sodium bicarbonate as Dakin's solution, or 0.5–5.25% in aqueous solution
Iodine
  Irrigating solution and short-term dressing: 2% I_2 in 5% KI aqueous solution
Field disinfection: 5% I_2 in tincture of alcohol

Phenols
Camphorated phenol
  Dressing: 30% phenol, 60% camphor, 10% ethanol
Para-mono-chlorophenol (PMCP)
  Irrigating solution: 2% aqueous solution
  Dressing: camphorated PMCP (CMCP); 65% camphor, 35% PMCP
Eugenol
  Dressing: full strength

Chlorhexidine
Chlorhexidine gluconate
  Field disinfection and irrigating solution: 0.12–2% aqueous solution

Calcium hydroxide
$Ca(OH)_2$
  Dressing: aqueous suspension/paste with varying amounts of salts added

give its monomer, formaldehyde; its toxic, allergenic and genotoxic properties are as for formaldehyde.

Halogens

Halogens include chlorine and iodine which are used in various formulations in endodontics. They are potent oxidizing agents with rapid bactericidal effects. Chlorine is released from sodium hypochlorite and from chloramine. The latter releases active chlorine at a lower rate, and has been used for short-term dressing of the root canal. Sodium hypochlorite is the current irrigating solution of choice; in concentrations 0.5–5.25% it has been used clinically, with bacteriological studies both *in vitro* and *in vivo* to support its application. Necrotic tissue and debris are dissolved by sodium hypochlorite [36], a property exploited in mechanical cleansing of root canals [57,72]. Its toxicity is low; however, its bleaching properties are a nuisance if spilled onto patients' clothes, its smell is objectionable to some patients, and it may cause severe symptoms if injected beyond the apex [9].

Iodine is used as iodine potassium iodide, and in iodophors, which are organic iodine-containing compounds that release iodine over time. It is also a very potent antibacterial agent of low toxicity, but may stain clothing if spilled. As iodoform it was used in a paste formulation to serve as a permanent root canal filling [98]. Its current applications are as an irrigating solution and short-term dressing, in a 2% solution of iodine in 4% aqueous potassium iodide. Some patients may be allergic to iodine compounds, and their use in these patients is contraindicated.

Phenols

While phenol itself is no longer used in endodontics because of its high toxicity-to-efficacy ratio, the derivative para-mono-chlorophenol has been a very popular component of dressings. It has been used as a dressing both in aqueous solution [88] and in combination with camphor (as camphorated mono-chlorophenol, CMCP); it was long recognized as the dressing of choice for infected teeth. Thymol similarly enjoyed widespread popularity.

Eugenol is frequently used as a dressing for temporary control of pain after vital pulp exposure [39]. It has a well-documented, but limited, antimicrobial effect and is applied primarily for its pain-relieving effect [45].

Chlorhexidine

Chlorhexidine would appear to have great potential as an intracanal medicament, but it has never enjoyed the popularity in endodontics that it has in periodontology [47]. Its substantivity (persistence in the area of interest), its relatively broad spectrum of activity and its low toxicity may make it well-suited for irrigation and dressing applications in endodontics. Results of recent studies point to the suitability of chlorhexidine in endodontics [41,42,46,65,94], but clinicobacteriological data are still largely lacking. Effective concentrations would be expected to be in the 0.2–2% range.

Calcium hydroxide

Calcium hydroxide has reached a unique position as a dressing in endodontics. After its successful clinical application for a variety of indications [40], multiple biological functions have been ascribed to this chemical compound [30]. Its primary function is probably antibacterial in most clinical situations, with added benefits from its cauterizing activity and high pH, and also from the paste consistency which physically restricts bacterial colonization of the canal space. Calcium hydroxide is applied as a thick, creamy suspension in sterile water, saline or salt solutions with or without other additives. Small, if any, differences have been reported in the efficacy of different preparations [49].

Resistance of oral microbes to medicaments

In some cases, bacteria persist and produce symptoms and/or apical periodontitis despite apparently optimal cleansing and disinfection procedures [14]. They may either be inaccessible to the cleaning instruments and/or to the medicaments, or they may be resistant to the medicaments used. Special interest has recently focused on enterococci in persistent infections; these have been shown to be relatively resistant to calcium hydroxide [13,34] and occur in high frequency in retreatment cases [54].

Concept of predictable disinfection in endodontics

Given the infectious nature of apical periodontitis, any clinical procedure should be based on the ability of each step to prevent contamination and to eliminate infection. A standard procedure should furthermore be based on a worst-case scenario, which would be the infected root canal with associated chronic apical periodontitis. Individual treatment steps have been assessed for their efficacy in eliminating bacteria from infected root canals [13–17,79, 81] (Figure 7.1).

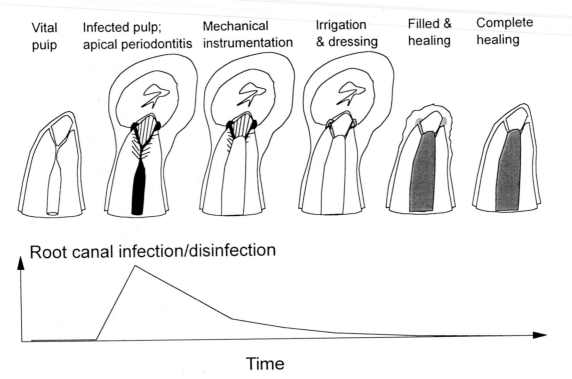

Figure 7.1 Apical periodontitis develops when the root canal system becomes infected. Treatment entails the reduction of bacteria by mechanical instrumentation and antibacterial irrigation. The antibacterial dressing, when effective, eliminates infection. Total disinfection allows for complete healing of the tooth with apical periodontitis following root canal filling.

Mechanical instrumentation

Even in the absence of an antibacterial irrigating solution and subsequent dressing, there is still a dramatic decrease in bacterial numbers in a root canal from mechanical cleansing alone [15,66]. However, in the majority of cases, bacteria which are left in the canal have the potential to multiply between appointments [15] and/or after filling [71].

Antibacterial effect of irrigation

The addition of sodium hypochlorite as an antibacterial irrigating solution increases the number of bacteria-free canals substantially [16]. The use of 5% rather than 0.5% sodium hypochlorite appears more effective, and the reduction in the number of infected teeth has been shown to be even greater when ethylenediaminetetraacetate (EDTA) was alternated with sodium hypochlorite [16,17], and

when ultrasonic instrumentation of the canal was performed [81].

Effect of antibacterial dressing

The number of bacteria-free canals may be increased to almost 100% when a dressing of calcium hydroxide is placed in fully instrumented canals between visits [13,21,66,73]. Calcium hydroxide has been found to be more effective than CMCP in comparative experiments [13].

Follow-up studies

Teeth treated as described above have been followed for periods up to 7 years, and the results have shown success rates (definite signs of healing of apical periodontitis) in more than 90% of cases [14]. While success rates from different studies may be difficult to compare, it appears that these clinical results are better than most, if not all, previous reports.

From controlled to predictable disinfection

Data, obtained clinically, furnish a rational approach to suggested guidelines for treatment of infected teeth. The clinical experiments document *controlled* disinfection by advanced bacteriological techniques. When applied to clinical practice, adherence to these principles of mechanical instrumentation, irrigation with sodium hypochlorite and EDTA, and dressing with calcium hydroxide, would be expected to produce *predictable* disinfection (bacteria-free canals) in almost 100% of cases, and in turn to produce clinical and radiographic evidence of healing apical periodontitis in over 90% of cases. Indeed, large series of follow-up studies using this treatment regimen for infected teeth have borne out the high success rate [27]. A need for routine chairside bacteriological control of procedures is not implied.

Treatment of non-infected teeth

None of the steps advocated for the treatment of the infected tooth place in jeopardy the success of treatment of a tooth with an initially non-infected pulp. Vital pulp extirpation followed by instrumentation with sodium hypochlorite and a dressing of calcium hydroxide give a clean pulp wound with minimal or no inflammation (Figure 7.2). Therefore, as a means of securing the absence of microbes in these cases, the same treatment principles should apply. One exception is when permanent root canal filling is possible at the first appointment; there is no need to have a period of canal dressing for the purpose of disinfection. Also, it may be questioned whether EDTA serves any purpose in the treatment of non-infected pulps.

Other principles of treatment may have a potential for equal or better efficacy and success rates. However, the extensive documentation with clinical bacteriological control, and clinical and radiological follow-ups make the above guidelines a standard of reference. Alternative methods and medicaments

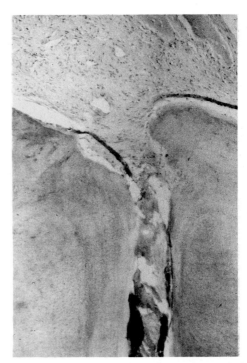

Figure 7.2 Inflammation-free extirpation wound of a mature monkey central incisor after 2 weeks of dressing with calcium hydroxide.

should be tested and compared with the elements of this method prior to general clinical acceptance.

Induction of hard-tissue formation

The process of creating a hard-tissue barrier at an open apex or at a grossly overinstrumented apex is termed apexification [24]. Through the use of calcium hydroxide in the long-term treatment of traumatized young permanent incisors, it was learned that when infection was controlled, a barrier of bone/cementum-like tissue was formed with varying degrees of completeness, but with a high degree of predictability [22] (Figure 7.3). This barrier serves as a mechanical point of compression of the root filling, and any toxic responses of the tissues to the filling materials are minimized by the intervening barrier. While it may not be essential that calcium hydroxide be used as a dressing for this

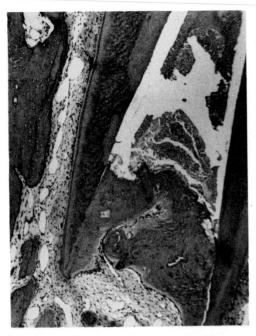

Figure 7.3 Formation of a hard tissue barrier at the apex of an immature mandibular central incisor (monkey). The pulp was extirpated and a dressing of calcium hydroxide placed for 3 weeks.

purpose, it has the best and most extensive clinical documentation. Similar principles apply in the formation of a hard-tissue barrier more coronally, e.g. at the line of a horizontal root fracture or at a pulpotomy wound surface.

Sources and control of pain

Endodontic pain is mainly associated with inflammation, which in turn is usually linked with infection [35,37,38,82]. The inflammatory responses to the trauma of pulp extirpation and instrumentation may elicit pain of lesser magnitude and duration than pain following bacterial activity. The rationale behind pain control by interappointment dressings is thus primarily to combat infection.

Pain during and after endodontic treatment is a highly multifaceted clinical phenomenon. The scientific approaches to manifestation of pain are also diverse in both scope and technique, and very few studies on pain in endodontics are comparable to each other. There are strong psychological components to the clinical expression of pain of endodontic origin [52]. Clinical pain is further confounded by the concomitant presence of microbial and iatrogenic sources. The quantification of pain clinically is also very difficult to standardize for comparative purposes.

The incidence of interappointment or posttreatment pain seems to be very much dependent on the criteria defining pain [61,89]. As an operative definition, the incidence of patients requiring an extra, non-scheduled visit following self-reported pain may have some merit. It would not include the discomfort sometimes or often associated with the practical necessities of the treatment itself (injection, clamp placement, severance of the pulp). By such criteria, no significant advantage of one medicament over another has been documented [29,92].

Due to the lack of precise knowledge of the source of pain in individual cases, the introduction of medicaments in dressings to alleviate inter- and posttreatment pain has been by theoretical considerations, and by trial and error, rather than by clinical research. Most interest has focused on the use of corticosteroids in the interappointment dressing; particularly, the use of Ledermix with triamcinolone has gained widespread acceptance and use [1,25,75]. Also other commercially available formulations contain corticosteroids. The use of steroids in endodontics was initially criticized as it was felt that they might interfere with the body's reactions to microbial invasion, and because local application could interfere with natural synthesis of steroids. It is doubtful whether these concerns are justified: there is no indication that harmful side-effects are associated with its use in dentistry, and the doses applied are rather small compared with other medical indications [2]. However, while concerns for side-effects may have been exaggerated, the clinical benefits, if any, over calcium hydroxide medication remain questionable. Non-steroidal anti-inflammatory drugs have also been tested clinically as intracanal dressings [59], but any clinical benefits again remain obscure.

For the control of pain, little seems to be gained either by the prophylactic addition to dressings or by the routine prescription of parenteral drugs [89]. It seems that endodontic pain may be better dealt with on a case-by-case approach, providing relief in doses of medication and by treatment appropriate for the individual patient.

Sources and control of exudation and bleeding

Purulent exudate is a clear sign of infection and is usually easily controlled by instrumentation and dressing with calcium hydroxide. A serous exudate ('the weeping canal') is a more elusive clinical condition. It may show no bacterial growth if cultured and can be resistant to control by conventional instrumentation and dressing. It is usually associated with a relatively large apical foramen or an overinstrumented, patent foramen. Dressing with calcium hydroxide for extended periods may be necessary to control the exudation. Sometimes the application for a few minutes of dry calcium hydroxide packed against the exudating surface succeeds in desiccating or necrotizing that surface to the point where seepage is controlled and treatment may continue.

To the extent that exudation is associated with inflammation, and inflammation may be reduced by local corticosteroids, it would be rational in these cases to include steroid-containing dressings [1]. Given the limited nature of this problem, clinical studies are hard to design and carry out, and data are lacking to support suggested modes of treatment.

Bleeding from the canal is usually easily controlled by simple occlusion of the bleeding surface by paper points, dry or moistened with 3% hydrogen peroxide. Packing of calcium hydroxide on to the bleeding surface also effectively stops bleeding within a few minutes.

Sources and control of resorption

Root resorption is a complication of root canal infection and trauma, in some instances with deleterious consequences to the tooth [8]. The apical, external root resorption associated with chronic apical periodontitis is self-

limiting and stops when the canal infection is adequately controlled. It is likely that this resorption occurs to eliminate necrotic and/or infected cementum and dentine.

Traumatic tooth injuries, particularly avulsions followed by replantation, frequently lead to resorptive processes. Surface resorption is self-limiting and entails repair of cemental damage induced by the trauma. Ankylosis or replacement resorption, however, may be progressive in nature and proceed irrespective of the treatment or of any medicament placed in the canal. Inflammatory resorption of the root surface occurs in response to a necrotic and infected root canal, and may be extremely rapid, causing tooth loss in months if left untreated. Root canal treatment is essential when inflammatory root resorption is evident or imminent, and calcium hydroxide is the current medicament of choice for this purpose [93]. Prolonged use of calcium hydroxide with multiple changes of the dressing may lead to necrosis of cells trying to recolonize the cementum surface. While this finding may suggest that the time of treatment with calcium hydroxide in these cases should be kept short (1–2 weeks), long-term placement of calcium hydroxide remains a clinically proven procedure in the treatment of resorption [93].

It has been suggested that because Ledermix inhibits the spread of dentinoclasts [69], it may provide added benefits in the control of inflammatory root resorption [70], particularly when mixed with calcium hydroxide [5]. More experimental is the use of calcitonin, a hormone which inhibits osteoclastic bone resorption, in canal dressings for inflammatory root resorption [68].

Distribution of medicaments applied to the root canal

There is limited knowledge on the actual distribution, in hard and soft tissues, of medicaments applied to the root canal [3,19,90]. There are several barriers to the penetration of chemical agents from the pulp canal through tooth structures and into the periapical tissues [4,34]. There is also limited knowledge on the localization of microorganisms, inflamed tissues and cells targeted by the medicaments [56,58].

Diffusion and solubility

The ability of a medicament to dissolve and diffuse in the predominantly aqueous periapical environment would seem essential for its successful action. Lipid-soluble substances may have difficulty reaching targets at a distance in the tissues. Amphipathic drugs may have particular benefits; it may not be coincidental that aldehydes and phenol derivatives have had clinical success [100]. Thus aqueous solutions of para-mono-chlorphenol may penetrate further and have greater antimicrobial activity than the more concentrated lipid solute [88]. The low but significant solubility in water of calcium hydroxide has the dual advantage of limiting its toxic effects while the depot of the compound in suspension at the same time provides continuous release of the agent.

Vaporizing agents have been advocated on the premise that the vapour would be more permeating than liquids [26]. On the contrary, limited antibacterial activity might be expected since the gas may or may not be antibacterial, and must still dissolve in tissue fluids to exert its effect.

Penetration of dentine

Studies *in vivo* have found the raised pH effect of calcium hydroxide to pervade the width of dentine [90], but to decrease rapidly in the tissues beyond. The application of calcium hydroxide on a dentine surface in turn significantly reduces its permeability [67]. However, it has been shown *in vitro* that calcium hydroxide is slower than many other medicaments in killing bacteria in experimentally infected dentinal tubules [34]. Similarly, the active ingredients in Ledermix show a decreasing gradient in dentine from the site of application to the cementum surface [5]. Eugenol, which occurs in several root canal sealer formulations, decreases in concentration by 100-fold over 1 mm of dentine [45]. Moreover, intact cementum appears to be an effective, if not complete, barrier to medicament penetration [4].

Effect of the smear layer

Bacteriological data, both *in vitro* [65] as well as *in vivo* [13], indicate that medicaments penetrate to act more effectively when applied in a root canal that has been treated to remove the smear layer. In infected teeth with chronic apical periodontitis one may assume that bacteria are lodged peripheral to the main canal where the medicaments are applied [78,95]. The removal of the smear layer through the use of EDTA seems prudent in these cases. Following complete disinfection, however, or in the treatment of a non-infected tooth, retention or recreation of the smear layer may be advantageous in adding to the sealing-off of the canal by the final root filling, although there are conflicting reports on the role of the smear layer in filling root canals [23].

It should also be recognized that a plug of dentine smear is frequently formed at the apical part of the instrumented canal (Figure 7.4). This may obviously impair the ability of any medicament to penetrate through the apex.

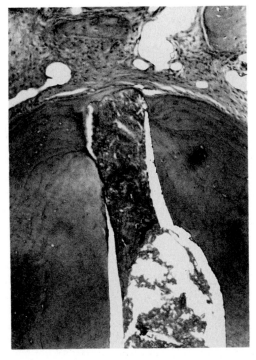

Figure 7.4 A plug of dentine and pulp debris separates the main canal from the apical orifice.

Tissue toxicity and biological considerations

Endodontic medicaments can cause tissue damage which will lead to inflammatory responses in soft tissues. These responses may interfere with the healing of apical periodontitis or serve as a locus for colonization by microorganisms to create a lesion where none existed. Any antiseptic will have a concentration gradient in the tissues with bactericidal and then bacteriostatic activity, but the cytotoxic effects will always be wider-ranging (Figure 7.5). Experiments with cell-culture techniques and toxicity tests in animals have aided in our selection among chemicals and medicaments for endodontic use [84]. Moreover, the allergenic and genotoxic properties of medicaments must form part of the selection criteria [62].

The very strong tissue toxicity, as well as the allergenicity and mutagenicity of aldehydes, has been part of the reason why these agents are no longer recommended for routine use. Similarly, phenols are strongly cytotoxic and are hardly recommendable for use by current standards [84]. Although toxicity is reduced by the addition of camphor, the toxicity/efficacy ratio is still very high.

In recommended concentrations, halogen compounds have high antibacterial activity combined with low tissue toxicity. This forms part of the reason why sodium hypochlorite is the irrigating solution of choice and why iodine potassium iodide has been an attractive alternative for short-term intracanal dressing [73]. Cases have been reported, however, of patients with extremely painful reactions to sodium hypochlorite inadvertently placed or injected into the periapical tissues [9].

Calcium hydroxide is, by virtue of its extremely high pH, potentially quite toxic. However, applied on vital tissue, the damage is limited to a narrow zone of superficial necrosis with a potential for complete regeneration [76].

Suggested clinical procedures

Mechanical reduction of bacteria

Mechanical instrumentation is the main factor in reducing most bacteria infecting root canals. Rubber dam is essential in preventing the root canal system from salivary infection. All efforts should be made to complete the mechanical phases of cleaning and shaping early in treatment, preferably at the first appointment. Any caries must be completely excavated, defective restorations removed, and the tooth and surrounding rubber dam surface thoroughly disinfected. All instrumentation should be done in the presence of an irrigating solution. The clinical studies with bacteriological control have employed master apical file sizes of ISO 40 or larger, which exceed the general recommendations in many current textbooks.

Application of medicaments

Irrigation

Sodium hypochlorite has the best clinical and laboratory documentation. It may be applied, as a 1–5% aqueous solution, in a sterile syringe with a short 12–25 mm needle with outer diameter as low as practical (0.4 mm). Every precaution should be taken to keep the needle from wedging in the canal so as to prevent accidental injection of sodium hypochlorite into the periapical tissues. Fresh

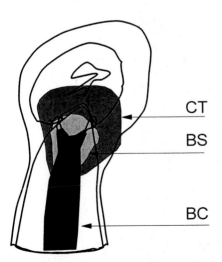

Figure 7.5 Theoretical zones of bactericidal (BC), bacteriostatic (BS) and cytotoxic (CT) activity from an antiseptic in the root canal.

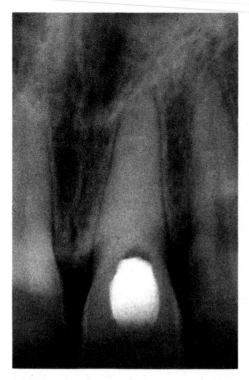

Figure 7.6. The radiopacity of a thick suspension of calcium hydroxide is close to that of dentine. An effective filling gives the appearance of a completely obturated canal.

solution is applied and the old suctioned off between each change of files. Syringes of 10 ml capacity are practical for the purpose. Alternatively sodium hypochlorite may be introduced using ultrasonic equipment.

Dressing

Prior to the application of a dressing to disinfect an infected root canal, the canal is flushed with a 15–17% neutral aqueous solution of EDTA. After allowing the chelating agent to act for 1–2 min, it is suctioned off and the canal is dried with paper points.

Calcium hydroxide has clearly the best documentation in most, if not all, indications. It, or any other dressing in paste form, may be applied with a spiral filler. Excess water may be sucked up by the blunt end of a paper point, and root canal pluggers of suitable dimensions may be used to ensure that the suspension or paste reaches, and is condensed, apically. More material may be added as needed with the spiral, and the

packing procedure repeated until a homogeneous filling is obtained (Figure 7.6).

Some commercially available products are available with injection syringes for the calcium hydroxide. In teeth with large pulp canals, as in very young maxillary incisors, the syringe may suffice for placement. In narrow canals, however, placement must be supplemented by spiral filler and compaction.

Temporary filling

The pulp chamber must be free of medicament and cleaned to receive the temporary filling. The dressing should be protected from saliva by a 3–4 mm thick layer sealing material, typically based on zinc oxide–eugenol (preferably fortified) or zinc sulphate. When the temporary filling is at particular risk of fracture or dislodgement, extra precautions should be considered. A dual filling ('the double seal') is then advisable: one internal, sealing the dressing and designed to remain even if the external part breaks off; and one external, designed for occlusal function and/ or aesthetic reasons (Figure 7.7). Should the temporary filling fail, the root canal is at risk of recontamination, so defeating the purpose of placing a medicament.

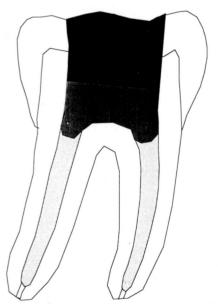

Figure 7.7. The dressing may be protected by a deeper, self-retained intermediate temporary filling supplemented by a coronal (or aesthetic) superficial part.

References

1. ABBOTT PV (1990) Medicaments: aids to success in endodontics. Part 2. Clinical recommendations. *Australian Dental Journal* **35**, 491–496.
2. ABBOTT PV (1992) Systemic release of corticosteroids following intra-dental use. *International Endodontic Journal* **25**, 189–191.
3. ABBOTT PV, HUME WR, HEITHERSAY GS (1989) The release and diffusion through human coronal dentine *in vitro* of triamcinolone and demeclocycline from Ledermix paste. *Endodontics and Dental Traumatology* **5**, 92–97.
4. ABBOTT PV, HUME WR, HEITHERSAY GS (1989) Barriers to diffusion of Ledermix paste in radicular dentine. *Endodontics and Dental Traumatology* **5**, 98–104.
5. ABBOTT PV, HUME WR, HEITHERSAY GS (1989) Effects of combining Ledermix and calcium hydroxide pastes on the diffusion of corticosteroid and tetracycline through human tooth roots *in vitro*. *Endodontics and Dental Traumatology* **5**, 188–192.
6. ABBOTT PV, HUME WR, PEARMAN JW (1990) Antibiotics and endodontics. *Australian Dental Journal* **35**, 50–60.
7. ANDO N, HOSHINO E (1990) Predominant obligate anaerobes invading the deep layers of root canal dentine. *International Endodontic Journal* **23**, 20–27.
8. ANDREASEN JO, ANDREASEN F (1992) Root resorption following traumatic dental injuries. *Proceedings of the Finnish Dental Society* **88**, 95–114.
9. BECKER GL, COHEN S, BORER R (1974) The sequelae of accidentally injecting sodium hypochlorite beyond the root apex. *Oral Surgery, Oral Medicine, Oral Pathology* **38**, 633–638.
10. BJORVATN K (1986) Scanning electron-microscopic study of pellicle and plaque formation on tetracycline-impregnated dentin. *Scandinavian Journal of Dental Research* **94**, 89–94.
11. BROOK I, FRAZIER EH, GHER ME (1991) Aerobic and anaerobic microbiology of periapical abscess. *Oral Microbiology and Immunology* **6**, 123–125.
12. BUCKLEY JP (1906) The rational treatment of putrescent pulps and their sequelae. *Dental Cosmos* **48**, 537–544.
13. BYSTRÖM A, CLAESSON R, SUNDQVIST G (1985) The antibacterial effect of camphorated paramonochlorophenol, camphorated phenol and calcium hydroxide in the treatment of infected root canals. *Endodontics and Dental Traumatology* **1**, 170–175.
14. BYSTRÖM A. HAPPONEN RP, SJÖGREN U, SUNDQVIST G (1987) Healing of periapical lesions of pulpless teeth after endodontic treatment with controlled asepsis. *Endodontics and Dental Traumatology* **3**, 58–63.
15. BYSTRÖM A, SUNDQVIST G (1981) Bacteriologic evaluation of the efficacy of mechanical root canal instrumentation in endodontic therapy. *Scandinavian Journal of Dental Research* **89**, 321–328.
16. BYSTRÖM A, SUNDQVIST G (1983) Bacteriological evaluation of the effect of 0.5 per cent sodium hypochlorite in endodontic therapy. *Oral Surgery, Oral Medicine, Oral Pathology* **55**, 307–312.
17. BYSTRÖM A, SUNDQVIST G (1985) The antibacterial action of sodium hypochlorite and EDTA in 60 cases of endodontic therapy. *International Endodontic Journal* **18**, 35–40.
18. CHONG BS, PITT FORD TR (1992) The role of intracanal medication in root canal treatment. *International Endodontic Journal* **25**, 97–106.
19. CIARLONE AE, PASHLEY DH (1992) Medication of the dental pulp: a review and proposals. *Endodontics and Dental Traumatology* **8**, 1–5.
20. COHEN ML (1994) Antimicrobial resistance: prognosis for public health. *Trends in Microbiology* **2**, 422–425.
21. CVEK M, HOLLENDER L, NORD CE (1976) Treatment of non-vital permanent incisors with calcium hydroxide. *Odontologisk Revy* **27**, 93–108.
22. CVEK M, SUNDSTRÖM B (1974) Treatment of non-vital permanent incisors with calcium hydroxide. V. Histologic appearance of roentgenographically demonstrable apical closure of immature roots. *Odontologisk Revy* **25**, 379–391.
23. CZONSTKOWSKY M, WILSON EG, HOLSTEIN FA (1990) The smear layer in endodontics. *Dental Clinics of North America* **34**, 13–25.
24. DYLEWSKI JJ (1971) Apical closure of nonvital teeth. *Oral Surgery, Oral Medicine, Oral Pathology* **32**, 82–89.
25. EHRMANN EH (1965) The effect of triamcinolone with tetracycline on the dental pulp and apical periodontium. *Journal of Prosthetic Dentistry* **15**, 144–152.
26. ELLERBRUCH ES, MURPHY RA (1977) Antimicrobial activity of root canal vapors. *Journal of Endodontics* **3**, 189–193.
27. ERIKSEN HM, ØRSTAVIK D, KEREKES K (1988) Healing of apical periodontitis after endodontic treatment using three different root canal sealers. *Endodontics and Dental Traumatology* **4**, 114–117.
28. FABRICIUS L, DAHLÉN G, ÖHMAN AE, MÖLLER ÅJR (1982) Predominant indigenous oral bacteria isolated from infected root canals after varied times of closure. *Scandinavian Journal of Dental Research* **90**, 134–144.
29. FAVA LR (1992) Human pulpectomy: incidence of postoperative pain using two different intracanal dressings. *International Endodontic Journal* **25**, 257–260.
30. FOREMAN PC, BARNES IE (1990) Review of calcium hydroxide. *International Endodontic Journal* **23**, 283–297.
31. FRANK AL, GLICK DH, WEICHMAN JA, HARVEY H (1968) The intracanal use of sulfathiazole in endodontics to reduce pain. *Journal of the American Dental Association* **77**, 102–106.
32. GENCO RJ (1991) Using antimicrobial agents to manage periodontal diseases. *Journal of the American Dental Association* **122**, (9), 31–38.

33. GROSSMAN LI (1951) Polyantibiotic treatment of pulpless teeth. *Journal of the American Dental Association* **43**, 265–278.

34. HAAPASALO M, ØRSTAVIK D (1987) *In vitro* infection and disinfection of dentinal tubules. *Journal of Dental Research* **66**, 1375–1379.

35. HAHN CL, FALKLER WA, MINAH GE (1993) Correlation between thermal sensitivity and microorganisms isolated from deep carious dentin. *Journal of Endodontics* **19**, 26–30.

36. HAND RE, SMITH ML, HARRISON JW (1978) Analysis of the effect of dilution on the necrotic tissue dissolution property of sodium hypochlorite. *Journal of Endodontics* **4**, 60–64.

37. HASHIOKA K, SUZUKI K, YOSHIDA T, NAKANE A, HORIBA N, NAKAMURA H (1994) Relationship between clinical symptoms and enzyme-producing bacteria isolated from infected root canals. *Journal of Endodontics* **20**, 75–77.

38. HASHIOKA K, YAMASAKI M, NAKANE A, HORIBA N, NAKAMURA H (1992) The relationship between clinical symptoms and anaerobic bacteria from infected root canals. *Journal of Endodontics* **18**, 558–561.

39. HASSELGREN G, REIT C (1989) Emergency pulpotomy: pain relieving effect with and without the use of sedative dressings. *Journal of Endodontics* **15**, 254–256.

40. HEITHERSAY GS (1975) Calcium hydroxide in the treatment of pulpless teeth with associated pathology. *Journal of the British Endodontic Society* **8**, 74–93.

41. HELING I, SOMMER M, STEINBERG D, FRIEDMAN M, SELA MN (1992) Microbiological evaluation of the efficacy of chlorhexidine in a sustained-release device for dentine sterilization. *International Endodontic Journal* **25**, 15–19.

42. HELING I, STEINBERG D, KENIG S, GAVRILOVICH I, SELA MN, FRIEDMAN M (1992) Efficacy of a sustained-release device containing chlorhexidine and Ca(OH)$_2$ in preventing secondary infection of dentinal tubules. *International Endodontic Journal* **25**, 20–24.

43. HERMANN BW (1930) Dentinobliteration der Wurzelkanäle nach Behandlung mit Calcium. *Zahnärztliche Rundschau* **39**, 888–899.

44. HESS JC (1986) Germes anaérobies et gangrènes pulpaires. Experience clinique du traitement local au Métronidazole. *Journal Dentaire du Quebec* **23**, 15–18.

45. HUME WR (1986) The pharmacologic and toxicological properties of zinc oxide-eugenol. *Journal of the American Dental Association* **113**, 789–791.

46. JEANSONNE MJ, WHITE RR (1994) A comparison of 2.0% chlorhexidine gluconate and 5.25% sodium hypochlorite as antimicrobial endodontic irrigants. *Journal of Endodontics* **20**, 276–278.

47. JOLKOVSKY DL, WAKI MY, NEWMAN MG *ET AL.* (1990) Clinical and microbiological effects of subgingival and gingival marginal irrigation with chlorhexidine gluconate. *Journal of Periodontology* **61**, 663–669.

48. KAKEHASHI S, STANLEY HR, FITZGERALD RJ (1965) The effects of surgical exposures of dental pulp in germ-free and conventional laboratory rats. *Oral Surgery, Oral Medicine, Oral Pathology* **20**, 340–349.

49. KIRK EE, LIM KC, KHAN MO (1989) A comparison of dentinogenesis on pulp capping with calcium hydroxide in paste and cement form. *Oral Surgery, Oral Medicine, Oral Pathology* **68**, 210–219.

50. MARKOWITZ K, MOYNIHAN M, LIU M, KIM S (1992) Biologic properties of eugenol and zinc oxide-eugenol. A clinically oriented review. *Oral Surgery, Oral Medicine, Oral Pathology* **73**, 729–737.

51. MILLER WD (1890) *Micro-organisms of the Human Mouth.* Philadelphia, PA, USA: SS White Dental Manufacturing Co.

52. MOHORN S, MAIXNER W, FILLINGIM R, SIGURDSSON A, BOOKER D (1995) Effect of psychological factors on preoperative and postoperative endodontic pain. *Journal of Dental Research* **74**, 43 (abstract 254).

53. MOLANDER A, REIT C, DAHLÉN G (1990) Microbiological evaluation of clindamycin as a root canal dressing in teeth with apical periodontitis. *International Endodontic Journal* **23**, 113–118.

54. MOLANDER A, REIT C, DAHLÉN G, KVIST T (1994) Microbiological examination of root filled teeth with apical periodontitis. *International Endodontic Journal* **27**, 104 (abstract).

55. MÖLLER ÅJR, FABRICIUS L, DAHLÉN G, ÖHMAN AE, HEYDEN G (1981) Influence on periapical tissues of indigenous oral bacteria and necrotic pulp tissue in monkeys. *Scandinavian Journal of Dental Research* **89**, 475–484.

56. MOLVEN O, OLSEN I, KEREKES K (1991) Scanning electron microscopy of bacteria in the apical part of root canals in permanent teeth with periapical lesions. *Endodontics and Dental Traumatology* **7**, 226–229.

57. MOORER WR, WESSELINK PR (1982) Factors promoting the tissue dissolving capability of sodium hypochlorite. *International Endodontic Journal* **15**, 187–196.

58. NAIR PN, LUDER HU (1985) Wurzelkanal- und periapikale Flora: eine licht- und elektronenmikroskopische Untersuchung. *Schweizerische Monatsschrift fur Zahnmedizin* **95**, 992–1003.

59. NEGM MM (1994) Effect of intracanal use of nonsteroidal anti-inflammatory agents on posttreatment endodontic pain. *Oral Surgery, Oral Medicine, Oral Pathology* **77**, 507–513.

60. NYGAARD-ÖSTBY B (1971) *Introduction to Endodontics.* Oslo, Norway: Universitetsforlaget.

61. OGUNTEBI BR, DESCHEPPER EJ, TAYLOR TS, WHITE CL, PINK FE (1992) Postoperative pain incidence related to the type of emergency treatment of symptomatic pulpitis. *Oral Surgery, Oral Medicine, Oral Pathology* **73**, 479–483.

62. ØRSTAVIK D (1988) Endodontic materials. *Advances in Dental Research* **2**, 12–24.

63. ØRSTAVIK D (1988) Antibacterial properties of endodontic materials. *International Endodontic Journal* **21**, 161–169.

64. ØRSTAVIK D, KEREKES K, ERIKSEN HM (1987) Clinical performance of three endodontic sealers. *Endodontics and Dental Traumatology* **3**, 178–186.

65. ØRSTAVIK D, HAAPASALO M (1990) Disinfection by endodontic irrigants and dressings of experimentally infected dentinal tubules. *Endodontics and Dental Traumatology* **6**, 142–149.

66. ØRSTAVIK D, KEREKES K, MOLVEN O (1991) Effects of extensive apical reaming and calcium hydroxide dressing on bacterial infection during treatment of apical periodontitis: a pilot study. *International Endodontic Journal* **24**, 1–7.

67. PASHLEY DH, KALATHOOR S, BURNHAM D (1986) The effects of calcium hydroxide on dentin permeability. *Journal of Dental Research* **65**, 417–420.

68. PIERCE A, BERG JO, LINDSKOG S (1988) Calcitonin as an alternative therapy in the treatment of root resorption. *Journal of Endodontics* **14**, 459–464.

69. PIERCE A, HEITHERSAY G, LINDSKOG S (1988) Evidence for direct inhibition of dentinoclasts by a corticosteroid/antibiotic endodontic paste. *Endodontics and Dental Traumatology* **4**, 44–45.

70. PIERCE A, LINDSKOG S (1987) The effect of an antibiotic/corticosteroid paste on inflammatory root resorption *in vivo*. *Oral Surgery, Oral Medicine, Oral Pathology* **64**, 216–220.

71. PITT FORD TR (1982) The effects on the periapical tissues of bacterial contamination of the filled root canal. *International Endodontic Journal* **15**, 16–22.

72. RUBIN LM, SKOBE Z, KRAKOW AA, GRON P (1979) The effect of instrumentation and flushing of freshly extracted teeth in endodontic therapy: a scanning electron microscope study. *Journal of Endodontics* **5**, 328–335.

73. SAFAVI KE, DOWDEN WE, INTROCASO JH, LANGELAND K (1985) A comparison of antimicrobial effects of calcium hydroxide and iodine-potassium iodide. *Journal of Endodontics* **11**, 454–456.

74. SANJIWAN R, CHANDRA S, JAISWAL JN, MATS AN (1990) The effect of metronidazole on the anaerobic microorganisms of the root canal – a clinical study. *Federation of Operative Dentistry* **1**, 30–36.

75. SCHROEDER A (1962) Cortisone in dental surgery. *International Dental Journal* **12**, 356–373.

76. SCHRÖDER U, GRANATH LE (1971) Early reaction of intact human teeth to calcium hydroxide following experimental pulpotomy and its significance to the development of hard tissue barrier. *Odontologisk Revy* **22**, 379–396.

77. SELTZER S, BENDER IB, EHRENREICH J (1961) Incidence and duration of pain following endodontic therapy: relationship to treatment with sulfonamides and to other factors. *Oral Surgery, Oral Medicine, Oral Pathology* **14**, 74–82.

78. SHOVELTON DS (1964) The presence and distribution of micro-organisms within non-vital teeth. *British Dental Journal* **117**, 101–107.

79. SJÖGREN U, FIGDOR D, SPÅNGBERG L, SUNDQVIST G (1991) The antimicrobial effect of calcium hydroxide as a short-term intracanal dressing. *International Endodontic Journal* **24**, 119–125.

80. SJÖGREN U, HAPPONEN RP, KAHNBERG KE, SUNDQVIST G (1988) Survival of *Arachnia propionica* in periapical tissue. *International Endodontic Journal* **21**, 277–282.

81. SJÖGREN U, SUNDQVIST G (1987) Bacteriologic evaluation of ultrasonic root canal instrumentation. *Oral Surgery, Oral Medicine, Oral Pathology* **63**, 366–370.

82. SKIDMORE AE (1991) Pain of dental origin. *Clinical Journal of Pain* **7**, 192–204.

83. SLOTS J, RAMS TE (1990) Antibiotics in periodontal therapy: advantages and disadvantages. *Journal of Clinical Periodontology* **17**, 479–493.

84. SPÅNGBERG L (1994) Intracanal medication. In: Ingle JI, Bakland LK (eds) *Endodontics*, 4th edn, pp. 627–640. Malvern, PA, USA: Williams and Wilkins.

85. STRINDBERG LZ (1956) The dependence of the results of pulp therapy on certain factors. An analytic study based on radiographic and clinical follow–up examinations. *Acta Odontologica Scandinavica* **14**, (suppl 21), 99–101.

86. SUNDQVIST G (1976) Bacteriological studies of necrotic dental pulps. Thesis no. 7. Umeå, Sweden: Umeå University.

87. SUNDQVIST G (1994) Taxonomy, ecology, and pathogenicity of the root canal flora. *Oral Surgery, Oral Medicine, Oral Pathology* **78**, 522–530.

88. TAYLOR GN, MADONIA JV, WOOD NK, HEUER MA (1977) *In vivo* autoradiographic study of relative penetrating abilities of aqueous 2% parachlorophenol and camphorated 35% parachlorophenol. *Journal of Endodontics* **2**, 81–86.

89. TORABINEJAD M, CYMERMAN JJ, FRANKSON M, LEMON RR, MAGGIO JD, SCHILDER H (1994) Effectiveness of various medications on postoperative pain following complete instrumentation. *Journal of Endodontics* **20**, 345–354.

90. TRONSTAD L, ANDREASEN JO, HASSELGREN G, KRISTERSON L, RIIS I (1981) pH changes in dental tissues after root canal filling with calcium hydroxide. *Journal of Endodontics* **7**, 17–21.

91. TRONSTAD L, KRESHTOOL D, BARNETT F (1990) Microbiological monitoring and results of treatment of extraradicular endodontic infection. *Endodontics and Dental Traumatology* **6**, 129–136.

92. TROPE M (1990) Relationship of intracanal medicaments to endodontic flare-ups. *Endodontics and Dental Traumatology* **6**, 226–229.

93. TROPE M (1995) Clinical management of the avulsed tooth. *Dental Clinics of North America* **39**, 93–112.

94. VAHDATY A, PITT FORD TR, WILSON RF (1993) Efficacy of chlorhexidine in disinfecting dentinal tubules *in vitro*. *Endodontics and Dental Traumatology* **9,** 243–248.

95. VALDERHAUG J (1974) A histologic study of experimentally induced periapical inflammation in primary teeth in monkeys. *International Journal of Oral Surgery* **3,** 111–123.

96. VAN JOOST T, DIKLAND W, STOLZ E, PRENS E (1986) Sensitization to chloramphenicol; a persistent problem. *Contact Dermatitis* **14,** 176–178.

97. WADE WG, MORAN J, MORGAN JR, NEWCOMBE R, ADDY M (1992) The effects of antimicrobial acrylic strips on the subgingival microflora in chronic periodontitis. *Journal of Clinical Periodontology* **19,** 127–134.

98. WALKHOFF O (1928) *Mein System der Medikamentösen Behandlung Schwerer Erkrankungen der Zahnpulpa und des Periodontiums*. Berlin, Germany: Hermann Meusser.

99. WENNBERG A (1980) Biological evaluation of root canal antiseptics using *in vitro* and *in vivo* methods. *Scandinavian Journal of Dental Research* **88,** 46–52.

100. WESLEY DJ, MARSHALL FJ, ROSEN S (1970) The quantitation of formocresol as a root canal medicament. *Oral Surgery, Oral Medicine, Oral Pathology* **29,** 603–612.

8

Root canal filling

P.M.H. Dummer

Introduction

The entire root canal system should be filled following cleaning and shaping. The objectives of obturation are:

1. To prevent percolation of periradicular exudate into the pulp space via the apical foramina and/or lateral and furcation canals.
2. To prevent percolation of gingival exudate and microorganisms into the pulp space via lateral canals opening into the gingival sulcus.
3. To prevent microorganisms left in the canal after preparation from proliferating and escaping into the periradicular tissues via the apical foramina and/or lateral canals.
4. To seal the pulp chamber and canal system from leakage via the crown in order to prevent passage of microorganisms and/or toxins along the root canal filling and into the periradicular tissues via the apical foramina and/or lateral canals.

The quality of canal obturation depends on the complexity of the canal system, the efficacy of canal preparation, the materials and techniques used and the skill and experience of the operator. Obturation of the canal system is not the final stage in root canal treatment as restoration of the clinical crown to prevent leakage of fluids and oral microorganisms into the pulp chamber is critical to the long-term success of treatment [159]. Indeed, there is some evidence to suggest that the quality of the final restoration is more important than the quality of canal obturation [147].

Over the years a number of materials and techniques have been used to obturate canals. At present, the material of choice is gutta-percha combined with a sealer, because it is versatile and can be used in a variety of techniques. It is essential that several filling techniques are mastered to undertake a range of cases. The aim of this chapter is to describe the fundamental principles of canal filling, to describe in detail canal filling techniques using gutta-percha and to give a brief overview of alternative methods of canal filling.

Canal anatomy

Pulp anatomy is complex, with the majority of canals having apical deltas, lateral canals and other aberrations; posterior teeth are noted for accessory canals, fins and anastomoses. These features, together with the results of physiological and pathological dentine deposition, resorptive processes and procedural accidents during preparation, provide a challenge for even the most experienced clinician. Clearly, the anatomy of the canal system will have a major influence on the techniques used to obturate canals and on the quality of the final canal filling.

Access and canal preparation

The aims of preparation are to clean and shape the canal system. Although access and preparation have been discussed in Chapters 3 and 6, it is worth emphasizing that meticulous attention to the preparation stage will facilitate obturation. The preparation stage should not only remove microorganisms and debris from within the canal system but also shape the canal to receive the root canal filling. Cleaning of the canal can often be achieved with irrigating fluids and minimal removal of dentine from canal walls; however, achieving the correct shape invariably requires additional effort to create the flowing flared preparation demanded by most methods of obturation. Inappropriate access and canal preparation can leave microorganisms, pulpal remnants and dentine debris on canal walls. These will invariably prevent proper adaptation of the filling to the walls, and affect the physical properties of the sealer which may be forced through the foramen during obturation. Furthermore, creation of an inappropriate shape will make it difficult to introduce material along the length of the canal, resulting in a poorly condensed filling with voids. Thus, the ability to fill canals predictably is dependent to a large degree on the quality of access and canal preparation.

Criteria for obturation

In the past canal obturation was delayed for one or more visits after preparation to give time for medicaments sealed into the canal to reduce or eliminate the microbial population and for the patient's signs and symptoms to resolve [22,24]. Unfortunately, delaying obturation can lead to other problems such as leakage of microorganisms or toxins along the interface of temporary filling and tooth, and even total loss of the temporary restoration. In addition, it is clear that most medicaments (other than calcium hydroxide) have only a limited antibacterial action [22] and are effective for only a short period after placement [124] so that there is little indication for their routine use. The problems inherent in delaying canal obturation and the fact that modern canal preparation is effective at eliminating microorganisms from the canal system has meant that many cases can be prepared and filled in one visit, provided that there is sufficient time for treatment [131].

In simple terms, those teeth with little or no problems can be prepared and filled in one visit, whereas more complex cases should be treated with more caution and obturation delayed. In fact, the success rates of root canal fillings completed in either one visit or in multiple visits are similar [131], and it could be argued that all cases could be completed in one visit given that sufficient time is available [195]. However, it would seem sensible to delay obturation of teeth in the following categories:

1. Teeth with signs of apical periodontitis, e.g. those with tenderness to apical palpation.
2. Teeth associated with radiographic signs of apical periodontitis.
3. Teeth with excessive exudate that cannot be stopped.
4. Teeth with a purulent discharge into the canal.
5. Teeth associated with a procedural accident, e.g. perforation.

These criteria are not rigid guidelines as it has been shown that some teeth with these problems can be treated successfully in one visit [129].

Materials used to fill root canals

A large number of materials have been used to obturate canals, ranging from orangewood sticks through precious metals to dental cements. Requirements for a canal filling material have been described for many years [19,58]. Most materials have been shown to be inadequate and rejected as impractical or biologically unacceptable.

Sealers

A root canal sealer (cement) is used in combination with root canal filling materials, e.g. gutta-percha. At one time it was thought that the sealer played a secondary role by simply cementing (binding, luting) the core filling material into the canal; however, it is now appreciated that the sealer has a primary role in sealing the canal by obliterating the irregularities between the canal wall and the core material. All modern obturating techniques make use of sealer to enhance the seal of the root canal filling [43,77,92,121]. However, assessment of sealing ability is not included in the requirements specified in the current International Standard covering sealers [2].

Functions of sealer

Root canal sealers are used in conjunction with core filling materials for the following purposes:

1. Cementing (luting, binding) the core material into the canal.
2. Filling the discrepancies between the canal walls and core material.
3. Acting as a lubricant to enhance the positioning of the core filling material.
4. Acting as a bactericidal agent.
5. Acting as a marker for accessory canals, resorptive defects, root fractures and other spaces into which the main core material may not penetrate.

The requirements and characteristics of an ideal sealer are [60]:

1. Non-irritating to periapical tissues.
2. Insoluble in tissue fluids.
3. Dimensionally stable.
4. Hermetic sealing ability.
5. Radiopaque.
6. Bacteriostatic.
7. Sticky and good adhesion to canal wall when set.
8. Easily mixed.
9. Non-staining to dentine.
10. Good working time.
11. Readily removable if necessary.

Inevitably, no single material satisfies all the requirements but several materials do function adequately in clinical practice. The choice of canal sealer is not only dependent on its ability to create a sound seal, but it must also be well-tolerated by the periradicular tissues and be relatively easy to manipulate so that its optimum physical properties can be achieved.

Sealers are toxic when freshly prepared [103,175]; however, their toxicity is substantially reduced after setting [137]. Thus, although sealers produce varying degrees of periradicular inflammation, it is normally only temporary and does not appear to prevent tissue healing [168].

Most sealers are absorbable to some extent when exposed to tissue fluid [134]. Thus, the volume of sealer must be kept to a minimum, with the vast majority of the filling being made up by the core material. In essence, the core material should force the less viscous sealer into inaccessible areas such as canal anastomoses and apical deltas and into irregularities along the canal walls created during preparation. Excess sealer should ideally flow backwards out of the canal orifice, although a number of gutta-percha techniques tend to force sealer apically and laterally via the foramina and accessory canals. Passage of sealer into the periradicular tissues is not encouraged; however, there is no evidence that such 'overfilling' reduces the success rate of treatment, provided that canal preparation and obturation have been carried out meticulously. Furthermore, clinical experience suggests that excess sealer forced into the periradicular region is absorbed relatively quickly.

Sealers in use today can be divided into four groups based on their constituents:

1. Zinc oxide–eugenol sealers.
2. Calcium hydroxide sealers.
3. Resin sealers.
4. Glass ionomer sealers.

Zinc oxide–eugenol sealers

Most of the zinc oxide–eugenol sealers are based on Grossman's formula [59] which is itself a modification of the original Rickert's sealer [151]. Commercial products include Tubliseal (Kerr, Romulus, MI, USA), Pulp Canal Sealer (Kerr) and the less readily available Roth sealer (Roth, Chicago, IL, USA). A number of products are available with extended working times.

Once set, zinc oxide–eugenol sealers form relatively weak, porous materials which are susceptible to decomposition in tissue fluids [192], particularly when forced into the periradicular tissues [184]. All zinc oxide–eugenol cements are cytotoxic and the response may last longer than those produced by other materials [137]. The materials have the potential for sensitization [78] and have been shown to be mutagenic in extremely high doses [198]. However, these problems are not apparent when the materials are used clinically. They are probably used more often than all the other sealers combined and give satisfactory results. The various products have a range of setting times and flow characteristics so that for each case some thought should be given to the choice of sealer. For example, difficult canals which need some time to fill require a sealer with an extended working time.

Calcium hydroxide sealers

Calcium hydroxide-based sealers have been developed on the assumption that they preserve the vitality of the pulp stump and stimulate healing and hard-tissue formation at the foramen. Commercial products include Sealapex (Kerr), a calcium hydroxide-containing polymeric resin, and Apexit (Ivoclar-Vivadent, Liechtenstein).

Laboratory research has demonstrated their sealing ability to be similar to zinc oxide–eugenol materials [87], although it remains to be seen whether during long-term exposure to tissue fluids the materials maintain their integrity since calcium hydroxide is soluble and may leach out and weaken the remaining cement [184].

Resin sealers

Resin-based materials have been available for many years [165] but remain less popular than zinc oxide–eugenol and calcium hydroxide sealers. The first resin sealer, AH26 (Dentsply, Konstanz, Germany), consisted of an epoxy resin base which set slowly when mixed with an activator. It had good sealing [108,130] and adhesive properties and antibacterial activity but gave an initial severe inflammatory reaction [137]. The initial reaction subsided after some weeks and the material was then tolerated well by the periradicular tissues [45,137]. The resin has a strong allergenic and mutagenic potential [166], and cases of contact allergy [83] and paraesthesia [6] have been reported. The material has also been shown to release formaldehyde [174]. Recently AH26 has been superseded by AH Plus (Dentsply), but there are no published reports on its biocompatibility or clinical performance.

Glass ionomer sealers

The ability of glass ionomer cement to adhere to dentine [193] would appear to provide a number of potential advantages over conventional sealers. Indeed, its endodontic potential was recognized not long after it became available commercially as a restorative material [143]. Initial evaluation of the material was confined to tests on cements designed for intracoronal restorations and it was many years before a product for specific endodontic use was formulated [146].

The physical, chemical and biocompatibility properties of glass ionomer cements have been reported extensively [189,194]. As with many other materials, unset glass ionomer cement has been found to be cytotoxic [36,95]. However, after setting cytotoxic reactions and inflammatory responses are reduced with time [12,26,89].

The physical properties of a new endodontic sealer (Ketac Endo, Espe, Seefeld, Germany) have been reported as superior to Grossman's sealer [146]. However, studies on the apical sealing properties of the material have been equivocal with some reports showing glass ionomers to be less effective than others [52,82,172], whilst others have shown no differences [18]. When using glass ionomer cements there would appear to be no differences in coronal leakage between techniques involving single points or lateral condensation [180], between presence or absence of smear layer [160] or between lateral condensation and obturation with heat-softened gutta-percha [160]. However, less coronal leakage has been demonstrated with a glass ionomer cement than with a proprietary zinc oxide–eugenol sealer [158]. Pilot studies have also demonstrated that the shear bond strength of gutta-percha to glass ionomer cement was similar to that with zinc oxide–eugenol sealers and that fluoride leached out of the cement and was taken up by dentine [161]. Use of glass ionomer cement to fill the pulp chamber of molar teeth following root canal obturation has been shown to reduce coronal leakage [27,157].

Of particular interest are the results of a recent clinical trial evaluating the performance of a glass ionomer sealer [49]. The results from this multicentre trial suggested that the outcome of root canal treatment with Ketac-Endo (Espe) was similar to those reported in previous studies using traditional sealers.

Smear layer

The smear layer is a layer of debris, comprised of both organic and inorganic components, found on canal walls after endodontic instrumentation [112,115,169]. It is made up largely of particulate dentine debris removed by endodontic instruments during canal preparation but may also contain pulpal remnants and microorganisms. With further instrumentation the material is forced against the canal walls forming a friable and loosely adherent layer. The smear layer is typically 1–2 μm thick, although it can also be found within the dentinal tubules for up to 40 μm [115].

The smear layer has received much attention recently [169], not only because it may harbour microorganisms already in the canal but also because it may create an avenue for leakage of microorganisms and act as a substrate for microbial proliferation [17,141]. It may also be broken down by bacterial toxins [35] to provide a pathway for leakage. The smear layer also has the potential to interfere with the adaptation of sealer against the canal walls and prevent tubular penetration, thereby increasing the likelihood of leakage [61,158,159]. Indeed, it has been shown that most leakage occurs between the root canal sealer and the wall of the root canal [84].

For these reasons removal of the smear layer prior to obturation appears to be desirable as it would eliminate microorganisms and allow for better adaptation of sealer. However, this procedure has been questioned since opening of the tubules might increase the diffusion of potentially irritant obturating materials through the tubules to the root surface [50], allow microorganisms trapped in the tubules to escape [39] or to proliferate within the tubules [128] and even increase leakage [47]. Thus, at the present time, no clear consensus has emerged about removal of the smear layer.

In laboratory studies a number of methods have been effective in removing the smear layer [169]. One involves the use of 17% ethylenediaminetetraacetic acid (EDTA) as a chelating agent, along with sodium hypochlorite to dissolve the organic portion [61]. Another involves use of 10–55% citric acid to dissolve the inorganic component, followed by rinsing with sodium hypochlorite [161]. Smear layer removal is easier in the coronal part of the canal compared with the apical part [161].

Gutta-percha

Gutta-percha has been used to fill root canals for over 100 years [14] and is the most widely used and accepted obturating material. Gutta-percha is a form of rubber obtained from a number of tropical trees. It is a *trans*-polyisoprene which, in its pure form, is hard, brittle and less elastic than *cis*-polyisoprene, natural rubber. It is mixed with a variety of other materials to produce a blend which can be used effectively within the root canal. Thus, the points of gutta-percha available commercially contain gutta-percha (19–22%), zinc oxide (59–75%) and various waxes, colouring agents, antioxidants and metal salts to provide radiopacity. The proportions of the constituents vary from brand to brand, with the result that there is considerable variation in the stiffness, brittleness and tensile strength of commercially available gutta-percha points [48].

Gutta-percha points have many advantages as they are:

1. Inert.
2. Dimensionally stable.
3. Non-allergenic.
4. Antibacterial.
5. Non-staining to dentine.
6. Radiopaque.
7. Compactible.
8. Softened by heat.
9. Softened by organic solvents.
10. Removable from the root canal when necessary.

As with all materials gutta-percha points have some disadvantages as they:

1. Lack rigidity.
2. Do not adhere to dentine.
3. Can be stretched.

Canal obturation with gutta-percha

The objective of canal obturation is to fill completely the canal system in an attempt to seal the canal from leakage in apical and coronal directions. Gutta-percha can be used in a variety of techniques because of its versatility; however, it must be emphasized that a sealer is always required to lute the material to the canal wall and to fill minor irregularities which cannot be filled by gutta-percha itself.

In recent years a large number of filling techniques have been described, often accompanied by unsubstantiated claims of greater efficacy, reduced leakage or improved economics. Although it is essential to strive for improved filling techniques, the clinician must be aware that 'newer' does not necessarily mean 'better'. Indeed, there is little evidence from clinical trials to suggest that any differences exist between the techniques in terms of the ultimate success or failure of

the procedure. In general terms, clinicians should be cautious in their approach to new filling techniques and await the outcome of laboratory and/or clinical studies before adopting a new regime.

Broadly speaking, techniques of filling canals with gutta-percha can be divided into three main groups:

1. Use of cold gutta-percha.
2. Use of heat-softened gutta-percha.
3. Use of solvent-softened gutta-percha.

Cold gutta-percha techniques

Cold gutta-percha techniques are generally simple to master as they are not complicated by needing to soften the material with heat or solvents; neither do they require expensive and often complicated devices or equipment. However, it should be clear that cold gutta-percha cannot be compacted into irregularities within the canal system, with the result that this role must be fulfilled entirely by sealer.

Cold gutta-percha can be used in a number of techniques:

1. Full-length single point.
2. Apical (sectional) single point.
3. Lateral condensation.

Full-length single point

With the advent of the standardized preparation technique [85], the method of filling canals with a single full-length gutta-percha point and sealer became popular. The theory behind the technique was simple and attractive; the canal was prepared to a round cross-sectional shape of standard size by use of reamers and then obturated by a gutta-percha point of matching diameter. However, it soon became apparent that a round canal shape was rarely achieved, especially in curved canals [76,91,164], and that single-point obturation was likely to be less than ideal as it would rely inevitably on substantial amounts of sealer to fill the gaps, resulting in increased leakage [7,10]. It was also clear that discrepancies in size [75,97] and taper [67] between points and equivalent numbered instruments were prevalent. Unfortunately, although some clinicians appreciated these problems and adopted alternative filling techniques, a large number of clinicians were oblivious to the research findings and continued to use the technique (Figure 8.1).

Current canal preparation techniques which aim to flare canals to produce a flowing conical funnel shape cannot be filled adequately with a single-point technique using zinc oxide or calcium hydroxide-based sealers, and therefore should not be attempted. The new range of glass ionomer sealers may reopen the debate about use of single points, although at this stage of their development it is too early to recommend their use in this way.

Apical (sectional) single point

In a tooth scheduled for restoration with a post crown, a substantial part of the canal must be available to accommodate the post. Because of the possibility of affecting the apical seal or of dislodging the entire gutta-percha point when removing the coronal part, the sectional point technique was described. The apical 4–5 mm of a point was

cut off and then mounted on the end of a file before being introduced into the canal. Once the gutta-percha point was seated at the end-point of preparation the file was rotated, detached from the gutta-percha and removed. The technique was unpredictable and suffered from the same problems as the full-length point technique in terms of lack of fit. Therefore, use of an apical (sectional) single point is not recommended.

Lateral condensation

Lateral condensation of cold gutta-percha is taught and practised throughout the world [40] and is the technique of choice for many clinicians. It is simple and rapid to carry out, can be used in virtually all cases and is the standard against which many new techniques are compared (Figure 8.2).

Lateral condensation involves the placement of a master (primary) point at the end-point of preparation followed by the insertion of additional (accessory) points alongside (Figure 8.3). The use of a standardized master point provides a predictable apical fit, whereas the accessory points obturate the space

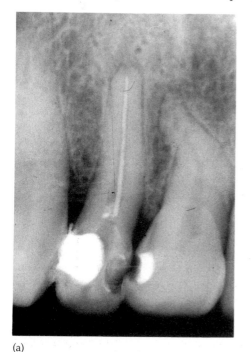
(a)

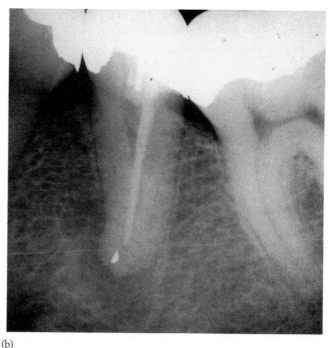
(b)

Figure 8.1 (a) Maxillary right lateral incisor filled with single gutta-percha point. (b) Mandibular left second premolar filled with single gutta-percha point. Note voids alongside fillings and periapical radiolucencies on both teeth.

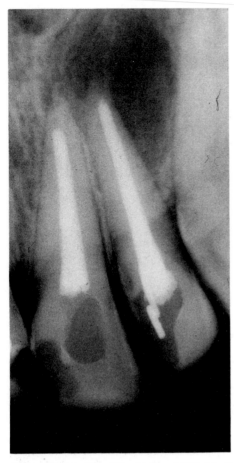

Figure 8.2 Maxillary left central and lateral incisors filled with laterallly condensed gutta-percha.

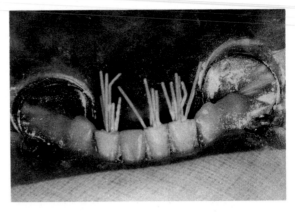

Figure 8.3 Mandibular incisors with gutta-percha points protruding from access cavities after lateral condensation (courtesy of Dr D.H. Edmunds).

produced as a result of the flared canal shape. The resultant filling consists of numerous points cemented together and to the canal wall by sealer; it does not result in a merging of the points into a homogeneous mass of gutta-percha.

A spreader is inserted alongside the master point to improve the adaptation of the master point at the end-point of preparation and to create the space for accessory points. When inserted to within 1 mm of the end-point of preparation, the spreader compacts effectively the master point apically [199] and laterally, resulting in considerably less leakage than if the spreader had only entered part-way into the canal [4]. In fact, the necessity to advance the spreader well into the canal is the only reason why canals are flared; a narrow, parallel canal shape would not allow

a spreader to advance sufficiently to influence the adaptation of the apical region of the master point. Narrow preparations also predispose to the unwanted removal of the master point upon withdrawal of the spreader as it tends to pierce the master point rather than lie alongside it.

The requirements for successful lateral condensation are therefore:

1. A flared canal preparation with a definite apical stop (Chapter 6).
2. A well-fitting master gutta-percha point of standard size and taper.
3. A series of spreaders of the appropriate size and shape.
4. An assortment of accessory points which match the size and taper of spreaders.
5. An appropriate sealer.

Well-fitting master point. The master point must fit to the full length of the preparation, be tight at the end-point of preparation, and it must be impossible to force it through the foramen.

The size of the master point is guided by the master apical file used in the final preparation of the apical stop or matrix. The selected point is held with tweezers at a length equivalent to the working distance and then inserted into the canal. Ideally, the point should:

1. Pass down to the full working distance so that the beaks of the tweezers touch the reference point.

2. Be impossible to push beyond this position, i.e. through the foramen.
3. Fit tightly at the end-point of preparation, giving some resistance to withdrawal (tugback).

The tweezers are squeezed slightly so as to notch the point and are then released leaving the point *in situ* (Figure 8.4). A radiograph is then exposed to confirm its position in relation to the end-point of preparation and the radiographic apex. Theoretically, if the original estimate of the working distance was correct, the point should be in the appropriate position and canal obturation can proceed. Some authorities condense the master point with a spreader prior to taking the radiograph in order to ensure that it reaches the end-point of preparation.

However, a number of problems can occur, either as a result of technical difficulties during canal preparation or because of size discrepancies in the gutta-percha points and/or instruments. Most of these problems can be overcome with little effort but they require some thought to ensure that the exact problem is identified.

Point reaches working distance but is loose. This may occur for a number of reasons.

1. The gutta-percha point was smaller than expected. During the manufacture of points a tolerance of ±0.05 mm is allowed at d_1 so that it is possible for the point

with the correct nominal size to be smaller than the equivalent file size and prepared canal width. The solution is to try-in a selection of other points of the same size in the hope that one of the correct size will be found; to remove 1 mm increments off the tip of the point with a sharp blade to increase the tip diameter; or to try-in a point of larger nominal diameter. If points are reduced in length, care should be taken to ensure that the tip has not been flattened before it is re-inserted into the canal.

2. The end-point of preparation was wider than expected. Just as the size of points may vary, so can the size of files. The tolerance of files can be ±0.02 mm at d_1 so that it is possible for the canal to be wider than anticipated. The solution is the same as described above.

   The canal can become wider than expected through inappropriate choice of instruments and/or preparation technique, leading to the removal of excess dentine from the outer wall of the canal apically. Should this problem be identified, then either a selection of points can be tried-in until one is found to fit, or an alternative filling method chosen.

Point passes beyond working distance through foramen. This can occur when the apical stop is inadequate or when the point is too small. If the stop is not sufficiently definite, then the point will pass more deeply into the canal and through the foramen. The solution is either to reprepare the canal with larger instruments until a distinct stop is created at the end-point of preparation or to remove 1 mm increments from the point until its diameter is sufficient to bind in the canal at the working distance. In general terms the creation of a definite apical stop is the solution of choice.

Point does not reach working distance. This is the most common problem which occurs with the positioning of the master point, and there are a number of reasons:

1. Straightening of curved canals. During the preparation of curved canals it is likely that some straightening of the curve will occur as the instruments tend to remove

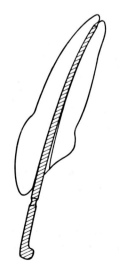

Figure 8.4 Master gutta-percha point notched at working distance corresponding to the level of incisal edge reference point.

more dentine from the outer curve apically and from the inner curve in the mid-root. Clearly, a straighter canal will become shorter as the files will pass along its length in a more direct manner to the end-point of preparation. The exact degree of straightening cannot be predicted with certainty and will vary depending on the curvature of the canal, when the canal length was measured and the suitability of the shaping procedure. However, it is likely that with most preparation techniques, approximately 0.5 mm of length will be lost in moderately and severely curved canals. It is obvious that this reduction in length should be taken into account during the preparation stage and at the time of obturation.

During the selection and try-in of a master apical point in a curved canal an adjustment should be made to the length in order to take account of this phenomenon and a radiographic check on position completed before any attempt is made to achieve the original working length through further canal preparation.

2. The point was larger than expected. Just as points can be smaller than the nominal size and appear loose, they can also be larger and not seat fully. Thus, if a point is a short distance (<2 mm) away from the end-point of preparation it may be possible to try a selection of points of the same nominal diameter in the hope of finding one that fits.

3. The canal was not widened sufficiently at the end-point of preparation. This is a common problem and occurs when the master apical file is either smaller than its nominal size or, more likely, that it was not used sufficiently to widen the canal fully. It is essential that the master apical file is manipulated until it can pass down freely to the end-point of preparation without any undue force being applied. With insufficient preparation it may be possible to force the master apical file to the working distance; however, if the same technique is adopted with a gutta-percha point then it will bind and buckle short of the expected length. The solution to this problem is to select a new file and reinstrument the canal to the working length until the file is loose.

4. Dentine debris is blocking the apical region of the canal. This is another common problem which occurs as a result of insufficient irrigation. Prevention is better than cure as many blockages are difficult to eliminate. Thus, during canal preparation copious volumes of irrigant should be used and canal preparation should include frequent and effective recapitulation at the end-point of preparation.

The solution to this problem is to irrigate the canal thoroughly and then to manipulate gently small files deep within the canal in an attempt to disrupt the compacted dentine and float out the debris in the irrigant. These small files can be rotated to improve their effectiveness but great care should be exercised to prevent the files creating their own canal and perforating the canal wall. This procedure is time-consuming and potentially dangerous in curved canals and the use of large inflexible files with *sharp* tips must be avoided. Endosonic devices enhance debris removal and are more likely to clear canal blockages.

Selection of spreaders and accessory gutta-percha points. Once the master apical point has been selected, it is important to select and try-in the spreader in order to ensure that it can pass down the canal to within 1 mm of the end-point of preparation. Spreaders should be precurved in curved canals and a rubber stop used to identify the length of insertion. To eliminate the risk of root fracture, excessive condensation pressures should be avoided by the use of finger spreaders [66].

Spreaders are either manipulated with fingers (like files) or have long handles. The working part can have a non-standardized taper or standardized International Organization for Standardization (ISO) 0.02 taper, the same as most files. Non-standardized spreaders have relatively small diameters at the tip but a range of tapers from extra-fine through fine, medium to large; some manufacturers use letters rather than words to denote the degree of taper, e.g. A–D. Spreaders with a standardized taper are manufactured with ISO diameters such as size 20 up to size 40.

The choice of spreader design, that is, with non-standardized or standardized taper, is determined by operator preference and the type of accessory points to be used. When non-standardized spreaders are used the points should be non-standardized; however, standardized spreaders require standardized accessory gutta-percha points. In this way the space created by the spreader will be filled by the point. It is important to realize that space created by a standardized spreader cannot be filled adequately with a non-standardized point. It is sound clinical practice to use spreaders and points from the same manufacturer to ensure compatibility.

The size of spreader, and thus points, is determined by the size of the canal. Large canals with substantial taper are more efficiently filled with more tapered points, whilst smaller canals with narrower tapers should be filled by finer points. On most occasions an extrafine or fine (A, B) spreader is required along with matching points.

Completion of lateral condensation

The initial phases of lateral condensation have already been described. After these preliminary stages, the filling procedure is relatively straightforward:

1. The master point, spreader, accessory points and sealer should be carefully arranged to ensure that they can be handled efficiently (Figure 8.5).

2. The canal should be dried thoroughly with paper points. Use of alcohol to promote effective drying is not recommended for inexperienced operators.

3. The sealer should be mixed, carried into the canal and smeared (buttered) onto the canal wall. Sealer application can be achieved using a hand file rotated anticlockwise, by coating a paper point and inserting into the canal, or by coating the master point itself. There is no need to apply a large volume of sealer with a spiral filler.

4. The master point should be buttered lightly with sealer and then inserted immediately to the full distance so that the notch made by the tweezers lies at the reference point.

5. The spreader is then placed alongside the point and pushed apically with controlled force until it reaches the appropriate depth, 1 mm from the end-point of preparation. The direction of force should be apical with no lateral rocking of the spreader to prevent root fracture. In straight canals the spreader can be rotated at the same time as being pushed apically; however, this is contraindicated in curved canals. Apical pressure should be applied in a constant manner for approximately 10 s to achieve the appropriate compaction of the gutta-percha in an apical and lateral direction. In curved

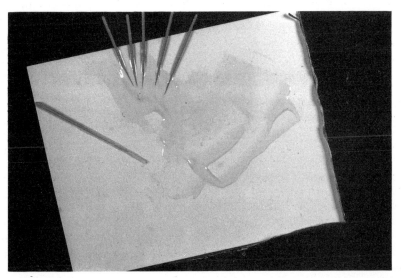

Figure 8.5 Master gutta-percha point and accessory points arranged on mixing pad with sealer in preparation for lateral condensation.

canals the spreader should be applied either lateral to or on the outer aspect of the master point; it should not be applied along the inner aspect of the curve or the spreader is likely to pierce the point and drag it out subsequently.

6. The first accessory point should be inserted into the space created by the spreader and seated fully.

7. The spreader is then cleaned and re-inserted immediately into the canal as described above. On this occasion the spreader will not enter the canal to the same length.

8. The second accessory point is inserted into the space.

9. The sequence of spreader application and point insertion continues until the canal is full. The number of additional points required will vary from case to case. Where a post-retained restoration is planned, lateral condensation need not continue along the whole length of the canal but can stop when the apical 5–6 mm have been filled.

10. If the final restoration is not post-retained, the excess gutta-percha emerging from the canal should be removed with a hot instrument and condensed vertically at the orifice with a plugger that fits the canal tightly to ensure a satisfactory coronal seal. In anterior teeth the gutta-percha should be reduced to below the gingival level in order to maintain the translucency of the crown and to prevent the possibility of sealer staining the dentine [185]; in posterior teeth the gutta-percha should be seared off at the canal orifice. When the final restoration is to be post-retained the gutta-percha can be removed immediately to the appropriate level within the canal, normally leaving approximately 4–5 mm of apical filling undisturbed [116,205]. Preparation of the post space at this stage is useful since the operator will be aware of the anatomy of the canal system and know what length of post is possible.

Lateral condensation is relatively simple to carry out, rapid, and has been used for many years with considerable success (Figures 8.6–8.8) [23,98]. However, since it is impossible for cold gutta-percha to flow into irregu-

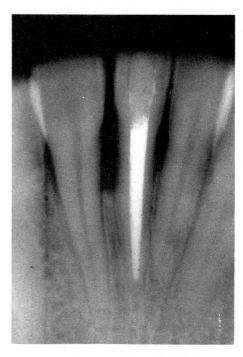

Figure 8.6 Mandibular right central incisor filled with laterally condensed gutta-percha.

larities within the canal system, parts of the canal must either remain unfilled or be filled only with sealer which has been forced into these regions by the pressure exerted through the insertion of spreaders and points. This perceived deficiency of lateral condensation has resulted in the development of techniques whereby gutta-percha is softened by heat or solvents, with the intention that the core material can be condensed more effectively into the irregularities. Some of these techniques rely on the predictability of cold lateral condensation in the apical region and use heat simply to facilitate filling in the coronal two-thirds whilst other techniques rely on heat to soften the gutta-percha throughout the whole length of the canal.

Heat-softened gutta-percha techniques

For many years the only technique which used heat-softened gutta-percha was that of warm vertical condensation [163]. More recently a large number of innovative methods of warming and condensing gutta-percha have been

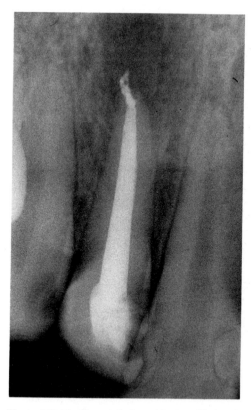

Figure 8.7 Maxillary right lateral incisor filled with laterally condensed gutta-percha. A small amount of sealer has escaped into the periradicular region.

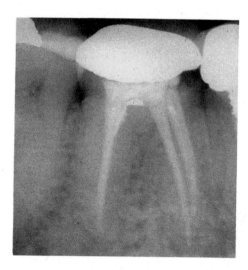

Figure 8.8 Mandibular right first molar filled with laterally condensed gutta-percha.

described. Some techniques involve placing cold gutta-percha into the canal and then warming it *in situ*; these can be referred to as intracanal heating techniques, whilst others rely on warming gutta-percha outside the canal before its placement – the extracanal heating techniques.

It must be emphasized that for most canals lateral condensation of gutta-percha is the method of choice. In general, the heat-softened techniques are technically more difficult and should be used with caution by inexperienced and non-specialist operators. Prior to use in patients the techniques must be practised in simulated canals and extracted teeth to ensure competency.

Intracanal heating techniques

These techniques include all those where cold gutta-percha is inserted into the canal and then heated within the canal so that it

becomes softened and condensable. All the techniques are used in conjunction with sealer. Intracanal heating techniques are not new, but their popularity was limited until Schilder [163] elegantly described his method for filling canals in three dimensions using warm vertical condensation.

Warm lateral condensation. Warm lateral condensation relies on a heated spreader to warm gutta-percha during lateral condensation and so achieve better adaptation of the material and a homogeneous mass of gutta-percha.

In its simplest form a conventional spreader can be heated in a glass bead heater or the cool part of a flame and then placed alongside the master apical point just as in the conventional cold technique. The heat softens the gutta-percha whilst the vertical and lateral action of the spreader creates space for additional points. Repeated insertion of the heated spreader should allow movement of the gutta-percha apically and laterally into irregularities whilst the additional points provide sufficient mass of material to obturate the entire system effectively. Some operators prefer to insert several cold accessory points prior to the use of heat. This technique can be difficult to master since gutta-percha tends to stick to the heated spreader and may become dislodged when the spreader is removed. Continual movement of the spreader is advocated to prevent this problem.

More refined techniques of warm lateral condensation involve the use of electrically heated spreaders. The first device for this purpose was the Endotec (Caulk Dentsply, Milford, DE, USA), a battery-operated system in which the application of heat was controlled by an activator button. The temperature of the spreader tip reached approximately 300°C in a matter of seconds and allowed the device to be advanced apically with only gentle force [122], causing the gutta-percha to spread apically and laterally. An accessory point was then inserted into the space created. Repeated use of the device allowed several additional points to be introduced with minimal effort to produce fillings of improved density [107], reduced apical leakage [99,111] and with gutta-percha in lateral canals [148]. The high temperature developed by the Endotec has caused some concern both for its potential deleterious effects on the cementum and periodontal ligament and on the integrity of gutta-percha, which is known to undergo partial decomposition at temperatures above 100°C. As a result of these concerns the Endotec has been discontinued. More recently, devices with temperature control systems have been introduced to allow safer, more controlled softening of gutta-percha (Touch 'n Heat or System B Heat Source, Analytic Technology, Redmond, WA, USA). The devices are battery-operated, rechargeable and portable, and accept an array of spreaders, pluggers and excavators.

Warm vertical condensation. Vertical condensation of warm gutta-percha was suggested by Schilder [163], who modified the Coolidge sectional gutta-percha technique [33]. The aim of this technique is to obliterate the canal with heat-softened gutta-percha packed with sufficient vertical pressure to force it to flow into the entire root canal system, including accessory and lateral canals. The traditional technique requires a widely flared canal preparation with a definite apical stop. The flared nature of the canal is necessary to accommodate the pluggers used to condense the gutta-percha, whilst the apical stop is essential to restrict movement of gutta-percha through the foramen. Excessive widening of the canal at the end-point is counterproductive and actually results in more apical leakage [200] and an increased incidence of overextensions [201].

Prior to obturation the appropriate pluggers must be selected and tried-in. In most cases three pluggers are used, one to fit in the coronal region, one in the middle and the smallest in the apical 3–4 mm. The pluggers should be used without binding on the canal wall to prevent undue pressure on the wall which might lead to root fracture.

A non-standardized gutta-percha point is then selected and the tip removed until it fits to within 2–3 mm of the end-point of preparation. Following sealer application the point is seated and the excess coronal gutta-percha in the access cavity and chamber removed with a hot instrument. A cold plugger is then used immediately to apply vertical pressure to the cut, softened end of the gutta-percha within the canal. A spreader is then heated and plunged into the gutta-percha to a depth of 3–4 mm and removed immediately to prevent adhesion of material. A cold plugger is then forced against the warmed surface and vertical pressure applied. In this early stage the middle and apical areas of the gutta-percha are not affected so the procedure is repeated with increasing depth of penetration of the heated spreader until first the middle and then the apical area is warmed and condensed vertically. In the process of reaching the apical region much of the gutta-percha is removed with the spreader so that the middle and coronal regions must be filled later with small increments of gutta-percha which are heated and condensed vertically as before.

The traditional warm vertical condensation technique produces homogeneous, compact fillings with gutta-percha flowing into irregularities, apical deltas and lateral canals [196]; signs of sealer and gutta-percha extrusion into the apical and lateral periodontal ligament are frequently observed. However, no significant improvement in apical [47] or coronal seal [101] has been demonstrated over cold lateral condensation.

Despite the use of very hot hand instruments the actual rise in temperature within the mass of gutta-percha is minimal [120], with no long-term effects which may endanger the integrity of the periodontium [69]. Unfortunately, the technique is time-consuming, demands substantial dentine removal during preparation and has been criticized for creating stresses during compaction. The technique is not recommended for non-specialists or inexperienced operators.

In recent years the traditional warm vertical condensation technique has been considerably simplified through the use of electrically heated spreaders and pluggers (Touch 'n Heat and System B Heat Source).

There has been a resurgence of interest in vertical condensation techniques by their effective obturation of complex canal systems [20,152]. One technique [152] consists of two stages – down-packing and back-packing. In down-packing a wave of warm gutta-percha is carried along the length of the master point starting coronally and ending in apical corkage. Essentially, this phase is identical to the initial stage of the traditional warm vertical condensation technique, except that the heat is generated electrically in the Touch 'n Heat rather than by heating an instrument in a flame. The apical and lateral movement of thermosoftened gutta-percha is referred to as a *wave of condensation.* Back-packing involves filling the middle and coronal regions of the canal and can be accomplished either in the traditional way or using thermoplastic delivery devices which can deposit increments of warm gutta-percha.

The other technique [20] is known as the *continuous wave of condensation technique* and uses the System B Heat Source. This monitors the temperature at the tip of the plugger, to maintain the right temperature throughout down-packing. The technique is simpler and more rapid than other techniques because down-packing is completed in a single continuous vertical movement. Essentially, the appropriate Buchanan Plugger is attached to the System B and then tried in the canal so that it stops some 5 mm from the end-point of preparation, a position termed the binding point. The pre-selected non-standardized point is cemented in place and the heated plugger driven down through the gutta-percha to within 3–4 mm of the binding point. The activating button is then released as the cooling plugger is pushed vertically for

some 10 s (sustained push) to counteract cooling shrinkage. Finally, the heat source is activated for a further second whilst apical pressure is maintained before the plugger is quickly withdrawn. Back-filling can be completed using the System B, gutta-percha plugs and Buchanan Pluggers, or with heated delivery devices.

These heated techniques appear simple but the skills necessary to achieve predictable results can be difficult to master. Considerable practice on extracted teeth is essential to avoid unnecessary clinical problems. No evidence is yet available to confirm whether the technique has a greater success rate.

Intracanal heating of gutta-percha with endosonic devices and even lasers [5] has also been described. However, reports of their efficacy are awaited.

Rotating condensor. The use of an engine-driven rotating compactor to soften and condense gutta-percha vertically and laterally was first described by McSpadden [114]. The technique was termed thermatic condensation and relied upon a rotating stainless-steel compactor generating sufficient frictional heat within the canal to plasticize the master point and then drive it apically. The original McSpadden compactors (Caulk Dentsply) were similar to Hedstrom files but with the blades directed towards the tip. They were later replaced with instruments resembling the Unifile (Caulk Dentsply), a hand file available at the time which had two grooves machined along its length rather than one. Compactors with other patterns were marketed as the Gutta-Condensor (Maillefer, Ballaigues, Switzerland), and the now-discontinued Engine Plugger (Vereinigte Dentalwerke, Munich, Germany).

The original technique demanded that the condensor was activated in the canal, alongside the master point, at approximately 12 000 rpm without apical pressure. After a matter of seconds the gutta-percha became softened and was driven apically by the controlled advance of the condensor to a point some 2 mm from the end-point of preparation. As the apical region filled with material, the condensor tended to back out of the canal, whereupon the instrument was slowly withdrawn while still rotating at the optimum speed. In large canals a second point was condensed in order to fill deficiencies in the middle and coronal regions.

Investigations of the technique provided mixed results. Some studies demonstrated improved apical sealing [28,133], superior radiographic appearance [100] and better replication of canal morphology [196] compared with lateral condensation, whereas others reported no improved sealing [11,156] or worse sealing [72,81].

Following concerns about the unpredictable nature of the technique, the original method was modified [179]. The so-called hybrid technique combined the predictability of lateral condensation in the apical region with the speed and efficacy of the rotating condensor in the middle and coronal areas. Thus, a master point was cemented and lateral condensation of accessory points completed in the apical 3–4 mm before undertaking thermal compaction.

Despite initial optimism, the use of compactors failed to gain universal acceptance. Although a variety of factors were responsible, the main problem was the training and experience required to master the technique. At the same time, the stiff stainless-steel instruments were prone to deformation and fracture, particularly if any attempt was made to negotiate curved canals. Perhaps of greatest importance was the rise in temperature associated with condensor rotation [70,71]. Considerable temperature rises were reported at the root surface which were in the range capable of damaging the cementum and periodontal ligament.

In recent years the design and manufacture of condensors have been modified along with the technique of using them. Modern condensors are manufactured from nickel–titanium, not stainless steel, and used with gutta-percha which has already been softened out of the mouth. These techniques will be described later under the extracanal heated techniques.

Precoated rotating condensor. The difficulties experienced with the first generation of rotating condensors led to the development of condensors which were precoated with gutta-percha (JS Quickfill, JS Dental, Ridgefield, CT, USA). The presence of a layer of gutta-percha on the condensor meant that a conventional point was not required and led to the hope that the frictional heat needed to soften the material would be less. Little has been published on the efficacy of these devices but the apical seal is similar to that of lateral condensation [140].

Extracanal heating techniques

These rely on gutta-percha being warmed and softened out of the mouth prior to its insertion within the canal. All the techniques are used with sealer.

Precoated carriers. An innovative approach to filling canals uses a stainless-steel file to carry thermally softened gutta-percha to the tooth [88]. The original carriers were endodontic files which were coated with gutta-percha. The gutta-percha coating the file was gently warmed in the cool part of a flame until it softened and then the whole unit was inserted into the canal to the appropriate length. That part of the file emerging from the canal orifice was then severed and removed, to leave the majority of the file embedded within the canal surrounded by gutta-percha and sealer. The efficacy of the technique was based on the flow characteristics of the gutta-percha and the ability of the carrier to transport and condense the material.

The technique was subsequently modified and made available commercially (Thermafil Endodontic Obturators, Tulsa Dental Products, Tulsa, OK, USA). The present series of carriers are made from nickel–titanium or plastic. Special gutta-percha coats the shaft of the device, making the warmed material sticky and adhesive but with excellent flow characteristics. The system now includes an oven to warm the obturators in a controlled and reproducible manner. In addition, a series of uncoated carriers is provided to check the diameter of the end-point of preparation and to simplify the selection of the appropriately sized obturator. Within the last few years a variety of similarly precoated carriers made by other companies has been marketed.

The technique for using precoated carriers is simple. Following preparation and drying of the canal, an uncoated carrier is inserted to the full working distance. If it passes down to the end-point of preparation without using force, the equivalent size of obturator is selected and the working distance marked with the silicone stop. The obturator is then placed in the heating chamber of the oven for the appropriate time. The canal is dried further, then coated with a small amount of sealer placed at the entrance to the orifice. The obturator is removed from the oven and immediately seated into the canal until it reaches the desired length. The excess gutta-percha in the chamber is removed and the remainder condensed vertically to enhance the coronal seal. After the gutta-percha has cooled, the shaft is severed with a bur and the handle discarded. The canal preparation is modified as less coronal flare is required.

A clear disadvantage of these devices, particularly when a post-retained restoration is planned, is the fact that the shaft of the carrier remains within the bulk of gutta-percha. Metal carriers cannot be reduced or partly removed, so the manufacturers have introduced plastic carriers which can be reduced with burs. However, although some studies have shown that this does not affect the apical seal [154,162], one has reported substantially more leakage after immediate post preparation [149].

The results of most laboratory studies on precoated carriers suggest the technique is significantly quicker than lateral condensation [41,42,63], produces fillings of similar radiographic quality [41,42] and an equivalent or better apical seal with both the metal [8,41,106,113] and plastic carriers [31,37, 42,64]. A minority of studies have reported that lateral condensation produced a better apical seal [30,65,105,145]. In laboratory studies the use of precoated carriers has been associated with an increased incidence of sealer and gutta-percha extrusion [31,41, 106,167]. However, no clinical reports have been published to confirm whether this phenomenon occurs *in vivo*. Studies have also reported that the carriers are often in direct contact with the canal wall and not embedded entirely within gutta-percha [31,90,105]. Concerns have also been expressed about the problems of removing carriers should retreatment be necessary [68,190,191]. No clinical study has been carried out to determine whether the use of precoated carriers results in a higher success rate compared with more conventional filling techniques (Figure 8.9).

Operator-coated carriers. Although precoated carriers are convenient, they are relatively expensive and cannot be customized easily for specific canals. A number of techniques are now available where the operator can coat the carrier with gutta-percha at the chairside prior to insertion. The SuccessFil technique (Hygenic, Akron, OH, USA) and the Alphaseal technique (NT Company, Chattanooga, TN, USA) provide syringes of gutta-percha which can be heated until softened and then applied to a carrier. The advantage of this customized technique is that the operator can place as much or as little of the softened gutta-percha onto the file to reflect the particular needs of the canal. There are no data on the efficacy of these carriers.

Thermoplastic delivery systems. This technique involves heating gutta-percha to a molten state and then forcing it under mechanical pressure (injection) into a relatively cool mould (the root canal) [202]. On dissipation of the heat, the material solidifies and retains the shape determined by the internal outline of the mould. The techniques used in endodontics for injecting softened gutta-percha are not true injection-moulding systems as

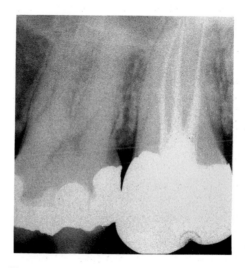

Figure 8.9 Maxillary left second molar filled by Thermafil obturators with metal carriers.

the pressure applied to the gutta-percha by the delivery systems is sufficient only to deposit the material into the canal; vertical condensation is then required to ensure adaptation of the gutta-percha to the canal wall and three-dimensional obturation of the canal system.

Injection of gutta-percha produces a seal comparable to lateral condensation [202], although extrusion of material may occur. The adaptation of gutta-percha to the canal walls has been confirmed [181]. In a commercially available delivery system [79], the gutta-percha was heated to 160°C and delivered through the needle tip at approximately 60°C [55]. The original device has been superseded by the Obtura II system (Obtura Corp., Fenton, MO, USA) with improved temperature control.

Criticism of the relatively high temperatures achieved by the Obtura led to the development of a low-temperature (70°C) system (Ultrafil System, Hygenic) [125]. Three gutta-percha formulations with a range of flow characteristics are available and the material emerges from the needle at approximately 40°C [55].

Both the high- and low-temperature systems have been thoroughly investigated. The high-temperature Obtura device has been shown to produce clinically acceptable results (Figure 8.10) [118,119,173], whilst a number of laboratory studies have demonstrated an apical seal as good as lateral condensation [43,47,77,170]. Warm injected gutta-percha can also penetrate dentinal tubules [61]. On the other hand, some studies have reported the apical seal to be less effective [15,102] and the incidence of gutta-percha under- or overextension to be high [43,117]. A clinical study of the low-temperature device reported an acceptable success rate [127]. Whilst a number of laboratory investigations have demonstrated acceptable apical seal [25,34, 38,125], good adaptation of gutta-percha to canal walls [126] and the filling of canal ramifications [93,94], other studies have revealed more apical leakage compared with lateral

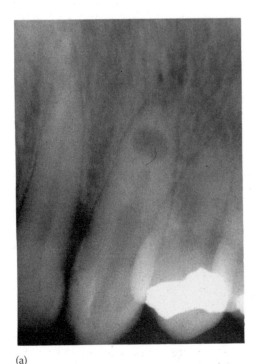
(a)

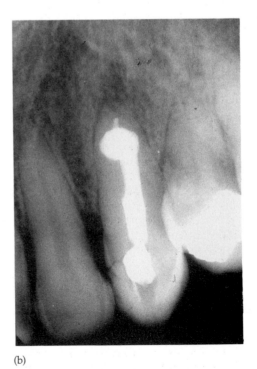
(b)

Figure 8.10 Maxillary left canine: (a) preoperative radiograph showing internal resorption in the apical part of the root canal. (b) Root canal and resorptive defect filled with warm gutta-percha using an injection delivery system (courtesy of Mr N. Claydon).

condensation [102], with unpredictable length control [21,94].

Clinical experience and the results of various laboratory studies have emphasized the need to limit enlargement of the foramen [150] and for the prepared canal to include a definite stop at the end-point of preparation [51,54,62]. The use of a sectional injection technique whereby the gutta-percha is deposited and condensed in several increments rather than in one has also been found to improve the apical seal as it allows better condensation of the material deposited apically [186,187]. Improvement of the apical seal has also been found when a conventional master gutta-percha point is cemented before injection of the heated gutta-percha [132]. Injection delivery systems can be used to back-fill the middle and coronal regions following lateral condensation [32] or vertical condensation [152].

Concerns about the condensation of injected gutta-percha at the end-point of preparation [188] because of either under-filling [21] or overextension [94] led to the development of the Trifecta technique (Hygenic). In this technique heat-softened gutta-percha from a syringe (SuccessFil, Hygenic) is placed on the tip of a file which is then used to carry the material to the end-point of preparation; anticlockwise rotation of the file deposits the gutta-percha, following which the file is removed. This first increment is then condensed apically before the remainder of the canal is filled with heat-softened gutta-percha from the Ultrafil injection delivery system. The technique has not been thoroughly evaluated. Concern has been expressed about the radiographic quality [56] and about extrusion of sealer and gutta-percha [109], but it is reported to seal the apical foramen [56,109]; no long-term clinical reports are yet available.

Operator-coated carrier-condensor. The original technique of thermatic condensation of gutta-percha used conventional gutta-percha points and a rotating condensor to generate heat [114]. Concerns about instrument fracture, inability to be used effectively in curved canals, heat generation and lack of predictability led to the development of a new generation of nickel–titanium condensors and a technique in which the condensor is coated with heat-softened gutta-percha prior to insertion into the canal. The special gutta-percha is available in two formulations, one relatively viscous and the other more fluid.

A number of methods can be used to obturate canals; one involves sealing a conventional master point into the canal followed by the immediate use of a condensor coated with heat-softened material. The heat generated by the rotating condensor plasticizes the conventional point which together with the already softened material, is forced apically and laterally by the action of the condensor. Under laboratory conditions this technique has been shown to produce a similar apical seal to lateral condensation [139,178]. Alternatively, the compactor can first be coated with the more viscous material and then with an additional layer of the more fluid material. Rotation of the condensor will further soften the gutta-percha and allow the more viscous material to force the thinner material into canal irregularities. In general, the more viscous material forms the bulk of the filling whilst the thinner material obturates the less accessible regions. No reports have so far been published on the use of this technique.

Solvent-softened gutta-percha

Chloroform-softened gutta-percha has a long tradition in endodontics, and associated filling techniques are still taught in many institutions and practised widely. The forerunner of the current methods was the Johnston–Callahan method of root canal filling. Following extensive drying of the canal with alcohol, it was filled with a solution of rosin (colophony) in chloroform into which was seated a gutta-percha master point. The chloroform softened the surface of the gutta-percha and made it swell, and the rosin acted as a glue to make the mass stick to the canal walls. This method is still taught with only minor modifications in Sweden, as the rosin–chloroform filling method.

The high degree of evaporation and the fluid nature of the rosin solution led to the development of chloro-percha. Primarily a thick suspension of fine carvings of gutta-percha in chloroform, chloro-percha was soon modified by the addition of zinc oxide and metal salts to act as much as a conventional sealer as merely softening the points. The Kloroperka of Nygaard-Östby, which has some 50% zinc oxide and 20% metal salts in addition to gutta-percha, Canada balsam and waxes, is the best-known formulation.

Chloroform is also used to aid in the production of custom-formed master points. This has been popularized as the chloroform dip technique [9,96]. In this method the apical 2–5 mm of the master gutta-percha point is dipped in chloroform for a few seconds (Figure 8.11) and inserted into the canal to the end-point of preparation. The point is then withdrawn and allowed to dry (Figure 8.12). The chloroform softens the outer layer of the gutta-percha so that when it is seated fully it takes up the shape of the apical portion of the canal. Because the volume of solvent is small and the thickness of gutta-percha affected is minimal, there is little shrinkage following solvent evaporation [104, 197]. The customized point is then cemented in place with a conventional sealer and the remainder of the canal filled with laterally condensed gutta-percha. The apical seal

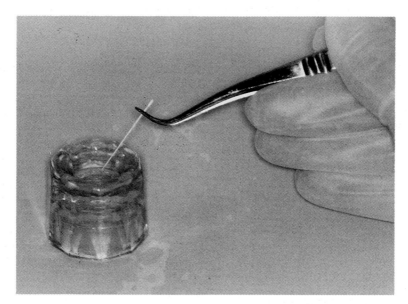

Figure 8.11 Apical 2 mm of gutta-percha point immersed in chloroform for 1–2 seconds in order to soften the surface.

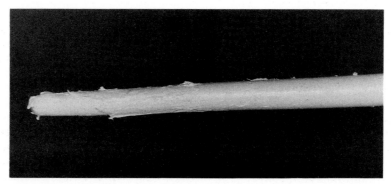

Figure 8.12 Apical portion of gutta-percha cone, following chloroform softening and insertion into the canal, showing canal wall irregularities.

obtained with this technique has been shown to be comparable with traditional cold lateral condensation [171].

Chloroform is a potent organic solvent with potentially undesirable biological effects. There are limits for the concentration in the working environment, and if chloroform is used injudiciously in the dental surgery, these may be exceeded. Other solvents with less potentially harmful side-effects have been tested as alternatives, some of which have found practical application.

Oil of eucalyptus has long been used as an alternative to chloroform in endodontics. It has a strong smell which may be less agreeable, and its ability to soften gutta-percha is much less than that of chloroform. Xylene and rectified turpentine also have substantially less dissolving ability compared with chloroform. Halothane, which is an inhalation anaesthetic agent, is bioacceptable and softens gutta-percha, even if not to the same extent as chloroform. Citrus extracts also have the ability to soften gutta-percha. Common to most, if not all, alternatives to chloroform is that, because of their lower vapour pressure, it takes longer for them to evaporate, and therefore their tissue-irritating properties last for longer.

Set specimens of Kloroperka or rosin–chloroform-softened gutta-percha are among the least irritating or cytotoxic endodontic materials. Further, histological examination of periapical tissues of teeth root-filled with Kloroperka shows a favourable response. These materials perform consistently poorly in leakage studies where dyes are used; this is because of the shrinkage caused by the evaporation of chloroform (or other solvent). Chloroform does not actually dissolve gutta-percha: its main effect is to cause a swelling of the resin structure. Even if massive shrinkage is prevented because the bulk of the gutta-percha points is unaffected, the 5–7% linear shrinkage at the interface of sealer and dentine may be sufficient to allow dye penetration. The clinical significance of this is unknown, and so far solvent-based filling methods have not been tested by bacterial leakage. These root canal fillings are dominant in Scandinavian studies on clinical performance of root canal treatment [23,57,177], and they appear successful.

Apical dentine plug

Problems with the biocompatibility of root canal filling materials and the potential for their extrusion through the foramen into the surrounding periradicular tissues led to the intentional use of an apical dentine plug during canal obturation. The apical dentine plug is built up from clean dentine filings packed into the apical foramen of the canal prior to obturation with conventional techniques. The rationale for this procedure is that dentine filings (shavings), when impinged on the vital apical pulp stump or periradicular tissue, act as a nidus for the deposition of cementum or intermediate-type hard tissue, while the plug acts as a barrier between the root canal filling material and connective tissue [123,142]. Studies in experimental animals revealed that packing uninfected shavings in the foramina stimulated the formation of cementum and bone at the apex [144,183]. On the other hand, use of infected dentine chips has a negative effect on healing [80,182]. Unfortunately, the results of investigations into the efficacy of apical dentine plugs have been contradictory. Some studies have reported more rapid healing [138] and that an effective barrier could be created [44], particularly when heat-softened gutta-percha techniques are used [167], whilst other studies have reported greater leakage [86] and the technique to be of dubious value [203].

Other methods of root canal filling

Although gutta-percha is the material of choice, the following brief historical review will clarify the position of other methods of obturation still used by some clinicians.

Silver points

Silver points made to standardized sizes were introduced in the 1930s as a method for filling fine tortuous canals. With the instruments and preparation techniques available at the time, such canals were difficult to enlarge adequately in order to accept gutta-percha points. The rigidity of silver points made it easier and quicker to complete the filling procedure since apical pressure on the points forced them down narrow canals to the end-point of preparation. Resultant radiographs invariably revealed a dense radiopaque filling which appeared to obturate the entire length of the canal (Figure 8.13). Unfortunately, because silver points could be forced down canals, many clinicians spent little time cleaning and shaping the canal system, with the result that pulpal debris and microorganisms were often left *in situ*. This abuse of silver points led to frequent failure as leakage of microorganisms and toxins into the periradicular tissues occurred over time.

Use of silver points is still not recommended today as they have a number of other inherent disadvantages. Silver points are round in cross-section and perform best when filling canals that have been prepared to a round cross-section of matching diameter. Unfortunately, a number of studies have shown that few canals are round or can be made round, particularly in more coronal regions [164]. Consequently, the seal in such circumstances relies heavily on relatively large volumes of the cement or sealer used to lute the silver point in place. A slender silver point in a flared canal is not able to force the sealer into the irregularities of the canal system leaving voids. Ultimately, tissue fluids will leak into the voids and dissolve the sealer. In due course, the combination of sealer dissolution and infection within the voids leads to failure. Silver points are also prone to corrosion when exposed to tissue fluids [16]. The corrosion products can leak into the periradicular tissues and compound the problems caused by simple sealer dissolution.

Finally, full-length silver points cannot be used in teeth where post-retained restorations are planned as the coronal portion of the point occupies the space required by the post. This led to the development of the apical or sectional silver-point technique whereby the silver point was notched with a disc approximately 3–5 mm from its end to create a weakened defect. The silver point was then introduced into the canal and with firm apical pressure the coronal portion of the point was rotated so as to sever the point at the defect, leaving the apical section in place (Figure 8.14).

Unfortunately, silver points do give a deceptively dense appearance on radiographs and some clinicians equate this with complete obturation of the canal system. The fact is that, although silver points may fill some canals and give successful results in those cases, they completely obturate the entire canal system less frequently and less predictably than techniques using gutta-percha. Their use today is contraindicated.

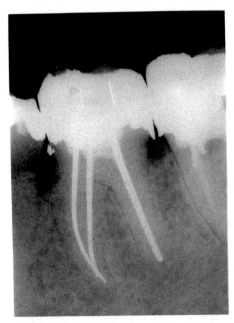

Figure 8.13 Mandibular left first molar filled with full length silver points.

Paste fillers

Paste fillers were introduced to simplify and speed up root canal treatment [155], just as silver points were introduced to facilitate obturation of difficult canals. The paste fillers should not be confused with sealers or cements designed to lute solid or semisolid materials into the canal. Rather, the paste fillers contain strong disinfectants (paraformaldehyde) and anti-inflammatory agents (corticosteroids) and were introduced in the belief that their use could bypass the accepted principles of canal preparation,

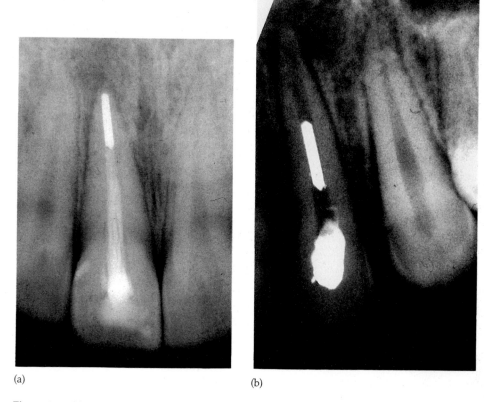

(a)   (b)

Figure 8.14 (a) Maxillary right central incisor filled with apical (sectional) silver point and gutta-percha in remainder of canal. (b) Maxillary left lateral incisor filled with apical (sectional) silver point. Note the silver point lodged halfway down canal.

disinfection and obturation. The proponents of paste fillers argued that the medicaments would allow canals to be treated without the need for thorough cleaning and shaping since the powerful disinfectants would eliminate microorganisms and because the anti-inflammatory agents would reduce the host response.

Unfortunately, the attraction of a rapid and simple method for root canal treatment found favour with many practitioners and numerous teeth were root filled using paste fillers (Figures 8.15 and 8.16). Not surprisingly, this concept resulted in repeated problems and some patients suffered permanent injury as a result of toxic materials being passed into the periradicular tissues and beyond [1,3]. Clearly, there is no place for these materials in modern practice and their use is contraindicated.

Paraformaldehyde

Most of the paste fillers (Endomethasone, Septodont, St Maur des Fosses, France; N2, Indrag Agsa, Locarno, Switzerland; SPAD, Quetigny, France) contain paraformaldehyde. If deposited in the periradicular tissues, this may give rise to severe inflammatory reactions and long-lasting or permanent injury, particularly if nerve bundles are affected [3,135].

The application of paraformaldehyde to vital tissue will result in the material or its components being spread throughout the body [13,184]. This is undesirable since not only can individuals show a hypersensitivity response [78,110] but the material may have both mutagenic and carcinogenic potency [136].

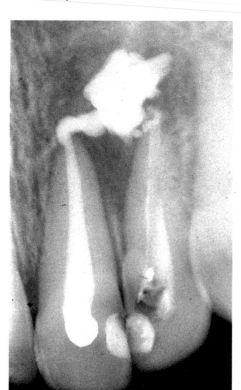

Figure 8.15 Maxillary left central and lateral incisors filled with paste. A substantial amount of paste has been extruded into the periradicular region.

Corticosteroids

Corticosteroid preparations severely affect the defence responses of the periradicular tissues by suppressing phagocytosis, providing the opportunity for microorganisms to multiply. Their use may possibly cause unwanted systemic side-effects [74,176].

Restoration of the root-filled tooth

The completion of the root canal filling does not mean that treatment has been completed. Considerable evidence now exists to support the concept of coronal leakage [159] and the necessity to restore the tooth with a good-quality coronal restoration [147]. Thus, following obturation the crown of the tooth must be restored permanently as soon as

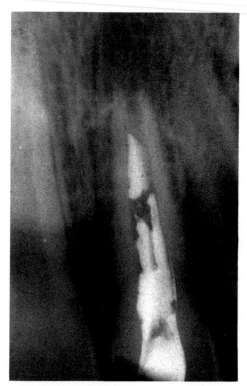

Figure 8.16 Maxillary left central incisor filled with paste. The filling is poorly condensed and contains numerous voids.

practicable to prevent the ingress of saliva and microorganisms into the chamber and along the root canal to the apical foramina.

Follow-up

Immediately following root canal preparation and filling, teeth may be tender and it is advisable to warn patients that this may occur [29,53]. Fortunately, the incidence of severe pain following root canal filling is low [73,204]. In most cases the pain is mild and transient and no active intervention is required. However, if an episode of severe pain occurs over an extended period then further investigation is necessary and a diagnosis should be established. In particular, the quality of treatment should be reviewed so that it can be established whether poor technique and/or procedural accidents have contributed to the problem. Once the cause has been identified then the correct treatment can be instituted; this may be root canal retreatment or surgical intervention.

Follow-up of root-filled teeth is important. The patient should be recalled and the tooth examined clinically and radiographically over an extended period. Because each case is different it is impossible to give firm guidelines for when recall should take place and when clinical examination should be supplemented by radiographic checks. However, it is essential that a radiograph should be taken straight after root canal filling to record the immediate postoperative condition. A further radiographic check at 1 year is advisable [46]. The strategy for further radiographic screening will depend on the case.

Criteria of success

Success of root canal treatment should be judged using a combination of clinical and radiographic criteria:

1. The tooth should be functional with no signs of swelling or sinus tract.
2. The patient should be free from symptoms.
3. The radiographic appearance of the periradicular tissues should either remain normal (if there was no evidence of bone involvement at the commencement of treatment) or return to normality as a result of the complete healing of any periradicular bone loss.

Success or failure cannot be judged immediately after treatment. For example, large areas of periradicular bone loss may take months and sometimes years to heal completely, whilst it can take many months for loss of bone in failing cases to become obvious radiographically.

References

1. ALANTAR A, TARRAGANO H, LEFEVRE B (1994) Extrusion of endodontic filling material into the insertions of the mylohyoid muscle. A case report. *Oral Surgery, Oral Medicine, Oral Pathology* **78**, 646–649.

2. ALIGHAMDI A, WENNBERG A (1994) Testing of sealing ability of endodontic filling materials. *Endodontics and Dental Traumatology* **10**, 249–255.

3. ALLARD KUB (1986) Paraesthesia – a consequence of a controversial root-filling material? A case report. *International Endodontic Journal* **19**, 205–208.

4. ALLISON DA, WEBER CR, WALTON RE (1979) The influence of the method of canal preparation on the quality of apical and coronal obturation. *Journal of Endodontics* **5**, 298–304.

5. ANIC I, MATSUMOTO K (1995) Comparison of the sealing ability of laser-softened, laterally condensed and low-temperature thermoplasticized gutta-percha. *Journal of Endodontics* **21**, 464–469.

6. BARKHORDAR RA, NGUYUEN NT (1985) Paraesthesia of the mental nerve after overextension with AH26 and gutta-percha: report of a case. *Journal of the American Dental Association* **110**, 202–203.

7. BEATTY RG (1987) The effect of standard or serial preparation on single cone obturation. *International Endodontic Journal* **20**, 276–281.

8. BEATTY RG, BAKER PS, HADDIX J, HART F (1989) The efficacy of four root canal obturation techniques in preventing apical dye penetration. *Journal of the American Dental Association* **119**, 633–637.

9. BEATTY RG, ZAKARIASEN KL (1984) Apical leakage associated with three obturation techniques in large and small root canals. *International Endodontic Journal* **17**, 67–72.

10. BEER R, GÄNGLER P, BEER M (1986) *In-vitro*-Untersuchungen unterschiedlicher Wurzelkanalfülltechniken und-materialien. *Zahn-, Mund-, und Kieferheilkunde mit Zentralblatt* **74**, 800–806.

11. BENNER MD, PETERS DD, GROWER M, BERNIER WE (1981) Evaluation of a new thermoplastic gutta-percha obturation technique using ^{45}Ca. *Journal of Endodontics* **7**, 500–508.

12. BLACKMAN R, GROSS M, SELTZER S (1988) An evaluation of the biocompatibility of a glass ionomer-silver cement in rat connective tissue. *Journal of Endodontics* **15**, 76–79.

13. BLOCK RM, LEWIS RD, HIRSCH J, COFFEY J, LANGELAND K (1983) Systemic distribution of [^{14}C]-labeled paraformaldehyde incorporated within formocresol following pulpotomies in dogs. *Journal of Endodontics* **9**, 176–189.

14. BOWMAN GA (1876) Root filling. *Missouri Dental Journal* **8**, 372–376.

15. BRADSHAW GB, HALL A, EDMUNDS DH (1989) The sealing ability of injection-moulded thermoplasticized gutta-percha. *International Endodontic Journal* **22**, 17–20.

16. BRADY JM, DEL RIO CE (1975) Corrosion of endodontic silver cones in humans: a scanning electron microscope and X-ray microprobe study. *Journal of Endodontics* **1**, 205–210.

17. BRÄNNSTRÖM M (1984) Smear layer: pathological and treatment considerations. *Operative Dentistry* (suppl 3), 35–42.

18. BROWN RC, JACKSON CR, SKIDMORE AE (1994) An evaluation of apical leakage of a glass ionomer root canal sealer. *Journal of Endodontics* **20,** 288–291.

19. BROWNLEE WA (1900) Filling of root canals in recently devitalized teeth. *Dominion Dental Journal* **12,** 254–256.

20. BUCHANAN LS (1994) The Buchanan continuous wave of condensation technique. A convergence of conceptual and procedural advances in obturation. *Dentistry Today* **October,** 80–85.

21. BUDD CS, WELLER RN, KULILD JC (1991) A comparison of thermoplasticized injectable gutta-percha obturation techniques. *Journal of Endodontics* **17,** 260–264.

22. BYSTRÖM A, CLAESSON R, SUNDQVIST G (1985) The antibacterial effect of camphorated paramonochlorophenol, camphorated phenol and calcium hydroxide in the treatment of infected root canals. *Endodontics and Dental Traumatology* **1,** 170–175.

23. BYSTRÖM A, HAPPONEN RP, SJÖGREN U, SUNDQVIST G (1987) Healing of periapical lesions of pulpless teeth after endodontic treatment with controlled asepsis. *Endodontics and Dental Traumatology* **3,** 58–63.

24. BYSTRÖM A, SUNDQVIST G (1981) Bacteriologic evaluation of the efficacy of mechanical root canal instrumentation in endodontic therapy. *Scandinavian Journal of Dental Research* **89,** 321–328.

25. CALLIS PD, PATERSON AJ (1988) Microleakage of root fillings: thermoplastic injection compared with lateral condensation. *Journal of Dental Research* **16,** 194–197.

26. CALLIS PD, SANTINI A (1987) Tissue response to retrograde root fillings in the ferret canine: a comparison of a glass ionomer cement and gutta-percha with sealer. *Oral Surgery, Oral Medicine, Oral Pathology* **64,** 475–479.

27. CARMAN JE, WALLACE JA (1994) An *in vitro* comparison of microleakage of restorative materials in the pulp chambers of human molar teeth. *Journal of Endodontics* **20,** 571–575.

28. CHAISRISOOKUMPORN S, RABINOWITZ JL (1982) Evaluation of ionic leakage of lateral condensation and McSpadden methods by autoradiography. *Journal of Endodontics* **8,** 493–496.

29. CHAPMAN CR (1984) New directions in the understanding and management of pain. *Social Science and Medicine* **19,** 1261–1277.

30. CHOHAYEB AA (1992) Comparison of conventional root canal obturation techniques with Thermafil obturators. *Journal of Endodontics* **18,** 10–12.

31. CLARK DS, ELDEEB ME (1993) Apical sealing ability of metal versus plastic carrier Thermafil obturators. *Journal of Endodontics* **19,** 4–9.

32. COLETTI P, BEATTY R, CAMPBELL J (1988) Effect of combined lateral condensation–injected warm gutta-percha obturations. *Journal of Dental Research* **67,** 219 (abstract 848).

33. COOLIDGE ED (1950) *Endodontia.* pp. 190–207. Philadelphia, USA: Lea and Febiger.

34. CZONSTKOWSKY M, MICHANOWICZ A, VAZQUEZ JA (1985) Evaluation of an injection of thermoplasticized low-temperature gutta-percha using radioactive isotopes. *Journal of Endodontics* **11,** 71–74.

35. CZONSTKOWSKY M, WILSON EG, HOLSTEIN FA (1990) The smear layer in endodontics. *Dental Clinics of North America* **34,** 13–25.

36. DAHL BL, TRONSTAD L (1976) Biological tests on an experimental glass ionomer (silicopolyacrylate) cement. *Journal of Oral Rehabilitation* **3,** 19–24.

37. DALAT DM, SPÅNGBERG LSW (1994) Comparison of apical leakage in root canals obturated with various gutta-percha techniques using a dye vacuum tracing method. *Journal of Endodontics* **20,** 315–319.

38. DEGROOD M, VERTUCCI F, NIXON C, PINK F (1990) Apical dye penetration associated with five root canal obturation techniques. *Journal of Dental Research* **69,** 176 (abstract 539).

39. DRAKE DR, WIEMANN AH, RIVERA EM, WALTON RE (1994) Bacterial retention in canal walls *in vitro*: effect of smear layer. *Journal of Endodontics* **20,** 78–82.

40. DUMMER PMH (1991) Comparison of undergraduate endodontic teaching programmes in the United Kingdom and in some dental schools in Europe and the United States. *International Endodontic Journal* **24,** 169–177.

41. DUMMER PMH, KELLY T, MEGHJI A, SHEIKH I, VANITCHAI JT (1993) An *in vitro* study of the quality of root fillings in teeth obturated by lateral condensation of gutta-percha or Thermafil obturators. *International Endodontic Journal* **26,** 99–105.

42. DUMMER PMH, LYLE L, RAWLE J, KENNEDY JK (1994) A laboratory study of root fillings in teeth obturated by lateral condensation of gutta-percha or Thermafil obturators. *International Endodontic Journal* **27,** 32–38.

43. ELDEEB ME (1985) The sealing ability of injection-molded thermoplasticized gutta-percha. *Journal of Endodontics* **11,** 84–86.

44. ELDEEB ME, NGUYEN TTQ, JENSEN JR (1983) The dentinal plug: its effects on confining substances to the canal and on the apical seal. *Journal of Endodontics* **9,** 355–359.

45. ERAUSQUIN J, MURUZABAL M (1968) Tissue reaction to root canal cements in the rat molar. *Oral Surgery, Oral Medicine, Oral Pathology* **26,** 360–373.

46. EUROPEAN SOCIETY OF ENDODONTOLOGY (1994) Concensus report of the European Society of Endodontology on quality guidelines for endodontic treatment. *International Endodontic Journal* **27,** 115–124.

47. EVANS JT, SIMON JH (1986) Evaluation of the apical seal produced by injected thermoplasticized gutta-percha in the absence of smear layer and root canal sealer. *Journal of Endodontics* **12,** 100–107.

48. FRIEDMAN CE, SANDRIK JL, HEUER MA, RAPP GW (1977) Composition and physical properties of gutta-percha endodontic filling materials. *Journal of Endodontics* **3,** 304–308.

49. FRIEDMAN S, LÖST C, ZARRABIAN M, TROPE M (1995) Evaluation of success and failure after endodontic therapy using a glass ionomer cement sealer. *Journal of Endodontics* **21,** 384–390.

50. GALVAN DA, CIARLONE AE, PASHLEY DH, KULILD JC, PRIMACK PD, SIMPSON MD (1994) Effect of smear layer removal on the diffusion permeability of human roots. *Journal of Endodontics* **20,** 83–86.

51. GATOT A, PEIST M, MOZES M (1989) Endodontic overextension produced by injected thermoplasticized gutta-percha. *Journal of Endodontics* **15,** 273–274.

52. GEE AJ DE, WU MK, WESSELINK PR (1994) Sealing properties of Ketac-Endo glass ionomer cement and AH26 root canal sealers. *International Endodontic Journal* **27,** 239–244.

53. GEORGE JM, SCOTT DS (1982) The effects of psychological factors on recovery from surgery. *Journal of the American Dental Association* **105,** 251–258.

54. GEORGE JW, MICHANOWICZ AE, MICHANOWICZ JP (1987) A method of canal preparation to control apical extrusion of low-temperature thermoplasticized gutta-percha. *Journal of Endodontics* **13,** 18–23.

55. GLICKMAN GN, GUTMANN JL (1992) Contemporary perspectives on canal obturation. *Dental Clinics of North America* **36,** 327–341.

56. GOLDBERG F, MASSONE EJ, ARTAZA LP (1995) Comparison of the sealing capacity of three endodontic filling techniques. *Journal of Endodontics* **21,** 1–3.

57. GRAHNEN H, HANSSON L (1961) The prognosis of pulp and root canal therapy. A clinical and radiographic follow-up examination. *Odontologisk Revy* **12,** 146–165.

58. GROSSMAN LI (1940) *Root Canal Therapy.* Philadelphia, PA, USA: Lea and Febiger.

59. GROSSMAN LI (1958) An improved root canal cement. *Journal of the American Dental Association* **56,** 381–385.

60. GROSSMAN LI, OLIET S, DEL RIO CE (1988) *Endodontics,* 11th edn, pp. 242–270. Philadelphia, PA, USA: Lea and Febiger.

61. GUTMANN JL (1993) Adaptation of injected thermoplasticized gutta-percha in the absence of the dentinal smear layer. *International Endodontic Journal* **26,** 87–92.

62. GUTMANN JL, RAKUSIN H (1987) Perspectives on root canal obturation with thermoplasticized injectable gutta-percha. *International Endodontic Journal* **20,** 261–270.

63. GUTMANN JL, SAUNDERS WP, SAUNDERS EM, NGUYEN L (1993) An assessment of the plastic Thermafil obturation technique. Part 1. Radiographic evaluation of adaptation and placement. *International Endodontic Journal* **26,** 173–178.

64. GUTMANN JL, SAUNDERS WP, SAUNDERS EM, NGUYEN L (1993) An assessment of the plastic Thermafil obturation technique. Part 2. Material adaptation and sealability. *International Endodontic Journal* **26,** 179–183.

65. HADDIX JE, JARRELL M, MATTISON GD, PINK FE (1991) An *in vitro* investigation of the apical seal produced by a new thermoplasticized gutta-percha obturation technique. *Quintessence International* **22,** 159–163.

66. HADDIX JE, OGUNTEBI BR (1989) Endodontic obturation with gutta percha: an update. *Florida Dental Journal* **60,** 18–26.

67. HAGA CS (1968) Microscopic measurements of root canal preparations following instrumentation. *Journal of the British Endodontic Society* **2,** 41–46.

68. HAMBURG L (1992) Current developments in the filling of root canals. *Ontario Dentist* **69,** 13–15.

69. HAND RE, HUGET EF, TSAKNIS PJ (1976) Effects of a warm gutta-percha technique on the lateral periodontium. *Oral Surgery, Oral Medicine, Oral Pathology* **42,** 395–401.

70. HARDIE EM (1986) Heat transmission to the outer surface of the tooth during the thermo-mechanical compaction technique of root canal obturation. *International Endodontic Journal* **19,** 73–77.

71. HARDIE EM (1987) Further studies on heat generation during obturation techniques involving thermally softened gutta-percha. *International Endodontic Journal* **20,** 122–127.

72. HARRIS GZ, DICKEY DJ, LEMON RR, LUEBKE RG (1982) Apical seal: McSpadden vs lateral condensation. *Journal of Endodontics* **8,** 273–276.

73. HARRISON JW, BAUMGARTNER JC, SVEC TA (1983) Incidence of pain associated with clinical factors during and after root canal therapy. Part 2. Postobturation pain. *Journal of Endodontics* **9,** 434–438.

74. HARTMANN F (1981) Clinical applications of corticoids. *International Dental Journal* **31,** 273–285.

75. HARTY FJ, SONDOOZI AE (1972) The status of standardised endodontic instruments. *Journal of the British Endodontic Society* **6,** 57–62.

76. HARTY FJ, STOCK CJR (1974) The giromatic system compared with hand instrumentation in endodontics. *British Dental Journal* **137,** 239–244.

77. HATA G, KAWAZOE S, TODA T, WEINE FS (1995) Sealing ability of thermoplasticized gutta-percha fill techniques as assessed by a new method of determining apical leakage. *Journal of Endodontics* **21,** 167–172.

78. HENSTEN-PETTERSEN A, ØRSTAVIK D, WENNBERG A (1985) Allergenic potential of root canal sealers. *Endodontics and Dental Traumatology* **1,** 61–65.

79. HERSCHOWITZ SB, MARLIN J, STIGLITZ MR (1981) US Patent no. 831714.

80. HOLLAND R, DE SOUZA V, NERY MJ, DE MELLO W, BERNABÉ PFE, OTOBONI FILHO JA (1980) Tissue reactions following apical plugging of the root canal with infected dentin chips. *Oral Surgery, Oral Medicine, Oral Pathology* **49,** 366–369.

81. HOPKINS JH, REMEIKIS NA, VAN CURA JE (1986) McSpadden versus lateral condensation: the extent of apical microleakage. *Journal of Endodontics* **12,** 198–201.

82. HORNING TG, KESSLER JR (1995) A comparison of three different root canal sealers when used to

obturate a moisture-contaminated root canal system. *Journal of Endodontics* **21,** 354–357.

83. HØRSTED P, SØHOLM B (1976) Overfølsomhed over for rodfyldnings materialet AH26. *Tandlaegebladet* **80,** 194–197.

84. HOVLAND EJ, DUMSHA TC (1985) Leakage evaluation *in vitro* of the root canal sealer cement Sealapex. *International Endodontic Journal* **18,** 179–182.

85. INGLE JI (1961) A standardized endodontic technique utilizing newly designed instruments and filling materials. *Oral Surgery, Oral Medicine, Oral Pathology* **14,** 83–91.

86. JACOBSEN EL, BERY PF, BEGOLE EA (1985) The effectiveness of apical dentine plugs in sealing endodontically treated teeth. *Journal of Endodontics* **11,** 289–293.

87. JACOBSEN EL, BEGOLE EA, VITKUS DD, DANIEL JC (1987) An evaluation of two newly formulated calcium hydroxide cements: a leakage study. *Journal of Endodontics* **13,** 164–169.

88. JOHNSON WB (1978) A new gutta-percha filling technique. *Journal of Endodontics* **4,** 184–188.

89. JONCK LM, GROBBELAAR CJ, STRATING H (1989) Biological evaluation of glass–ionomer cement (Ketac-O) as an interface material in total joint replacement. A screening test. *Clinical Materials* **4,** 201–224.

90. JUHLIN JJ, WALTON RE, DOVGAN JS (1993) Adaptation of Thermafil components to canal walls. *Journal of Endodontics* **19,** 130–135.

91. JUNGMANN CL, UCHIN RA, BUCHER JF (1975) Effect of instrumentation on the shape of the root canal. *Journal of Endodontics* **1,** 66–68.

92. KAPSIMALIS P, EVANS R (1966) Sealing properties of endodontic filling materials using radioactive polar and nonpolar isotopes. *Oral Surgery, Oral Medicine, Oral Pathology* **22,** 386–393.

93. KARAGÖZ-KÜÇÜKAY I (1994) Root canal ramifications in mandibular incisors and efficacy of low-temperature injection thermoplasticized gutta-percha filling. *Journal of Endodontics* **20,** 236–240.

94. KARAGÖZ-KÜÇÜKAY I, BAYIRLI G (1994) An apical leakage study in the presence and absence of the smear layer. *International Endodontic Journal* **27,** 87–93.

95. KAWAHARA H, IMANISHI Y, OSHIMA H (1979) Biological evaluation of glass ionomer cement. *Journal of Dental Research* **58,** 1080–1086.

96. KEANE KM, HARRINGTON GW (1984) The use of chloroform-softened gutta-percha master cone and its effect on the apical seal. *Journal of Endodontics* **10,** 57–63.

97. KEREKES K (1979) Evaluation of standardized root canal instruments and obturating points. *Journal of Endodontics* **5,** 145–150.

98. KEREKES K, TRONSTAD L (1979) Long-term results of endodontic treatment performed with a standardized technique. *Journal of Endodontics* **5,** 83–90.

99. KERSTEN HW (1988) Evaluation of three thermoplasticized gutta-percha filling techniques using a

100. KERSTEN HW, FRANSMAN R, THODEN VAN VELZEN SK (1986) Thermomechanical compaction of gutta-percha. II. A comparison with lateral condensation in curved root canals. *International Endodontic Journal* **19,** 134–140.

101. KHAYAT A, LEE SJ, TORABINEJAD M (1993) Human saliva penetration of coronally unsealed obturated root canals. *Journal of Endodontics* **19,** 458–461.

102. LACOMBE JS, CAMPBELL AD, HICKS ML, PELLEU GB (1988) A comparison of the apical seal produced by two thermoplasticized injectable gutta-percha techniques. *Journal of Endodontics* **14,** 445–450.

103. LANGELAND K (1974) Root canal sealants and pastes. *Dental Clinics of North America* **18,** 309–327.

104. LARDER TC, PRESCOTT AJ, BRAYTON SM (1976) Gutta-percha: a comparative study of three methods of obturation. *Journal of Endodontics* **2,** 289–294.

105. LARES C, ELDEEB ME (1990) The sealing ability of the Thermafil obturation technique. *Journal of Endodontics* **16,** 474–479.

106. LEUNG SF, GULABIVALA K (1994) An *in vitro* evaluation of the influence of canal curvature on the sealing ability of Thermafil. *International Endodontic Journal* **27,** 190–196.

107. LIEWEHR F, KULILD JC, PRIMACK PD (1993) Improved density of gutta-percha after warm lateral condensation. *Journal of Endodontics* **19,** 489–491.

108. LIMKANGWALMONGKOL S, ABBOTT PV, SANDLER AB (1992) Apical dye penetration with four root canal sealers and gutta-percha using longitudinal sectioning. *Journal of Endodontics* **18,** 535–539.

109. LLOYD A, THOMPSON J, GUTMANN JL, DUMMER PMH (1995) Sealability of the Trifecta technique in the presence or absence of a smear layer. *International Endodontic Journal* **28,** 35–40.

110. LONGWILL DG, MARSHALL FJ, CREAMER RH (1982) Reactivity of human lymphocytes to pulp antigens. *Journal of Endodontics* **8,** 27–32.

111. LUCCY CT, WELLER RN, KULILD JC (1990) An evaluation of the apical seal produced by lateral and warm lateral condensation techniques. *Journal of Endodontics* **16,** 170–172.

112. MCCOMB D, SMITH D (1975) A preliminary scanning electron microscopic study of root canals after endodontic procedures. *Journal of Endodontics* **1,** 238–242.

113. MCMURTREY LG, KRELL KV, WILCOX LR (1992) A comparison between Thermafil and lateral condensation in highly curved canals. *Journal of Endodontics* **18,** 68–71.

114. MCSPADDEN J (1980) *Self-study Course for the Thermatic Condensation of Gutta Percha.* York, PA, USA: Dentsply.

115. MADER CL, BAUMGARTNER JC, PETERS DD (1984) Scanning electron microscopic investigation of the smeared layer on root canal walls. *Journal of Endodontics* **10,** 477–483.

leakage model *in vitro. International Endodontic Journal* **21,** 353–360.

116. MADISON S, ZAKARIASEN KL (1984) Linear and volumetric analysis of apical leakage in teeth prepared for posts. *Journal of Endodontics* **10**, 422–427.

117. MANN SR, MCWALTER GM (1987) Evaluation of apical seal and placement control in straight and curved canals obturated by laterally condensed and thermoplasticised gutta-percha. *Journal of Endodontics* **13**, 10–17.

118. MARLIN J (1986) Injectable standard gutta-percha as a method of filling the root canal system. *Journal of Endodontics* **12**, 354–358.

119. MARLIN J, KRAKOW AA, DESILETS RP, GRON P (1981) Clinical use of injection-molded thermoplasticized gutta-percha for obturation of the root canal system: a preliminary report. *Journal of Endodontics* **7**, 277–281.

120. MARLIN J, SCHILDER H (1973) Physical properties of gutta-percha when subjected to heat and vertical condensation. *Oral Surgery, Oral Medicine, Oral Pathology* **36**, 872–879.

121. MARSHALL FJ, MASSLER M (1961) Sealing of pulpless teeth evaluated with radioisotopes. *Journal of Dental Medicine* **16**, 172–184.

122. MARTIN H, FISCHER E (1990) Photoelastic stress comparison of warm (Endotec) versus cold lateral condensation techniques. *Oral Surgery, Oral Medicine, Oral Pathology* **70**, 325–327.

123. MAYER A, KETTERL W (1958) Dauererfolge bei der Pulpitisbehandlung. *Deutsche Zahnärztliche Zeitung* **13**, 883–898.

124. MESSER HH, CHEN RS (1984) The duration of effectiveness of root canal medicaments. *Journal of Endodontics* **10**, 240–245.

125. MICHANOWICZ AE, CZONSTKOWSKY M (1984) Sealing properties of an injection-thermoplasticized low-temperature (70°C) gutta-percha: a preliminary study. *Journal of Endodontics* **10**, 563–566.

126. MICHANOWICZ AE, CZONSTKOWSKY M, PIESCO NP (1986) Low-temperature (70°C) injection gutta-percha: a scanning electron microscopic investigation. *Journal of Endodontics* **12**, 64–67.

127. MICHANOWICZ AE, MICHANOWICZ JP, MICHANOWICZ AM, CZONSTKOWSKY M, ZULLO TD (1989) Clinical evaluation of low-temperature thermoplasticized injectable gutta-percha: a preliminary report. *Journal of Endodontics* **15**, 602–607.

128. MICHELICH VJ, SHUSTER GS, PASHLEY DH (1980) Bacterial penetration of human dentin *in vitro*. *Journal of Dental Research* **59**, 1398–1403.

129. MULHERN JM, PATTERSON SS, NEWTON CW, RINGEL AM (1982) Incidence of postoperative pain after one-appointment endodontic treatment of asymptomatic pulpal necrosis in single-rooted teeth. *Journal of Endodontics* **8**, 370–375.

130. OGUNTEBI BR, SHEN C (1992) Effect of different sealers on thermoplasticized gutta-percha root canal obturations. *Journal of Endodontics* **18**, 363–366.

131. OLIET S (1983) Single-visit endodontics: a clinical study. *Journal of Endodontics* **9**, 147–152.

132. OLSON AK, HARTWELL GR, WELLER RN (1989) Evaluation of the controlled placement of injected thermoplasticized gutta-percha. *Journal of Endodontics* **15**, 306–309.

133. O'NEILL KJ, PITTS DL, HARRINGTON GW (1983) Evaluation of the controlled placement of injected thermoplasticised gutta-percha. *Journal of Endodontics* **9**, 190–197.

134. ØRSTAVIK D (1983) Weight loss of endodontic sealers, cements and pastes in water. *Scandinavian Journal of Dental Research* **91**, 316–319.

135. ØRSTAVIK D, BRODIN P, AAS E (1983) Paraesthesia following endodontic treatment: survey of the literature and report of a case. *International Endodontic Journal* **16**, 167–172.

136. ØRSTAVIK D, HONGSLO JK (1985) Mutagenicity of endodontic sealers. *Biomaterials* **6**, 129–132.

137. ØRSTAVIK D, MJÖR IA (1988) Histopathology and X-ray microanalysis of the subcutaneous tissue response to endodontic sealers. *Journal of Endodontics* **14**, 13–23.

138. OSWALD RJ, FRIEDMAN CE (1980) Periapical response to dentin fillings. *Oral Surgery, Oral Medicine, Oral Pathology* **49**, 344–355.

139. PAGE ML, HARGREAVES KM, ELDEEB M (1995) Comparison of concentric condensation technique with laterally condensed gutta-percha. *Journal of Endodontics* **21**, 308–313.

140. PALLARÉS A, FAUS V (1995) A comparative study of the sealing ability of two root canal obturation techniques. *Journal of Endodontics* **21**, 449–450.

141. PASHLEY DH (1984) Smear layer: physiological considerations. *Operative Dentistry* (suppl 3), 13–29.

142. PETERSSON K, HASSELGREN G, PETERSSON A, TRONSTAD L (1982) Clinical experience with the use of dentine chips in pulpectomies. *International Endodontic Journal* **15**, 161–167.

143. PITT FORD TR (1979) The leakage of root fillings using glass ionomer cement and other materials. *British Dental Journal* **146**, 273–278.

144. PITTS DL, JONES JE, OSWALD RJ (1984) A histological comparison of calcium hydroxide plugs and dentin plugs used for the control of gutta-percha root canal filling material. *Journal of Endodontics* **10**, 283–293.

145. RAVANSHAD S, TORABINEJAD M (1992) Coronal dye penetration of the apical filling materials after post space preparation. *Oral Surgery, Oral Medicine, Oral Pathology* **74**, 644–647.

146. RAY H, SELTZER S (1991) A new glass ionomer root canal sealer. *Journal of Endodontics* **17**, 598–603.

147. RAY HA, TROPE M (1995) Periapical status of endodontically treated teeth in relation to the technical quality of the root filling and the coronal restoration. *International Endodontic Journal* **28**, 12–18.

148. READER CM, HIMEL VT, GERMAIN LP, HOEN MM (1993) Effect of three obturation techniques on the filling of lateral canals and the main canal. *Journal of Endodontics* **19**, 404–408.

149. RICCI ER, KESSLER JR (1994) Apical seal of teeth obturated by the laterally condensed gutta-percha, the Thermafil plastic and Thermafil metal obturator techniques after post space preparation. *Journal of Endodontics* **20,** 123–126.

150. RICHIE GM, ANDERSON DM, SAKUMURA JS (1988) Apical extrusion of thermoplasticized gutta-percha used as a root canal filling. *Journal of Endodontics* **14,** 128–132.

151. RICKERT UG, DIXON CM (1931) The controlling of root surgery. *Proceedings of Eighth International Dental Congress* Paris, France. **IIIa,** 15–22.

152. RUDDLE CJ (1994) Three dimensional obturation: the rationale and application of warm gutta-percha with vertical condensation. In: Cohen S, Burns RC (eds) *Pathways of the Pulp*, 6th edn, pp. 243–247. St Louis, MO, USA: Mosby-Year Book.

153. RUSSIN TP, ZARDIACKAS LD, READER A, MENKE RA (1980) Apical seals obtained with laterally condensed, chloroform-softened gutta-percha and laterally condensed gutta-percha and Grossman's sealer. *Journal of Endodontics* **6,** 678–682.

154. RYBICKI R, ZILLICH R (1994) Apical sealing ability of Thermafil following immediate and delayed post space preparations. *Journal of Endodontics* **20,** 64–66.

155. SARGENTI A, RICHTER SL (1965) *Rationalized Root Canal Treatment.* New York, NY, USA: AGSA.

156. SAUNDERS EM (1989) The effect of variation in thermomechanical compaction techniques upon the quality of the apical seal. *International Endodontic Journal* **22,** 163–168.

157. SAUNDERS WP, SAUNDERS EM (1990) Assessment of leakage in the restored pulp chamber of endodontically treated multirooted teeth. *International Endodontic Journal* **23,** 28–33.

158. SAUNDERS WP, SAUNDERS EM (1992) The effect of smear layer upon the coronal leakage of gutta-percha root fillings and a glass ionomer sealer. *International Endodontic Journal* **25,** 245–249.

159. SAUNDERS WP, SAUNDERS EM (1994) Coronal leakage as a cause of failure in root canal therapy: a review. *Endodontics and Dental Traumatology* **10,** 105–108.

160. SAUNDERS WP, SAUNDERS EM (1994) Influence of smear layer on the coronal leakage of Thermafil and laterally condensed gutta-percha root fillings with a glass ionomer sealer. *Journal of Endodontics* **20,** 155–158.

161. SAUNDERS WP, SAUNDERS EM, HERD D, STEPHENS E (1992) The use of glass ionomer as a root canal sealer – a pilot study. *International Endodontic Journal* **25,** 238–244.

162. SAUNDERS WP, SAUNDER EM, GUTMANN JL, GUTMANN ML (1993) An assessment of the plastic Thermafil obturation technique. Part 3. The effect of post space preparation on the apical seal. *International Endodontic Journal* **26,** 184–189.

163. SCHILDER H (1967) Filling root canals in three dimensions. *Dental Clinics of North America* **11,** 723–744.

164. SCHNEIDER SW (1971) A comparison of canal preparations in straight and curved root canals. *Oral Surgery, Oral Medicine, Oral Pathology* **32,** 271–275.

165. SCHROEDER A (1954) Mitteilungen über die Abschlussdichtigkeit von Wurzelfüllmaterialen und erster Hinweis auf ein neuartiges Wurzelfüllmittel. *Schweizer Monatschrift Zahnärztliche* **64,** 921–931.

166. SCHWEIKL H, SCHMALZ G, STIMMELMAYR H, BEY B (1995) Mutagenicity of AH26 in an *in vitro* mammalian cell mutation assay. *Journal of Endodontics* **21,** 407–410.

167. SCOTT AC, VIRE DE (1992) An evaluation of the ability of a dentin plug to control extrusion of thermoplasticized gutta-percha. *Journal of Endodontics* **18,** 52–57.

168. SELTZER S, SOLTANOFF W, SMITH J (1973) Biologic aspects of endodontics. V. Periapical tissue reactions to root canal instrumentation beyond the apex and root canal fillings short of and beyond the apex. *Oral Surgery, Oral Medicine, Oral Pathology* **36,** 725–737.

169. SEN BH, WESSELINK PR, TÜRKÜN M (1995) The smear layer: a phenomenon in root canal therapy. *International Endodontic Journal* **28,** 141–148.

170. SKINNER RL, HIMEL VT (1987) The sealing ability of injection-molded thermoplasticized gutta-percha with and without the use of sealers. *Journal of Endodontics* **13,** 315–317.

171. SMITH JJ, MONTGOMERY S (1992) A comparison of apical seal: chloroform versus halothane-dipped gutta-percha cones. *Journal of Endodontics* **18,** 156–160.

172. SMITH MA, STEIMAN HR (1994) An *in vitro* evaluation of microleakage of two new and two old root canal sealers. *Journal of Endodontics* **20,** 18–21.

173. SOBARZO-NAVARRO V (1991) Clinical experience in root canal obturation by an injection thermoplasticized gutta-percha technique. *Journal of Endodontics* **17,** 389–391.

174. SPÅNGBERG LSW, BARBOSA SV, LAVIGNE GD (1993) AH26 releases formaldehyde. *Journal of Endodontics* **19,** 596–598.

175. SPÅNGBERG LSW, LANGELAND K (1973) Biologic effects of dental materials. 1. Toxicity of root canal filling materials on Hela cells *in vitro*. *Oral Surgery, Oral Medicine, Oral Pathology* **35,** 402–414.

176. SPECTOR RG (1981) Pharmacological properties of the glucocorticoids. *International Dental Journal* **31,** 152–155.

177. STRINDBERG LZ (1956) The dependence of the results of pulp therapy on certain factors. An analytic study based on radiographic and clinical follow–up examinations. *Acta Odontologica Scandinavica* **14,** (suppl 21), 1–175.

178. TAGGER M, KATZ A, TAMSE A (1994) Apical seal using the GPII method in straight canals compared with lateral condensation, with or without sealer. *Oral Surgery, Oral Medicine, Oral Pathology* **78,** 225–231.

179. TAGGER M, TAMSE A, KATZ A, KORZEN BH (1984) Evaluation of apical seal produced by a hybrid root

canal filling method combining lateral condensation and thermatic compaction. *Journal of Endodontics* **10,** 299–303.

180. TIDSWELL HE, SAUNDERS EM, SAUNDERS WP (1994) Assessment of coronal leakage in teeth root filled with gutta-percha and a glass ionomer root canal sealer. *International Endodontic Journal* **27,** 208–212.

181. TORABINEJAD M, SKOBE Z, TROMBLY PL, KRAKOW AA, GRØN P, MARLIN J (1978) Scanning electron microscopic study of root canal obturation using thermoplasticized gutta-percha. *Journal of Endodontics* **4,** 245–250.

182. TORNECK CD, SMITH JS, GRINDALL P (1973) Biologic effects of procedures on developing incisor teeth. II. Effect of pulp injury and oral contamination. *Oral Surgery, Oral Medicine, Oral Pathology* **35,** 378–388.

183. TRONSTAD L (1978) Tissue reactions following apical plugging of the root canal with dentin chips in monkey teeth subject to pulpectomy. *Oral Surgery, Oral Medicine, Oral Pathology* **45,** 297–304.

184. TRONSTAD L, BARNETT F, FLAX M (1988) Solubility and biocompatibility of calcium hydroxide-containing root canal sealers. *Endodontics and Dental Traumatology* **4,** 152–159.

185. VAN DER BURGT TP, ERONAT C, PLASSCHAERT AJM (1986) Staining patterns in teeth discolored by endodontic sealers. *Journal of Endodontics* **12,** 187–191.

186. VEIS A, BELTES P, LIOLIOS E (1989) Sealing ability of thermoplasticized gutta-percha in root canal obturation using a sectional vs a single-phase technique. *Endodontics and Dental Traumatology* **5,** 87–91.

187. VEIS A, LAMBRIANIDIS T, MOLYVDAS I, ZERVAS P (1992) Sealing ability of sectional injection thermoplasticized gutta-percha technique with varying distances between needle tip and apical foramen. *Endodontics and Dental Traumatology* **8,** 63–66.

188. VEIS AA, MOLYVDAS IA, LAMBRIANIDIS TP, BELTES PG (1994) *In vitro* evaluation of apical leakage of root canal fillings after *in situ* obturation with thermoplasticized and laterally condensed gutta percha. *International Endodontic Journal* **27,** 213–217.

189. WALLS AWG (1986) Glass polyalkenoate (glass-ionomer) cements: a review. *Journal of Dentistry* **14,** 231–246.

190. WILCOX LR (1993) Thermafil retreatment with and without chloroform solvent. *Journal of Endodontics* **19,** 563–566.

191. WILCOX LR, JUHLIN JJ (1994) Endodontic retreatment of Thermafil versus laterally condensed gutta-percha. *Journal of Endodontics* **19,** 115–117.

192. WILSON AD, CLINTON DJ, MILLER RP (1973) Zinc oxide-eugenol cements: IV. Microstructure and hydrolysis. *Journal of Dental Research* **52,** 253–260.

193. WILSON AD, KENT BE (1971) The glass-ionomer cement: a new translucent dental filling material. *Journal of Applied Chemistry and Biotechnology* **21,** 313–318.

194. WILSON AD, MCLEAN JW (1988) *Glass-ionomer Cement.* Chicago, IL, USA: Quintessence.

195. WOLCH I (1975) One appointment endodontic treatment. *Journal of the Canadian Dental Association* **41,** 613–615.

196. WONG M, PETERS DD, LORTON L (1981) Comparison of gutta-percha filling techniques, compaction (mechanical), vertical (warm), and lateral condensation techniques, part 1. *Journal of Endodontics* **7,** 551–558.

197. WONG M, PETERS DD, LORTON L, BERNIER WE (1982) Comparison of gutta-percha filling techniques: three chloroform-gutta-percha filling techniques, part 2. *Journal of Endodontics* **8,** 4–9.

198. WOOLVERTON CJ, FOTOS PG, MOKAS J, MERMIGAS ME (1986) Evaluation of eugenol for mutagenicity by the mouse micronucleus test. *Journal of Oral Pathology* **15,** 450–453.

199. YARED GM, BOU DAGHER FE (1993) Elongation and movement of the gutta-percha master cone during initial lateral condensation. *Journal of Endodontics* **19,** 395–397.

200. YARED GM, BOU DAGHER FE (1994) Apical enlargement: influence on the sealing ability of the vertical compaction technique. *Journal of Endodontics* **20,** 313–314.

201. YARED GM, BOU DAGHER FE (1994) Apical enlargement: influence on overextensions during *in vitro* vertical compaction. *Journal of Endodontics* **20,** 269–271.

202. YEE FS, MARLIN J, KRAKOW AA, GRON P (1977) Three-dimensional obturation of the root canal using injection-molded, thermoplasticized dental gutta-percha. *Journal of Endodontics* **3,** 168–174.

203. YEE RDJ, NEWTON CW, PATTERSON SS, SWARTZ ML (1984) The effect of canal preparation on the formation and leakage characteristics of the apical dentin plug. *Journal of Endodontics* **10,** 308–317.

204. YESILOY C, KOREN LZ, MORSE DR, RANKOW H, BOLANUS OR, FURST ML (1988) Post-endodontic obturation pain: a comparative evaluation. *Quintessence International* **19,** 431–438.

205. ZMENER O (1980) Effect of dowel preparation on the apical seal of endodontically treated teeth. *Journal of Endodontics* **6,** 687–690.

9

Surgical endodontics

J.L. Gutmann

Introduction

Whilst a high degree of success is achievable with root canal treatment, surgery may be necessary to remove aetiological factors that may impair tooth retention. These include the inability to clean, shape and obturate the root canal system satisfactorily, the removal of aberrant root anatomy, the elimination or repair of clinician errors, the joint management of periodontal or restorative problems, and the potential need for a biopsy should periradicular disease fail to heal following good-quality non-surgical treatment.

Recent assessment of the terminology used in endodontic surgery has attempted to clarify and codify the terms used [6]. Likewise, research into endodontic surgery has helped to expand current clinical practice based on scientific concepts. The most common endodontic surgical procedure (periradicular surgery) consists of periradicular curettage, root-end resection (apicectomy), root-end preparation and root-end filling. Other procedures identified with endodontic surgery include perforation repair, root and tooth resection, crown-lengthening, intentional replantation, incision and drainage and cortical trephination. This chapter will focus primarily on the essentials of periradicular surgery, with only reference to more detailed sources [11,25,48].

Indications for periradicular surgery

Most texts on endodontic surgery list multiple, 'cook-book'-type indications for surgical intervention [10, 56]. These often include instrument separation, apical fracture, inadequate root canal filling, presence of a cyst. Clinical experience in the delivery of good-quality non-surgical root canal treatment and the ability to retreat root canal systems non-surgically have eliminated the routine need for surgery. Studies on the success and failure of non-surgical root canal treatment versus surgical intervention have clearly shown a higher success rate with high-quality non-surgical intervention [119]. Periradicular tissues heal at predictable levels following the elimination of all aetiological factors from the root canal, and the prevention of further contamination [72,116]. Additionally, the main cause for failure following surgical treatment is the failure to clean, shape and obturate properly the root canal system [111]. Therefore the routine choosing of surgical intervention without fully assessing the specific needs of each case, in particular the status of the root canal system, is unwarranted. Similarly, surgery for the convenience of the clinician is considered unacceptable.

With these concepts foremost in the mind of the clinician, it must be recognized that few true indications exist for surgery. These indications must always be in the best interest of the patient and within the realm of the clinician's understanding and expertise [45]. First, if there is a strong possibility of failure with non-surgical treatment, surgery may be indicated, e.g. calcified canals with concomitant patient signs and/or symptoms. Second, if failure has resulted from non-surgical treatment, and retreatment is impossible or would not achieve a better result, surgery may be indicated, e.g. non-negotiable canal, ledges with concomitant patient signs and/or symptoms. Third, if a biopsy is necessary at or near the root apex, surgery will be indicated, e.g. periradicular lesions not due to apparently adequate root canal treatment. Contraindications to surgery are very few and are usually limited to patient (psychological and

systemic), clinician (experience and expertise) and anatomical (extremely unusual bony or root configurations and complete lack of surgical access). Few cases, however, will not be amenable to surgical intervention.

Preoperative assessment

The quality of endodontic surgery, and in many respects the final successful outcome, is dependent on proper patient assessment, diagnosis and treatment planning. It is during this process that the facts surrounding the case in question must be obtained and integrated into a meaningful diagnosis and treatment plan [14]. Contraindications involving the patient's psychological or systemic make-up can be identified as well as patient acceptance of, and cooperation with, the anticipated surgical procedure. Often this will include procedures to minimize stress with patients who are particularly susceptible to pain and anxiety [48]. Oral soft- and hard-tissue conditions, including patient compliance with oral hygiene practices, can be ascertained and reinforced.

General patient systemic factors, which usually require medical consultation, are listed in Table 9.1. Review of drug regimens presently used or anticipated may alert the clinician to the potential use of stress-control measures, along with local considerations during surgical intervention. The reader is referred for further discussion of relevant medical concerns [48].

Local patient factors focus on the nature of the previous root canal treatment, if any, and the ultimate management of both soft and hard tissues during surgical entry and wound closure. These include the potential need to remove previous dental restorations which

Table 9.1 General medical conditions

Hypertension	Coronary atherosclerotic disease
Stable angina	Myocardial infarction
Infective endocarditis	Chronic obstructive pulmonary disease
Asthma	Cerebrovascular accident
Epilepsy	Diabetes
Adrenal insufficiency	Steroid therapy
Organ transplant	Impaired hepatic or renal function

are failing and to attempt non-surgical retreatment as part of overall management. The removal of leaking crowns, restorations with deep decayed margins, poorly adapted interproximal restorations and root fillings of silver cones or pastes is common. Favourable results have been obtained when root canal systems are retreated prior to surgical management [39,64].

Radiographic examination is also essential, using prior radiographs if available, along with additional films exposed at the consultation visit [14]. When posterior teeth are involved, it is common to take several radiographs from different angles, identifying the number, curvature and angle of the roots requiring surgery. Likewise, anatomical structures which may impair surgical or visual manipulation of the surgical site are identified, such as the mental foramen, zygomatic process, anterior nasal spine and external oblique ridge.

Crucial to the success of the surgical procedure will be communication with the patient concerning the need for surgery, the prognosis, the use of preoperative medication or mouth rinses, the actual procedures to be performed, the potential for postoperative discomfort, the use of postoperative palliative procedures, the need for suture placement and removal, follow-up care and long-term assessment [48]. It is recommended that the following pretreatment regimens be considered:

1. A periodontal examination should be performed prior to surgery and, if necessary, scaling and/or root planing performed. The patient's oral hygiene practices should be assessed and reinforced.
2. Patients can be placed on chlorhexidine rinses 1 day before surgery, to continue for 2–3 days afterwards.
3. Patients can begin taking a non-steroidal anti-inflammatory medication 1 day before surgery, or at the latest one dose 1 h beforehand.
4. Patients should be advised to refrain from smoking.
5. If sedative premedication is to be used, the patient must bring an accompanying person, who will be responsible for escorting home and compliance with postoperative instructions.

Surgical kit

Basic instruments for surgical intervention have changed little in the past century. Many manufacturers have attempted to duplicate or enhance these instruments, but few major changes exist. Rather than citing specific companies or numbered instruments, it would be far better for the clinician to become familiar with the different types of instruments, and how and why they are beneficial in the performance of endodontic surgery. It is well accepted that there is more than one way to achieve high quality in the delivery of surgery. Therefore, instruments must be chosen which best allow the surgeon to perform as well as possible. Instruments must be sharp, undamaged and permit total control of the surgical site. Back-up instrument support for indispensable items must also be considered. Table 9.2 lists key instruments and their general use.

Table 9.2 Surgical kit

Presurgical assessment

Mirror and curved explorer
Straight and curved periodontal probes

Soft-tissue incision, elevation and reflection

Sharp scapels – numbers 15, 15c, 11 and 12
Broad-based periosteal elevator
Broad-based periosteal retractor
Tissue forceps
Surgical aspirator
Irrigating syringes and needles

Periradicular curettage

Straight and angled bone curettes
Small endodontic spoon curette
Periodontal curettes
Fine, curved mosquito forceps
Small, curved surgical scissors

Bone removal and root-end resection

Surgical length round and tapered fissure burs
Straight and angled bone curettes
Straight handpiece
Contra-angled handpiece/slow and high

Table 9.2 (*continued*)

Root-end preparation/placement of root-end filling/finish of resected root end

Miniature contra-angle or ultrasonic unit; sonic handpiece

Burs – very small inverted cone or round; angled ultrasonic or sonic tips

Root-end filling material

Haemostatic agent (avoid bone wax)

Miniature material carriers and condensers

Small ball burnisher

Paper points or fine aspirator tip

Citric acid 10–50% and sterile cotton pellets

Small, fine explorer

Suturing and soft-tissue closure

Surgical scissors

Haemostat or fine needle holders

Various suture types and sizes (3-0 to 5-0)

Sterile gauze for soft-tissue compression

Miscellaneous (or readily available)

Adequate aspiration equipment

Additional light source

Magnification

Root canal filling materials

Anaesthetic syringes and anaesthetic

Surgical technique

Tissue anaesthesia and haemostasis

Crucial to the successful performance of endodontic surgery is the ability to achieve profound anaesthesia and tissue haemostasis in the surgical site. Not only do they stop patient discomfort during the procedure and for a significant period thereafter, but they also improve vision in the surgical site, minimize surgical time, enhance surgery (root-end resection, preparation and filling), and reduce surgical blood loss, postsurgical haemorrhage and postsurgical swelling [48]. To achieve these objectives, an anaesthetic solution containing a vasoconstrictor is essential [57].

The choice of the anaesthetic–vasoconstrictor combination is dependent on the health status of the patient and surgical needs. When no systemic impediments are present,

further criteria for selection depend on the complexity and definitive nature of the surgical procedure. While multiple combinations of drugs can be used, 2% lignocaine with adrenaline has long been recognized as an excellent anaesthetic agent for endodontic surgery because of its clinical success in producing profound and prolonged analgesia [29,74]. Although several studies support the efficacy of 2% lignocaine with 1:200 000 to 1:100 000 concentrations of adrenaline for profound anaesthesia [40,62,66], clinical usage suggests that a 1:50 000 concentration provides better haemostasis [22,29]. The use of the 1:50 000 adrenaline results in easier visualization of the surgical site, reduced surgical time and improved postsurgical haemostasis, in addition to decreased blood loss [29].

While it is accepted that the lowest concentration of a drug to produce a given effect is always the treatment of choice, and in the patient's best interest to prevent systemic complications, consideration must be given to the twofold goal of *anaesthesia and haemostasis* required for successful endodontic surgery. Therefore, careful assessment of the patient's systemic status is essential prior to the use of 2% lignocaine with 1:50 000 adrenaline. Where 2% lignocaine with 1:50 000 is unavailable, 1:80 000 is clinically acceptable. This is especially important because lignocaine with adrenaline can elevate systemic plasma levels of the vasoconstrictor [134], although the haemodynamic response to this increase is still controversial [52,67]. This potential rise in adrenaline concentration suggests that high-risk patients should be carefully monitored. It also implies that great care should be taken during injection to prevent intravascular placement of the solution [57].

While 2% lignocaine with 1:100 000 is recommended for regional nerve blocks prior to endodontic surgery, this level of vasoconstrictor does not suffice for local haemostasis at the surgical site. Haemostasis must also be established at the surgical site [16], by additional injections supraperiosteally using 2% lignocaine with 1:50 000 [46]. In healthy patients a dose of 2–4 ml is recommended. In the maxilla achievement of both anaesthesia and haemostasis can be accomplished simultaneously. This requires multiple injections, depositing the solution throughout the entire submucosa superficial to the periosteum at the level of the root apices in the surgical site. The needle, with the bevel toward the bone, is advanced to the target site and, following aspiration, 0.5 ml of solution is slowly deposited (Figure 9.1). The needle may be moved peripherally and similar small amounts of solution deposited. If warranted, additional mucosal penetrations can be made to ensure that the entire surgical field has been injected. Slow, peripheral supraperiosteal infiltration into the submucosa promotes maximum diffusion, through the gingival tissues, periosteum and bone (Figure 9.2).

In the mandible, it is essential that the anaesthetic–vasoconstrictor solution be slowly infiltrated adjacent to the root apices, in addition to the block injection of the inferior alveolar nerve. Coupled with thorough localized infiltration, incisions which are made in alignment with the long axis of the supporting supraperiosteal vascular and tissues which are carefully elevated and reflected will minimize haemorrhage in the surgical site [48].

The amount of anaesthetic solution containing 1 : 50 000 adrenaline necessary to achieve anaesthesia and haemostasis is dependent on the surgical site, but 1.5–2.0 ml will generally suffice. The rate of injection can also influence the degree of haemostasis and anaesthesia obtained, with a rate of 1–2 ml/min recommended [109]. Injecting at rates exceeding this amount results in the localized pooling of solution, delayed and limited diffusion into the adjacent tissues, minimal

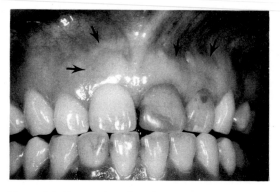

Figure 9.2 Slow and careful infiltration of the anaesthetic solution provides widespread and effective tissue haemostasis (delineated by arrows) for treatment of left maxillary central incisor.

effect on the microvasculature of the soft tissues and bone, and less than optimal anaesthesia and haemostasis. Rapid injection rates result in the potential for producing a systemic blood concentration in excess of toxic levels. The only predictable time to achieve haemostasis is prior to any incisions. Later attempts during surgery generally fail. Therefore, once the injection has been given, sufficient time must elapse before the initial incision (5–10 min), to allow for proper vascular constriction throughout the surgical site.

Soft-tissue incision and reflection

Good surgical access requires the incision and elevation of the soft tissue from the underlying bone. The design of this tissue flap is crucial not only to surgical entry and management of the root structure, but also healing of the surgical wound. The design of soft-tissue flaps has received wide and varied attention over the past century. For years the semilunar flap (Partsch incision) in the apical loose alveolar mucosa was recommended. Whilst still popular and successful in carefully planned cases, newer flap designs have been advocated based on a biological approach to tissue management and wound healing. Table 9.3 outlines the range of contemporary surgical flap designs [48]. There are compelling biological reasons to consider the use of full mucoperiosteal tissue flaps whenever possible. While they may be slightly more

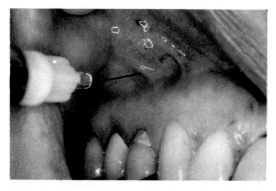

Figure 9.1 Placement of anaesthetic solution around the root apex of the tooth to be treated surgically.

Table 9.3 Periradicular surgical soft-tissue flap designs

Type of flap	Advantages/disadvantages
Full mucoperiosteal tissue flaps	
Triangular	Maintains intact vertical blood supply
Rectangular	Minimizes haemorrhage
Trapezoidal	Primary wound closure and rapid healing
Horizontal (envelope)	Allows survey of bone and root structure
	Excellent surgical orientation
	Minimal postoperative sequelae
	May have loss of tissue attachment
	May have loss of crestal bone height
	Possibility of tissue flap dislodgement
	Possible loss of interdental papilla integrity
Limited mucoperiosteal flaps	
Submarginal curved (semilunar)	Marginal and interdental papilla intact
Submarginal retangular (Luebke-Ochsenbein)	Unaltered soft-tissue attachment
	Adequate surgical access – may be compromised in posterior cases or cases with lateral root defects
	Good healing potential
	Disruption of blood supply
	Possibility of tissue shrinkage
	Delayed secondary healing/scarring
	Limited orientation to apical region
	Very limited in posterior surgery

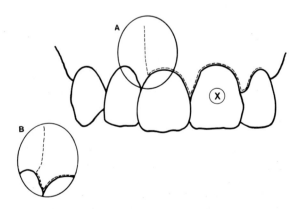

Figure 9.3 Triangular tissue flap design with single vertical releasing incision. The vertical releasing incision can be performed in different ways. Either (A) the incision leaves the interdental papilla intact or (B; insert) the incision includes the interdental papilla. In either case the incision line should meet the tooth at 90°.

difficult to use, mastery can be attained and the benefits realized by both clinician and patient (Table 9.3). Figures 9.3–9.8 diagrammatically detail each design while the following text gives a brief description of their application.

Full mucoperiosteal tissue flap – incision, reflection and retraction

The horizontal incision begins in the gingival sulcus, extending through the gingival fibres to the crestal bone. The scalpel blade is held in a near vertical position (Figure 9.9). In the interdental region, the incision should pass through the mid-col area, separating the buccal and lingual papillae, and severing the gingival fibres to the depth of the interdental crestal bone (Figure 9.10). This is critical to prevent sloughing of the papillae due to a

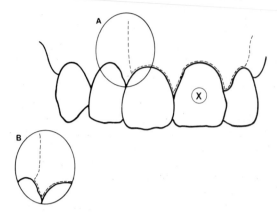

Figure 9.4 Rectangular tissue flap design with double vertical releasing incisions. As with the triangular flap design, variations can be used with the vertical incisions (A and B); a description has been included in Figure 9.3.

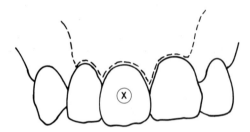

Figure 9.5 Trapezoidal tissue flap design. Note vertical releasing incisions are angled towards the base of the flap.

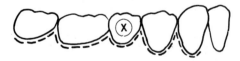

Figure 9.6 Horizontal tissue flap design. No vertical releasing incisions are used initially but they can be added later to enhance surgical access if necessary.

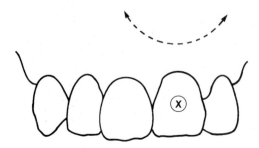

Figure 9.7 Semilunar tissue flap design. Note that the scope of this flap limits extension if necessary.

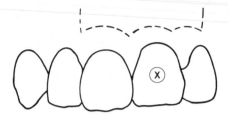

Figure 9.8 Luebke-Ochsenbein (submarginal) tissue flap design. This flap may have one or two vertical releasing incisions, or may be limited to a horizontal incision, only if sufficient surgical and visual access can be obtained.

compromised blood supply. Because of the shape of the embrasure space, incision in this area often requires the use of a number 11 or 12 scalpel blade to follow the interproximal tooth contours (Figure 9.10). Vertical (releasing) incisions are used in the triangular and rectangular flap designs (Figures 9.3 and 9.4), and are vertically oriented, passing between the roots of adjacent teeth and coursing parallel to the long axes of the roots. The incision should be over intact bone and be to the depth of the bone. Vertical incisions terminate at the mesial or distal-line angles of teeth, and never in papillae or in the mid-root area.

The trapezoidal flap design (Figure 9.5) incorporates angled releasing incisions and is not considered biologically acceptable for endodontic surgery because it cuts across the vertically positioned supraperiosteal vasculature and tissue-supportive collagen fibres. The horizontal or envelope flap design (Figure 9.6) is often used for maxillary or mandibular molars, or palatal flaps. However,

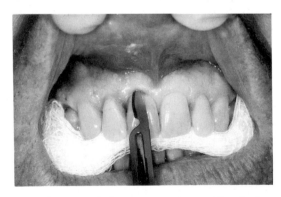

Figure 9.9 Intrasulcular incision with a no. 15 scalpel blade. Note the vertical position of the scalpel as it cuts through and releases the crestal fibres.

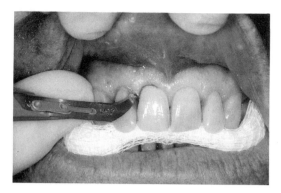

Figure 9.10 Use of a no. 12 scalpel blade to release the fibres of the interdental papilla. Note the depth and angulation of the blade.

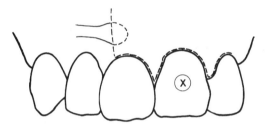

Figure 9.11 The periosteum is initially elevated by applying force against the cortical bone in the region of the attached gingival tissues.

some type of releasing incision is generally incorporated, albeit not as long as that used with triangular or rectangular flaps.

Tissue reflection always begins in the attached gingiva of the vertical incision. The periosteal elevator is positioned to apply reflective forces in a lateral direction against the cortical bone, while elevating the tougher fibrous-based tissue of the gingiva (Figure 9.11). This also elevates the periosteum and its superficial tissues from the cortical plate.

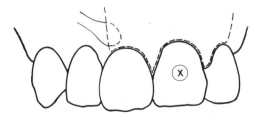

Figure 9.12 The periosteal elevator is subsequently moved coronally to elevate the previously released interdental papilla.

Subsequently, the elevator is directed coronally (Figure 9.12) to elevate the marginal and interdental gingiva with minimal traumatic force (Figure 9.13). All reflective forces should be applied to the bone and periosteum, with minimal forces on the gingival elements. This is referred to as undermining elevation [48].

After tissue reflection, bleeding tissue tags are often seen on the cortical surface in the crestal region and between root eminences (Figure 9.14). Because these tissue tags play an important role in healing they should not be removed during surgery.

Adequate retraction of the tissue flap is essential for surgical access to the periradicular and radicular tissues. The retractor must always rest on sound bone with light but firm pressure. Pinching of the soft-tissue flap with the retractor must be avoided to minimize tissue damage and untoward postsurgical sequelae (Figure 9.15). If this is not possible the reflected tissue must be elevated further or the tissue flap extended to release its attachment from the bone.

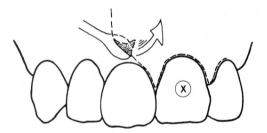

Figure 9.13 The entire tissue flap is elevated with minimal force being directed on the marginal and interdental gingival tissues.

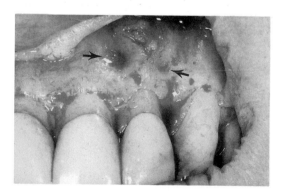

Figure 9.14 Tissue tags remain on the cortical bone after flap elevation (arrows).

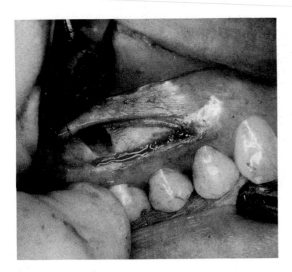

Figure 9.15 Pinching of the mucosal tissue with the periosteal retractor should be avoided during surgery.

Limited mucoperiosteal tissue flap – incision, reflection and retraction

These tissue flaps do not include the marginal and interdental gingiva. The horizontal incisions of these flaps should be in the attached gingiva, with the vertical incision or vertical component involving both the attached gingiva and alveolar mucosa. It is critical that there is an absolute minimum of 2 mm of attached gingiva from the depth of the gingival sulcus before this flap design is chosen. However, a very narrow isthmus for safe incision exists between the sulcular depth and the mucogingival junction in most patients, especially in the mandible [1].

Historically the semilunar or curved submarginal flap design has been favoured. It is formed by a single curved incision beginning in alveolar mucosa, extending coronally into attached gingiva, and curving back into alveolar mucosa (Figure 9.7).

The rectangular submarginal flap design (Luebke-Ochsenbein flap) is formed by a scalloped horizontal incision in the attached gingiva and two vertical releasing incisions (Figure 9.8). Scalloping reflects the contour of the marginal gingivae and provides an adequate distance from the depths of the gingival sulci. Here also, the vasculature and collagen fibres are severed. It may be used in maxillary anterior or posterior teeth in which reflection of marginal and interdental gingivae is contraindicated because of tissue inflammation or aesthetic concerns with extensive fixed prostheses. Often, soft or osseous tissue anatomy negates the use of a limited mucoperiosteal flap design.

Osseous entry and root identification

Prior to root-end resection and removal of diseased soft tissue which may surround the root, bone may need to be removed to gain visual access to the surgical site. Removal of bone is usually accomplished with a large round bur (International Organization for Standardization (ISO) size 018 or 024), using a low- or high-speed handpiece. The bone is removed in a brush-stroke fashion [126] with copious irrigation, creating a window over the root apex. In many cases the approach may need to be from a coronal position on the bone, moving apically once the root structure has been identified. Entry as close to the apex, however, is recommended, with the angle of entry facilitating visibility and surgical access. This requires measuring the approximate length of the root on the bone.

The apex may also be identified during osseous palpation after soft-tissue reflection. Where the bone is thin, or the root apex is prominent, a straight bone curette can be used in a rotating motion to penetrate the cortical plate and identify the root structure (Figure 9.16). Once exposed, the bur can be used to create a greater window to outline the root apex. In those cases where the bone is thick, the same type of initial osseous penetration can be made and a radiopaque object placed in the small hole. A radiograph will provide information on the location of the root apex.

Root structure can be identified from bone by texture (smooth and hard), lack of bleeding upon probing, outline (presence of periodontal ligament, PDL), and colour (yellowish) [11]. Its perimeter (PDL) may also be identified by painting 1% methylene blue on the surface [24].

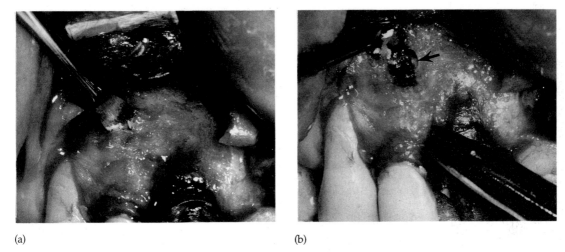

(a)   (b)

Figure 9.16 (a) Use of a straight curette to peel away the surface cortical bone. (b) Penetration through the bone with a curette alone to expose the root (arrow). Note bony chips on curette.

Removal of diseased soft tissue (periradicular curettage)

This procedure can often be performed before or in conjunction with root-end resection. The purpose is to remove the bulk of the soft tissues which may be present at various root canal orifices on the root surface. This adverse tissue response has been described as reactive or protective [123]. Therefore, omitting to remove every remnant of soft tissue will not lead to failure, as the tissue elements in the periphery of these lesions are often productive in nature and contain fibroblasts, vascular buds, new collagen and bone matrix. In those cases in which the soft-tissue mass is exposed upon flap reflection or initial bone removal, curettage can proceed prior to root-end resection. In other cases resection is necessary to gain access to most of the tissue.

Straight and angled surgical bone curettes are necessary, along with angled periodontal curettes (Figure 9.17). At times it may be necessary to inject 0.5 ml of anaesthetic solution to control haemorrhage and ensure patient comfort if the lesion is extensive. Initially the bone curettes are used to peel the soft tissue from the lateral borders of the bony crypt. This is accomplished with the concave surface of the curette facing the bony wall, applying pressure only against the bone (Figure 9.18) [43]. Care must be taken to

avoid penetration of the soft tissue which may shred the tissue, sever the vascular network, and increase local haemorrhage. Once the tissue is freed along the lateral margins, the bone curettes can be turned and used in scraping fashion along the deep walls of the crypt. This will detach the soft tissue from its lingual or palatal base. Once loosened, tissue forceps are used to grasp gently the tissue which is teased from its position with a bone curette. The tissue sample is placed directly into a bottle of 10% neutral buffered formalin for biopsy. In those cases which require root-end resection prior to curettage, make sure that the root structure is sufficiently exposed to minimize shredding of the soft tissues during resection.

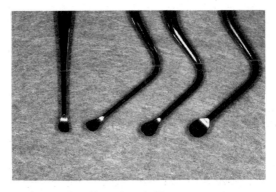

Figure 9.17 Straight and angled bone curettes are essential.

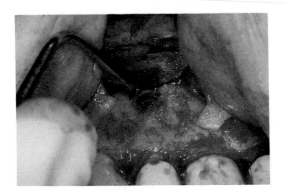

Figure 9.18 Use of the bone curette to peel the soft-tissue lesion from the bone cavity.

In the presence of large lesions, care must be exercised during curettage of the lateral surfaces of the bony crypt to avoid exposure of adjacent roots and their pulpal vasculature. Presurgical radiographs should reveal this possibility, and tissue in these areas may need to be left in position. Caution must also be exercised when close to the maxillary antrum, mental foramen or mandibular canal to prevent damage to vital structures. When soft tissue is adherent either lingually to the root or in the furcation region, periodontal curettes are essential for thorough removal.

Whilst retention of root structure is necessary for tooth stability and strength, rarely should periradicular surgery be limited to just curettage [47]. Therefore root-end resection is usually needed.

Root-end resection

The term root-end resection refers specifically to the removal of the apical portion of the root. There are many indications for resection of the root end during periradicular surgery, each designed to eliminate aetiological factors and to enhance the sealing of the root canal at the resected root surface [49]. These indications vary from case to case, but support the stated purpose.

The technique of root-end resection usually uses a lingual to labial bevel, angled to the coronal aspect of the tooth. This is designed for surgical access and visibility. Angles for root bevels have in the past been suggested to range from 30° to 45° in the line of sight,

although variables in each case determine the exact degree of cut [24,47,71,110]. From the anterior to the posterior, the angle of the bevel will gradually change from a direct coronal–buccal cut to one that is accentuated coronally and mesiobuccally placed. These angles of resection and their use will also be determined by the root inclination and curvature, number of roots, thickness of bone and position of the root in the bone and arch. Current evidence suggests that bevels more perpendicular to the long axis of the root may be desirable to minimize dentinal tubule exposure and to ensure exposure of all orifices from the canal system [25].

The root end can be resected and bevelled in one of two ways. Once the root end has been exposed, the bur (narrow straight-fissure) in a handpiece (straight or contra-angle) is positioned at the desired angle and the root is shaved away, beginning from the apex, cutting coronally (Figure 9.19a). The bur is moved from mesial to distal at the desired angle, shaving the root smooth and flat, and exposing the entire canal system and root outline. This approach allows for continual observation of the root end during cutting.

The second technique of resection is to predetermine the amount of root end to be resected. This approach, however, may remove more root structure than is necessary. The bur and handpiece are positioned at the chosen angle and the apex is resected by cutting through the root from mesial to distal (Figure 9.19b,c). Once the apex is removed, the root face is gently shaved with the bur to smooth the surface and ensure complete resection and visibility of the root face. This technique works well when an apical biopsy is desired or to gain access to significant amounts of soft tissue located lingual to the root.

The appearance of the root face following root-end resection will vary, based upon the type of bur used, the external root anatomy, the anatomy of the canal system exposed at the particular angle of resection, and the nature and density of the root canal filling material. Various types of burs have been recommended for root-end resection, such as round burs, straight fissure burs, diamond burs, and cross-cut fissure burs [48]. Each will leave a characteristic anatomical imprint

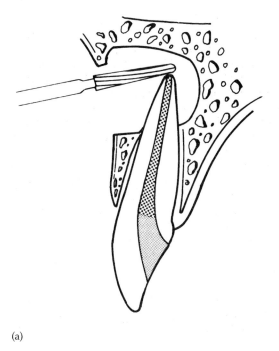

(a)

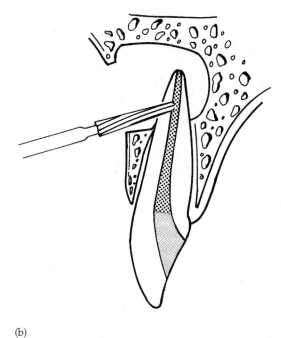

(b)

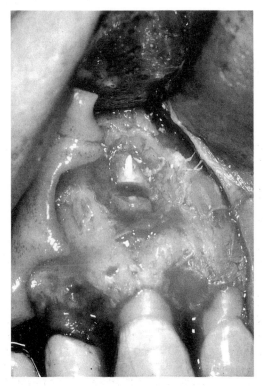

(c)

Figure 9.19 Diagrammatic representation of (a) root-end resection from the apex coronally; (b) root-end resection when the amount of root to be resected has been determined. (c) Clinical case of root-end resection in which a predetermined amount of the root has been resected.

on the root face, from rough-grooved and gouged to regularly grooved and smooth [82]. To date, no study has clearly defined the advantages of one type of bur over the other, although for years clinical practice has favoured a smooth flat root surface [44,81,122,132].

The extent to which the removal of the root end should occur will be dictated by the following factors [48]:

1. Access and visibility to the surgical site.
2. Position and anatomy of the root within the alveolar bone.
3. Anatomy of the cut root surface relative to the number of canals and their configuration.
4. Need to place a root-end filling into sound root structure.
5. Presence and location of procedural error, e.g. perforation.
6. Presence of an intra-alveolar root fracture.
7. Presence of any periodontal defects.
8. Anatomical considerations, e.g. proximity of adjacent teeth, or level of remaining crestal bone.
9. Presence of significant accessory canals; roots with such anatomical aberrances would be likely to receive more extensive resection.

Regardless of the rationale for the extent of root-end removal, there is no reason to resect the root to the base of a large periradicular lesion, as was previously advised. Likewise, resection to the point where little (<1 mm) or no crestal bone remains covering the buccal aspect of the root may very well doom the tooth to failure (Figure 9.20). On the other hand, failure to remove sufficient root structure to be able to inspect the resected root surface and establish an apical seal may also contribute to failure. In this case, root canals may be missed, or they may be so extensive that they cannot be properly managed within the confined space.

The complete root face must be identified and examined subsequent to resection. The examination is done with a fine, sharp probe, e.g. DG 16, guided around the periphery of the root and the root canal. The external root anatomy will determine the ultimate shape of the cut root end, as oval, round, dumbbell-shaped, kidney bean-shaped, or teardrop-

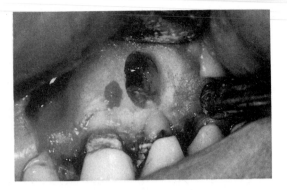

Figure 9.20 Severely angled resections, often coupled with large periradicular lesions, compromise the amount of remaining crestal bone. Note poor margins of restorations.

shaped (Figure 9.21). Outlines will vary depending on the tooth, angle of the bevel and position of the cut on the root. Once cut, however, the entire surface must be visible. If visibility or access is impaired, or the root possesses an unusual cross-sectional outline, 1% methylene blue dye can be placed on the

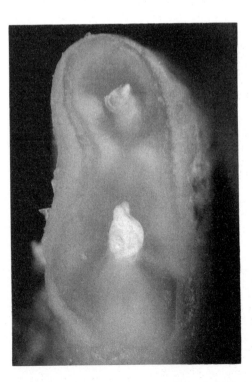

Figure 9.21 Resected root outline. Note the kidney bean shape along with position of the canals. No canal anastomosis is visible.

root surface to help identify the periodontal ligament that surrounds the root [24]. A small cotton pellet containing dye is wiped over the root face for 5–10 s. Subsequently the area is flushed with sterile water or saline. The dye will stain the periodontal ligament dark blue, highlighting the root outline. A potential drawback to this technique may be the deposition of cotton fibres on the resected surface or on bone. Residual remnants of cotton fibres have been shown to induce a foreign-body reaction in healing tissues [48].

The shape of the exposed canal system will vary depending on the angle of the bevel and the canal anatomy at the level of the cut. Canal systems will generally assume a more elongated and accentuated shape as the angle of the bevel is increased buccally (Figure 9.22). Often, canal systems will be irregular and extend further than anticipated.

Also visible on most resected root ends is the presence of a root canal filling material. Variations in quality of the filling will be seen in both the type of filling material, e.g. gutta-percha, silver cones, pastes, and the nature of the obturation technique, e.g. lateral con-

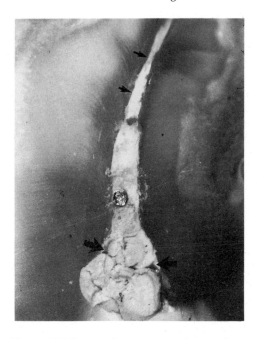

Figure 9.23 Root-end resection reveals a poorly condensed gutta-percha filling. Voids are present between the gutta-percha cones (large arrows), a broken instrument is present in the centre of the canal and the upper part of the canal is filled with root canal sealer (small arrows).

densation, vertical condensation or thermoplastic filling (Figure 9.23). Likewise, the different burs advocated for resection will create discrepancies in the surface of the filling material and adaptation to the canal walls. For example, coarse diamond burs will tend to rip and tear at the gutta-percha root canal filling, spreading the gutta-percha over the edge of the canal aperture and onto the resected root face (Figure 9.24). Invariably this will create gaps between the originally adapted gutta-percha and the root canal wall. Similar findings are noted with metal burs [48]. In order to prevent this, surface finishing with an ultrafine diamond is recommended (Figure 9.25; Ultrafine no. 862-012 diamond bur, Brasseler, Savannah, GA, USA).

The presence of additional foramina, anastomoses between foramina, fracture lines and the quality of the apical adaptation of the root canal filling must be checked on the resected root surface (Figure 9.26). If methylene blue has been used, it will also have a tendency to stain the periphery of the canal system and highlight fracture lines.

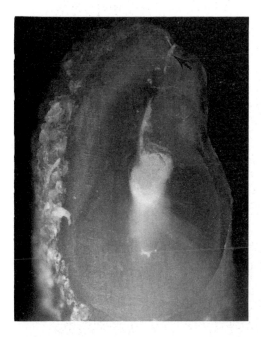

Figure 9.22 Angled resection reveals an extended canal space. Removal of additional root palatally will be necessary to manage the uppermost part of the canal system (arrow).

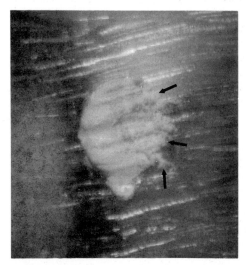

Figure 9.24 Rough surface of resected root after being cut with a coarse diamond. Note the gutta-percha has been dragged across the surface of the root (arrows).

Nitromersol, a dental disinfectant which stains reddish-brown, can also be used when examining the root face or a fibreoptic light can be aimed at or behind the root end to enhance visibility [10]. If these methods do not work, it may be necessary to remove additional root structure to identify the canal system or, in the case of a fracture line, to enhance its direction and extent.

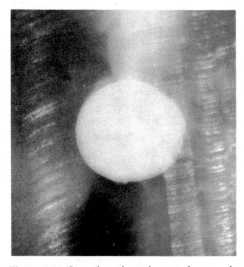

Figure 9.25 Smooth surface of resected root and root filling created with an ultrafine diamond and waterspray. Note the adaptation of the filling material to the outline of the canal.

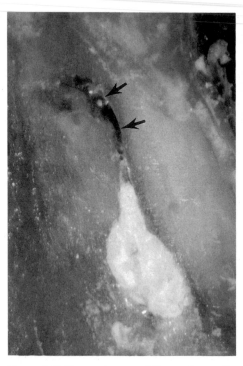

Figure 9.26 Resected root end. The main canal has been obturated but the canal extension contains necrotic debris (arrows). A root-end preparation and filling must be performed.

A major area of concern following root-end resection and dentinal tubule exposure is the possibility that these tubules may serve as a direct source of contamination from uncleaned root canals into the periradicular tissues, especially if there is coronal leakage. Root ends resected from 45° to 60° have as many as 28 000 tubules/mm^2 at a point immediately adjacent to the canal [128]. At the dentinocemental junction, an area which may communicate with the root canal even in the presence of a root-end filling, an average of 13 000 tubules/mm^2 are found. Likewise, due to angular changes in the tubules at the apex, there could be patent communication with the main canal if the depth of the root-end preparation in the buccal aspect of the cavity is insufficient to compensate for these anatomical variations [13,135]. Root-end resections in older teeth have shown less leakage than that seen in teeth from younger patients [55]; this corroborates the findings of sclerosis and reduced patency in apical dentinal tubules [26]. It has been suggested that, if the apical ramifications commonly found in

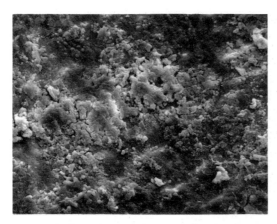

Figure 9.27 Smear layer on the resected root end.

young teeth are dismissed as a rationale for root-end resection, then resection would be inadvisable due to the patency of the apical dentinal tubules.

Another concern following root-end resection is the presence of a contaminated smear layer, containing tissue debris and possibly microorganisms, over the resected root end (Figure 9.27). This *may* serve as a source of irritation to the periradicular tissues, primarily preventing the intimate layering of cementum against the resected tubules. A thicker smear layer is usually created by cutting without waterspray than with a heavy air–waterspray [93], or by using coarse diamond burs than tungsten carbide burs [21]. Therefore it is recommended that root-end resection be performed under constant irrigation, which assists the partial removal of the dentinal smear layer from the surface. Also, if diamond burs are used to resect the root, a medium grit is preferred, followed by a fine or ultrafine grit diamond. If there is a gutta-percha root canal filling, resection without irrigation should be avoided as it may promote the lodging of dentine chips in the gutta-percha, which would serve as a source of irritation if contaminated. These chips may not be removable during the elimination of the smear layer with a dentinal cleanser [49].

Root-end cavity preparation

In order to seal the potential avenues of communication from the resected root end to the canal system adequately, a root-end preparation should be made into the root to the coronal extent of the resected apical tubules [41, 135]. This will vary from case to case, but generally a depth of 2–4 mm is sufficient [12,110] depending on the angle of the resection. Ideally this preparation is made in the long axis of the root, is parallel to the anatomical outline of the root, possesses adequate retention form and encompasses all exposed orifices of the root canal system. If this is the case, then the depths indicated will be sufficient in all aspects of the preparation. If, however, the resection is angled then the depth of the buccal aspect of the cavity preparation must be slightly deeper than the buccal extent of the root resection in order to fill behind all dentine tubules on the resected root face which might otherwise communicate with the canal system. The optimum depths for a root-end cavity, measured from the buccal aspect of the cavity, are 1.0, 2.1 and 2.5 mm for a 90°, 30° and 45° angle of resection, respectively [41].

The final outline of the preparation will depend mainly on the anatomy of the exposed canal space, and in some cases, the nature of the root outline. For example, in maxillary central incisors the shape of the root-end preparation will generally be round to oval in shape. In premolars or molars it may be very elongated and narrow in conjunction with oval or round shapes.

Root-end preparations can either be made with a bur, e.g. inverted cone or round bur (ISO size 008) at high or low speed, or with specially angled tips adapted for use on an ultrasonic unit or sonic handpiece (Figure 9.28). These approaches to root-end preparation make it possible to use any of the newer root-end filling materials, e.g. super EBA, intermediate restorative material (IRM), glass ionomer cement, Diaket or dentine-bonded composite resin.

Recent enhancements in apical root-end preparation have resulted from the development of ultrasonic cutting tips (Figure 9.29) [25]. These small, angled tips have been advocated for the ultrasonic shaping of apical preparations parallel to the long axis of the root after minimal root-end resection (Figure 9.30a). Their use in the debridement and enlargement of canal anastomoses and irregularities commonly found in molar roots has been recommended (Figure 9.30b,c) [25],

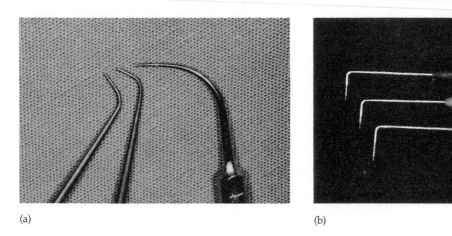

(a)   (b)

Figure 9.28 (a) Various ultrasonic tips for preparing a root-end cavity. (b) Sonic tips for root-end cavity preparation.

and the ability of this technique to achieve cleaner root-end preparations as opposed to bur preparations has recently been highlighted [50,125,142]. Further advances in the creation of clean, good-quality root-end preparations have been seen with the use of sonic tips for apical root cavities [38,70] and clinical experience would support the routine use of either of these newer techniques for root-end cavity preparation as opposed to burs.

After root-end preparation the cavity should be irrigated with sterile saline or water. Small suction tips, made from 20- or 18-gauge needles which can be bent and adapted to a high-speed suction device, are used to remove fluid and debris from the cavity. Some clinicians prefer using paper points to dry the preparation. Although flushing the cavity with citric acid has been recommended to remove the smear layer [25], recent studies have indicated that this may

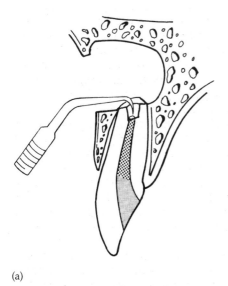

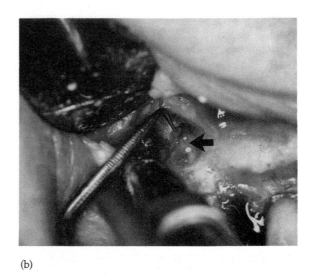

(a)   (b)

Figure 9.29 (a) Diagrammatic representation of root-end cavity preparation along the root axis using an ultrasonic tip. (b) An ultrasonic tip near the resected root end. Note good access and two canals (identified by gutta-percha) united by a thin white line; anastomosis (arrow). Preparation of the anastomosis is essential.

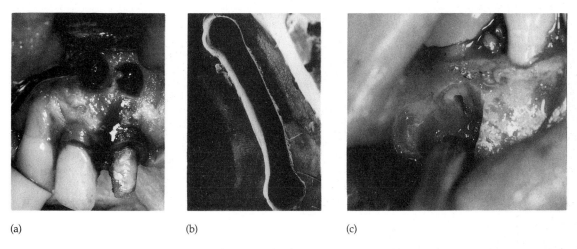

(a)   (b)   (c)

Figure 9.30 (a) Preparing a root-end cavity with an ultrasonic tip. (b) Root-end cavity prepared in a molar root uniting the two mesial canals through the anastomosis (SEM). (c) Ultrasonic root-end preparation in the mesial root of a mandibular molar.

actually enhance the amount of leakage after root-end filling [96,117]. Although citric acid creates cleaner root-end cavity walls and assists in debris removal, its regular use is questionable. Following drying of the cavity, it must be inspected to ensure that it is clean and encompasses all the canal orifices; this is aided by special small mirrors.

Root-end cavity obturation

To clean and obturate the root canal before root-end resection or to do it at the time of surgery has been controversial for many years. Some authors have found greater success when the canal is obturated in conjunction with surgery, less often when a previous root canal filling was left in place, and least often when the canal was filled immediately prior to surgery [5,76,86,110]. On the other hand a better prognosis has been identified when the root is cleaned and filled prior to surgery [64,75]. Favourable results with root canal obturation either before or during surgery have been demonstrated [39]. In a recent evaluation of the surgical management of non-surgical endodontic failures, cleaning, shaping and obturation of the root canal prior to surgery resulted in the highest rate of success [80]. In the cases that could be managed this way the root end was not resected, and surgical procedures were limited to curettage.

Cases in which root-end resection was performed and a root-end filling placed resulted in a higher number of failures. What is important is that the canal system is cleaned and sealed as well as possible. In many respects this necessitates that old root canal fillings should be redone as well as possible. Under these circumstances many cases may be successful without the use of a root-end filling.

In some cases in which a radiolucency exists and time is a factor, or cases in which there are persistent exacerbations between visits or failing root canal treatment which has been treated non-surgically in an assumed optimal manner, canal repreparation and refilling can be done at the time of surgery. A tissue flap is reflected, the root apex exposed and resected. The canal preparation is performed with the file tips protruding through the resected root end (Figure 9.31a). Small aspirators can be placed next to the apical opening to prevent root canal irrigant (0.5–2.5% sodium hypochlorite) entering the bony cavity. After adequate preparation, the canal is dried with paper points. Obturation should follow with gutta-percha and sealer condensed from the coronal access apically (Figure 9.31b). Any condensation technique is acceptable; however, the master gutta-percha point should not be pulled through the apex, as point retraction may occur. The excess gutta-percha can be removed with an

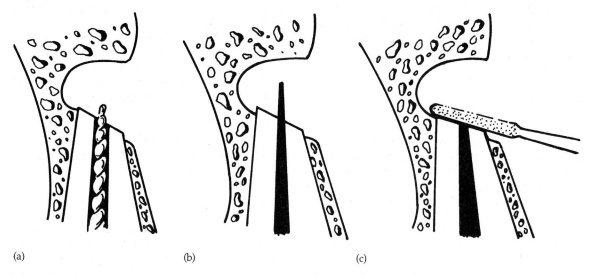

(a)   (b)   (c)

Figure 9.31 (a) Cleaning and shaping of the root canal with file tips through the resected root end. (b) Condensation of the gutta-percha filling with the tip through the root-end. (c) Removal of excess filling material and finishing of the root surface with an ultrafine diamond bur.

ultrafine bur (Figure 9.31c) which usually creates a well-adapted root canal filling on the resected surface. In these situations the placement of a root-end filling will usually be unnecessary. This is common with gutta-percha fillings, especially those placed immediately before or at the time of surgery. An ultrafine diamond bur or composite finishing bur can be run over the root surface with a sterile water or saline spray (Figure 9.25). If the canal is properly obturated the result will be a very smooth, well-adapted root canal filling. Paste fillings are unacceptable because of frequent voids, the irritating nature of most pastes and the potential for paste dissolution. Metal fillings (e.g. silver points) are also unacceptable because of poor adaptation and the potential for corrosion.

When a root-end cavity is to be obturated, it must be isolated to ensure moisture control. This is usually done with a haemostatic collagen-based agent, such as Hemofibrine or Hemocollagene (Figure 9.32; Septodont), which can remain in the osseous cavity or be removed prior to closure [48]. Also used is a solution of ferric sulphate which must be removed from the bone cavity prior to tissue closure [58,68].

Presently there are no commercially available materials which will provide a perfect seal, therefore the materials that are used

must be carefully prepared and placed to ensure the best possible adaptation to the root cavity walls. Current materials and their requirements are covered in the following section.

Coupled with the attempt to seal the apical end of the canal system, attention must also be directed to the coronal end [116]. It is illogical to place a filling material which is imperfect at the root end of the tooth and neglect the potential for coronal leakage

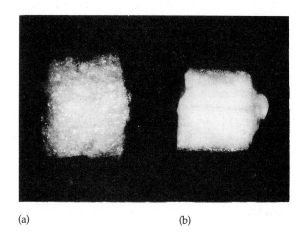

(a)   (b)

Figure 9.32 Collagen sponge materials for haemorrhage control in the apical bony cavity: (a) Hemofibrine; (b) Hemocollagene.

around root canal fillings and coronal restorations with carious lesions, imperfect margins, or through exposed dentinal tubules in the cervical area.

Root-end filling materials

The purpose of the root-end filling is to seal the canal system apically. The materials are the same as those used in restorative dentistry and non-surgical endodontics. A complete list of these materials is available along with a detailed historical, biological and clinical perspective on each material [48].

When using modern materials as root-end fillings, adherence to manufacturers' recommendations in preparation, manipulation and placement is important. Table 9.4 lists current materials that are recommended for root-end filling. Although there is a reasonable history of success with amalgam root-end fillings, problems have always existed with its long-term success, such as corrosion, persistence of apical inflammation and tissue argyria. Coupled with concerns over the mercury component, it is recommended that more bioinductive materials be used; therefore clinical studies support other materials [35,59,143].

Super EBA

This material is a modified zinc oxide–eugenol cement that has high compressive and tensile strengths, neutral pH and low solubility. It adheres to the walls of the root-end preparation even in the presence of moisture. The *in vitro* short-term seal obtained with super EBA has been shown to be affected minimally by blood contamination [130], whilst its *in vivo* sealing ability as a root-end filling material to microorganisms has been shown to be better than amalgam [99]. There is evidence of osseous tissue

Table 9.4 Current root-end filling materials

Super EBA
IRM
Glass ionomer
Diaket
Composite resin (dentine-bonded)

repair following its use as a bone implant [88] and periradicular tissue repair when used as a root-end filling material [91]. A clinically high success rate (95%) has been reported over a long period of evaluation [35]. When used in bur- or ultrasonically prepared root-end cavities in which the smear layer had either been retained or removed, leakage was observed [87,117]: In spite of some of the variables seen with this material, its widespread use as a root-end filling material has been advocated.

Glass ionomer cement

Glass ionomer cements bond physicochemically to dentine and enamel. Their biocompatibility enhances with setting, and marginal adaptation and adhesion to dentine have been shown to be improved with the use of acid conditioners and protective varnishes [102,103]. The sealing ability of glass ionomer cements has been demonstrated in recent studies of their use for root-end filling [2–4,28,92]. Antibacterial activity is acceptable [27] and sealing ability is better than those of amalgam, heat-sealed gutta-percha and zinc polycarboxylate cements [27,89]. Bone healing in intimate contact with glass ionomer cements has been shown when used for root-end filling [23,34,100,143]. Clinical studies support the use of glass ionomer cements for root-end filling [53,59,65,144]. Although these materials are moisture-sensitive, the occasional blood or saliva contamination does not appear to affect adversely healing of teeth with these materials as root-end fillings over a 5-year period [59]. The careful use of glass ionomer cements, according to manufacturers' directions, as root-end fillings can be recommended.

Dentine-bonded composite resin

There has been limited use but promising results with dentine-bonded composite resin root-end fillings. Key to their success appears to be a combination of minimal toxicity of the dentine-bonding agent, placement in a moisture-free environment and good adhesion to the underlying dentine with minimal polymerization contraction [114]. A clinical and radiographic evaluation of 388 human teeth over a 1-year period showed healing with dentine-bonded composite resin root-end fillings to be much better than with amalgam [113].

Histological and scanning electron microscopic assessment of this technique in both monkeys and humans has indicated reformation of the periodontium adjacent to the composite resin, including reformation of a lamina dura, insertion of Sharpey's fibres and cementum deposited in intimate contact with the composite resin [8,9]. Whilst these findings would suggest that ideal healing can be achieved with this material, further long-term studies are warranted before widespread use can be recommended.

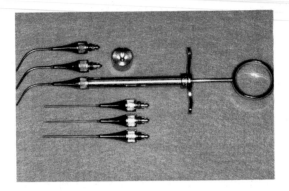

Figure 9.33 Messing carrier used to carry small increments of root-end filling material.

IRM

This material is a modified zinc oxide–eugenol which has been shown to seal better than amalgam, especially against microorganisms [98]. Healing of the periradicular tissues in the presence of IRM root-end fillings has been quite favourable [60,98]. Likewise, clinical studies have shown enhanced success with IRM root-end fillings (91%) compared with amalgam (75%) over long periods [35]. When using this material as a root-end filling, the clinician is cautioned to use a high powder-to-liquid ratio, for ease of placement, decreased setting time, reduced toxicity and reduced solubility [33]. Therefore the use of IRM as a root-end filling material can be recommended when mixed in a higher powder-to-liquid ratio than that for temporary restorations; a drawback is a significant reduction in clinical working time.

Diaket

Primarily a root canal sealer, this polyvinyl resin has been used as a root-end filling material for a number of years with a high level of empirical success. Diaket has excellent sealing ability [61,136] with a highly favourable tissue response in bone and periradicular tissues [83,140]. Histologically there is a suggestion that cementum can form immediately adjacent to or in intimate contact with Diaket, or with Diaket–tricalcium phosphate paste [140]. As with IRM, it is imperative that this material is mixed at a higher powder-to-liquid ratio than that for a root canal sealer [83,127]; a suggested ratio is at least 2 parts powder to 1 portion liquid [140]. This can be done on a glass slab 20–30 min before use, without risk of the material setting. It can be carried to the apical cavity with a small carrier, such as a Messing carrier (Figure 9.33), condensed and burnished similarly to amalgam. If the material cannot be used in this manner, it indicates an improper mix.

Experimental materials

The most promising experimental material for root-end filling is mineral trioxide aggregate (MTA) [129,131]. This material has been shown to have excellent sealing properties, not to be affected by saliva or blood contamination, and to allow for periradicular tissue repair when used as a root-end filling. It is not yet available commercially.

A self-setting apatite cement has also received initial assessment as a root-end filling material. An experimental material provided a comparable root-end seal to amalgam and super EBA [73]. The material is highly biocompatible and future research may provide further promise for this entity.

Lasers have also been used in an attempt to seal the root end [141]. However, laser application to hard tissue is in its infancy and presently lasers do not appear to have a viable role in the complete seal of the apical root canal system during periradicular surgery.

Treatment of the root face

In common with procedures in operative dentistry and periodontics, removal of the smear layer and exposure of the apical collagen fibres is recommended after root-end resection, primarily to remove potentially contaminated debris and to enhance the healing environment for cemental deposition. However, the nature of the dentine cleanser to achieve this ideal is uncertain, as various agents have been recommended, such as phosphoric acid [42,94], ethylenediamine-tetraacetic acid (EDTA) [19], hydrochloric acid [105,115], and citric acid [18,32,106]. Also, times of exposure and demineralization have been highlighted, as has been the optimal pH for activity. The optimal exposure of collagen and demineralization occurs with a burnishing application of citric acid (pH 1.0) for 3 min [30]. Longer applications result in collagen denaturation. The peak activity pH of citric acid is 1.42 [124].

Demineralization of resected root ends with a 2-min burnishing of 50% citric acid at pH 1.0 results in a rapid and predictable layering of a cementoid type of material on the resected surface of dogs' teeth after 45 days [31]. No direct application to human teeth under similar circumstances has been studied, although the omission of an acid cleaner does not preclude the formation of a viable cementum layer [77].

What appears to be crucial to ultimate healing and cemental deposition is the stabilization of the exposed dentinal collagen fibres along with minimal demineralization. Failure to do so may account for the discrepancies seen regarding the use of different concentrations of citric acid at various times in periodontal applications. Likewise, the exact benefits of citric acid are still considered speculative and in need of further research [84]. In essence, all that may be necessary to accomplish ideal healing at the resected root end is removal of the smear layer and retention of smear plugs, as proposed for coronal cavities [20]; however, this may be difficult to achieve clinically [93].

Studies have identified the use of the Fe^{3+} ion, as an aqueous solution of 10% citric acid and 3% ferric chloride (10:3), to stabilize dentine collagen during the demineralization process [78, 138]; however, applications were <30 s, as longer exposure increased demineralization and denaturation of the collagen. This approach has enhanced the bonding which occurs with restorative materials, and may also stimulate adhesion of the exposed, intact collagen with fibrin and fibronectin [101] and the splicing of collagen with newly formed collagen fibrils [108] during the wound-healing process. Further work on the resected root end is warranted.

The following treatment regimen is indicated for the resected root face after placement of a root-end filling, or root-end resection in which a well-condensed gutta-percha root filling is in place:

1. Surface finishing with an ultrafine diamond or 30-flute tungsten carbide composite-resin finishing-bur [25,49] (Figure 9.34).
2. Gentle burnishing of the surface with a weak acid cleaner (10%) for a short period (30 s) [49] (Figure 9.35).

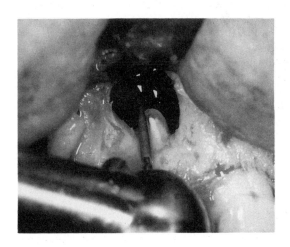

Figure 9.34 Smoothing of the resected root end with an ultrafine diamond.

These procedures achieve the desired result of a smooth root face without root-end-filling material covering the edges of the cavity surface interface, yet removal of the surface smear layer (Figure 9.36).

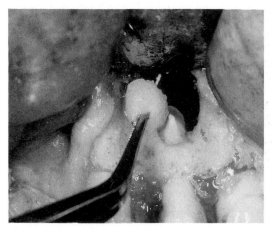

Figure 9.35 Burnishing of the resected root end with 10% citric acid.

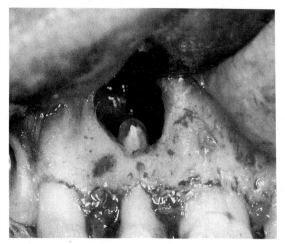

Figure 9.36 Finished root end prior to tissue closure. Note the smooth appearance of the root and root-end filling material.

Closure of the surgical site

When periradicular surgery has been performed and there is a stable buccal cortical plate of bone to protect the root structure and no evidence of marginal periodontitis, tissue closure is relatively straightforward. Intimate approximation of the healthy soft tissues and bone with sutures will suffice and healing will occur uneventfully. When there has been loss of the cortical bone, especially in the crestal region, or the presence of periodontal disease, the chances for long-term success are highly guarded.

The detection of bony dehiscences or large fenestrations should be made before surgery so that an alternative approach, e.g. guided tissue regeneration, is used (Figure 9.37) [63,95,97]. Endodontic surgery in the presence of marginal periodontitis also has a doubtful prognosis. The extensive use of root planing and curettage followed by acid conditioning is questionable in view of long-term success. Persistent periradicular inflammation following root-end surgery has been linked to the presence of marginal periodontitis at the time of surgery [111].

Prior to tissue-flap repositioning, the underside of the reflected tissue, the surrounding bone and the periradicular bone cavity should be inspected for debris. The surgical site is carefully flushed with saline. A radiograph is taken to ensure a clean surgical site and that the goals of surgery have been accomplished. Final irrigation with saline is often warranted, followed by tissue repositioning to the wound edges to ensure primary closure. Many clinicians will also apply gentle pressure to the repositioned tissue at this time to remove residual blood and to begin the intimate reattachment process.

Suturing will be necessary in all cases, with differing stitching available, e.g. interrupted, mattress, continuous or sling. Suturing always begins in the unattached mucosa and is carried into the attached tissues. Whilst there is no one formula for the number of sutures and their position, the clinician must

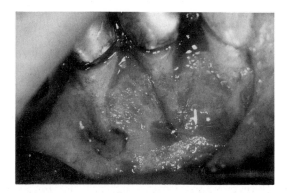

Figure 9.37 Loss of buccal cortical bone over the roots of two mandibular premolars with periradicular lesions. Correct treatment planning should be able to determine these defects prior to endodontic surgery.

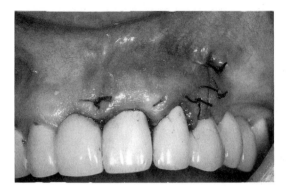

Figure 9.38 Close tissue flap approximation with minimal suturing and tissue damage.

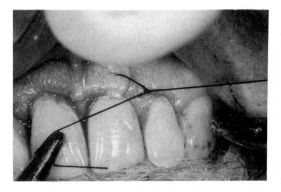

Figure 9.39 Suture knots must be kept away from the incision line to minimize infection of the wound.

exercise judgement in their placement to ensure adequate and stable positioning, especially in the crestal region. Vertical incisions may require anywhere from one to three sutures depending on the length and nature of the tissue (Figure 9.38).

Suture materials vary, with each having its own advantages and disadvantages. For years silk sutures have been favoured; the only disadvantage is the possibility of bacterial colonization. However, with proper suture placement, adequate cleaning of the surgical site by the patient and timely suture removal in 48–72 h, this problem is avoided. Gut sutures can also be used, but their handling characteristics can be a challenge. Recommended guidelines for soft-tissue closure following periradicular surgery include:

1. Silk sutures or synthetic sutures are universally acceptable.
2. Several needle sizes and shapes are often necessary due to osseous contours and tissue thickness. No single needle shape or radius is ideal for every situation. Thin tissue is often found along the vertical releasing incision and requires a small radius needle. Larger-radius needles are generally used in the horizontal incision.
3. Suture material size 4-0 is preferred; 3-0 may be too large and 5-0 may rip through the tissue.
4. Suture knots should always be placed away from the incision line to minimize microbial colonization in that area (Figure 9.39).

5. Sutured tissue should be routinely cleaned by the patient with chlorhexidine or warm saline rinses.
6. All sutures should be removed in 48–72 h.
7. Following suturing, the tissue must be compressed with firm finger pressure for 3–5 min to ensure correct tissue position, and a thin hiatus between the wound edges and a minimal blood clot between the bone and tissue flap (Figure 9.40). During this time, the patient can be given postoperative instructions.

Postoperative radiographic assessment

As previously indicated, a postoperative radiograph should be taken before closure of

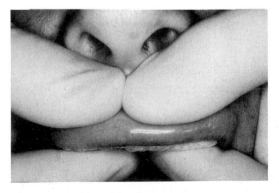

Figure 9.40 Compression of the tissue flap with gauze and light pressure is essential to minimize blood clot between tissue and cortical bone.

the surgical site. Mistakes can be rectified and procedures altered more easily at this point. In some cases, especially posterior teeth, several angled radiographs should be considered. Radiographs taken with specific film-holding devices are preferred. When review examination radiographs are taken with the same device, healing can be assessed more accurately. Some points for the clinician to consider are:

1. Is there scattered radiopaque material within the surgical site?
2. Are the correct root ends surgically obturated?
3. Do the root-end fillings appear adequate in depth and adaptation?
4. Are the fillings well condensed?
5. Is there unresected root structure, or have the wrong roots been inadvertently damaged?
6. Has root-end filling material been pushed into the maxillary sinus or mandibular canal?
7. Is there a fracture visible that was not seen clinically?

Postoperative patient instructions

When the soft tissues are properly managed and surgical time is minimized, healing is generally uneventful. Careful attention to postoperative instructions, however, is essential for patient comfort and tissue healing during the next few days. Postoperative instructions should be given verbally and supported in writing for the patient's easy reference:

1. Strenuous activity should be avoided, along with drinking alcohol and smoking.
2. An adequate diet consisting of fruit juices, soups, soft foods and liquid food supplements should be consumed. Avoid hard, sticky or chewy foods.
3. Do not tug at or unnecessarily lift the facial tissues.
4. Oozing of blood from the surgical site is normal for the first 24 h. Slight and transient facial swelling and bruising may be experienced.
5. Postsurgical discomfort is minimal but the surgical site will be tender and sore.

The use of analgesics for 24–48 h will help to alleviate this occurrence. Normally, continue with the analgesics given presurgically.
6. For the first day place ice packs with firm pressure directly on the face over the surgical site for 20 min and remove for 20 min. Repeat until retiring that evening.
7. The day following surgery and for the next 3–4 days, chlorhexidine rinses are used twice daily. Alternatively warm salt-water rinses are used every 1–2 h if possible (half a teaspoon of salt in a glass of water).
8. Sutures will be removed in 48–72 h.
9. Brushing of the surgical site is not recommended until the sutures are removed. Prior to that the surgical area can be cleaned using a large cotton puff or ball saturated with warm salt solution.
10. Telephone numbers are provided for your convenience should complications arise.

Postoperative examination and review

Re-examination of the patient, both clinically and radiographically, is normally scheduled at 6 months and 1 year. In most cases osseous repair is virtually complete at 1 year. Evidence of this as well as clinical healing has been considered as a valid criterion for continued success. Therefore, no additional follow-up may be necessary [51,59,112]. Failure to observe complete repair or delayed healing should warrant additional evaluation for as long as 4 years [107], until repair is evident, or signs and symptoms indicate failure.

Radiographic interpretation is highly variable and can easily be influenced by the quality and angulation of the film and processing irregularities. Therefore, the clinician should use a film-holding device for all follow-up radiographs. Likewise, familiarity with radiographic classifications of healing (success–failure) is essential [48,79,112]. This will enable case outcomes to be based on a sound, logical and consistent decision-making process [45].

Periradicular surgery of particular teeth

Maxillary anterior teeth

Surgical access to maxillary anterior teeth is relatively straightforward due to root position relative to the labial cortical bone. The lateral incisor may pose more of a challenge due to its common distopalatal root inclination and curvature. Deep osseous penetration is often necessary and the root apex may impinge on the palatal cortical plate of bone. Common also in this region is the excessively long canine that requires extensive soft-tissue elevation for access to the root end. Anatomical cross-sections after root-end resection usually reveal a round, oval or slightly oblong root outline with canals placed centrally on the root surface. Because the lateral incisor is commonly positioned to the palatal, both the buccal and palatal cortical plates of bone may be destroyed from advancing periradicular disease or surgical intervention. This usually leads to a greater frequency of scar tissue (incomplete healing) as opposed to complete bony repair.

Maxillary premolars

Surgical access to single-rooted premolars is also straightforward, with a minimal thickness of cortical plate covering the root apex. Complications generally occur when multiple roots are present, widely divergent in a bucco-palatal dimension, and/or the position of the maxillary sinus is such that penetration into the sinus cannot be avoided. Often, these roots have apices which have fenestrated the buccal cortex and access is relatively simple.

Resected root outlines are oval, oblong, dumbbell-shaped or round. In multiple-rooted premolars, canals are centrally placed and generally oval or circular on the resected root surface. In a two-canal, single-rooted premolar, two oval or round canals can be expected with a joining anastomosis. In this situation, the root-end cavity must encompass not only the canal openings but also the anastomosis, for which ultrasonic or sonic root-end preparation is indicated.

Maxillary molars

When buccal fenestrations exist, surgical access to the buccal roots of maxillary molars is easy. Depending on the position of the inferior border of the zygomatic process, extensive removal of bone may be necessary. Root outlines after resection are usually oval or circular for the distobuccal root and oblong, teardrop-shaped, figure-of-eight-shaped, or narrow and curved for the mesio-buccal root. This root has a high incidence of two canals with a joining anastomosis and therefore, all orifices on the resected root face must be identified. The mesiobuccal root is often thin in a proximal dimension, therefore care must be taken to avoid perforation during root-end cavity preparation.

Palatal root surgery is similar to the buccal, with some exceptions. Soft-tissue management is more difficult in reflection and retraction due to thickness of the palatal flap and an irregular surface of the cortical plate. Palatal roots have a tendency to curve to the buccal and the root is seldom fenestrated at the apex. This often implies that large amounts of bone must be removed in a site which has restricted access and visibility. Penetration into the sinus is not uncommon. The greater palatine nerve and vessels will invariably be encountered on the palatal root of a second molar. Resected root outlines are generally oval, round or oblong, with the canal placed centrally on the root surface.

Mandibular anterior teeth

Surgical access to the root apices of mandibular anterior teeth is often difficult because of lingual tooth inclination, wide buccolingual roots, thick cortical bone apically with increased amounts of cancellous bone between the cortex and root, and root dehiscences in the coronal half of the root. It is common for the root apices of mandibular incisors to be in close proximity to each other, which may pose problems in root-end management. Resected root outlines are narrow, oblong or figure-of-eight-shaped, with canal space on the resected root usually narrow mesiodistally and wide buccolingually. The incidence of two canals or joining canals on the root surface is high after root-end resection.

Mandibular premolars

Surgical access to mandibular premolars is usually direct, except for the occasional presence of significant muscle attachments in the soft tissues and the mental foramen in the bone. Surgical entry is often from a superior direction to avoid the foramen, which is most commonly close to the second premolar. The thickness of the cortical bone overlying the root apices is variable depending on tooth inclination in the arch. Root outlines are generally oval to oblong in a buccolingual dimension, with a small incidence of multiple canals exiting on the resected root surface; preoperative radiographs should warn of this possibility.

Mandibular molars

Surgical entry through the cortical plate to mandibular molars can be straightforward, but is more often complicated by limited access, shallow vestibule, thick cortical plates, external oblique ridge, root length, root position and inclination. Although the apices of molar roots are inclined buccally [10], the roots are often housed within thick cortical plates of bone. Additionally, individual root variations and curvatures often place the apices in positions difficult to reach. Therefore, these anatomical problems must be considered during treatment planning. Radiographic assessment is essential; the location of the mandibular canal must be identified through the use of angled films in a superior or inferior direction. Likewise proximally angled films will provide information about the number and curvature of roots.

Root outlines after resection are oval, dumbbell-shaped, oblong and wide in a buccolingual dimension. Canals often have joining anastomoses in both mesial and distal roots. The use of staining is strongly advised. Root-end cavities, by necessity, are oblong, encompassing the entire canal system as it exits on the resected root surface (Figure 9.30). Sonic or ultrasonic preparation of apical cavities is highly recommended.

General anatomical considerations

It is uncommon to penetrate the maxillary sinus during periradicular surgery. If this occurs, however, the opening must be protected to prevent the pushing of debris into the cavity during the management of the root end (Figure 9.41). This can be done with collagen-based haemostatic agents as previously mentioned. Bone wax should not be used because it can be pushed into the sinus and evoke a significant foreign-body giant-cell reaction along with delayed healing [37]. The postsurgical need for antibiotics or antihistamines has not been established [48]. Since primary closure can be achieved with soft-tissue repositioning and suturing, an effective seal is obtained, avoiding the need for drug therapy.

The mental foramen also poses a challenge for many clinicians. Discussion with the patient in the treatment-planning stage is essential to disclose the nature of the problem, the methods used to manage it and the potential for untoward postoperative sequelae. The best way to manage this entity is first to identify its position; second, to plan surgical entry away from it; third, to use the periosteal retractor to protect the foramen and its contents during surgery; fourth, to avoid pinching the soft tissues with the retractor.

An additional concern with all periradicular surgery is the presence of fenestrations and dehiscences, along with large penetrating periradicular lesions which have destroyed buccal and lingual cortical plates of bone [63,95,97]. Previous studies have identified less than favourable results when the surrounding bone has been compromised [54,112,121]. Management of these osseous defects often requires a guided tissue/bone regenerative procedure, which is becoming more popular. These situations should be diagnosed and treatment planned carefully; and when appropriate, consider help from experienced specialists.

Repair of perforation

Non-surgical repair of root perforations is reasonably successful [15,17,133,137], but

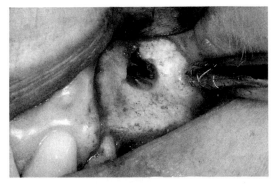

(a)

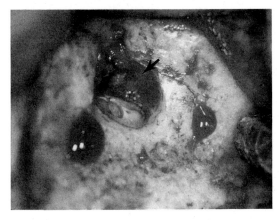

(b)

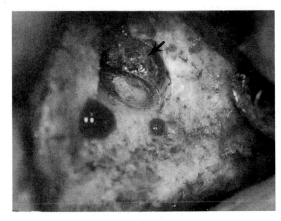

(c)

Figure 9.41 (a) Penetration into the maxillary sinus apical and distal to a premolar. (b) Blocking of the sinus perforation with a collagen sponge (arrow). Note root-end preparation and haemorrhage control around the resected apex. (c) Placement of the root-end filling (Diaket) in a moisture-free environment. Note that the collagen sponge is still in place (arrow). Collagen was left in place to serve as a matrix for closure of the sinus perforation.

when it fails or is impractical, surgery is necessary.

The surgical repair of root perforations is generally more difficult than root-end procedures. Perforations pose greater radiographic difficulties in identification, diagnosis and postsurgical assessment. Surgical management of perforated roots depends on access to the defect and the relationship of the perforation to crestal bone and the epithelial attachment.

Perforations occurring in the apical third pose the least problem in surgical management and are generally amenable to root-end resection [85,90,120]. Perforative defects to the mesial, distal or buccal can easily be seen and removed by root-end resection. If the perforation is to the palatal, sufficient root must be removed to eliminate the defect.

Mid-root perforations present a different set of challenges. Typically they are not in line with the coronal aspect of the canal, and may be identified by radiographs taken from different angles. Once identified surgically, they can be managed like any root end (Figures 9.42 and 9.43). Access to the defect margins, however, is more difficult when the perforation is located on the proximal surface of the root, and it is necessary to ensure complete marginal adaptation of the obturating material while preventing its placement into the surrounding bone (Figure 9.43). Access to lingual perforations is almost impossible on most teeth and other courses of treatment must be considered.

A common cause of perforation is due to post space preparation and placement. Often the post must be removed prior to root repair and a shorter post placed. In some cases the post may be ground down so that it lies inside the root. This is followed by placing a filling material. Because these types of perforations generally occur in anterior teeth, the use of amalgam to seal the perforation is not recommended because of tissue staining.

The prognosis for surgically repaired root perforations is based on a number of factors, similar to those for non-surgical repair of root perforations. Success is highly dependent on the following factors:

1. With any perforation in close proximity to the gingival sulcus, especially furcation perforations, the prognosis is very poor

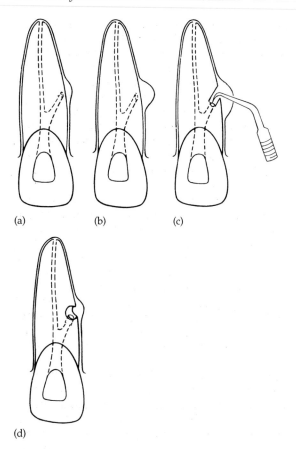

(a)   (b)   (c)

(d)

Figure 9.42 Access to a midroot proximal perforation. (a) Perforation; (b) access improved by careful removal of overlying bone; (c) creation of a cavity with an ultrasonic tip; (d) if necessary additional bone can be removed to enhance access to the defect.

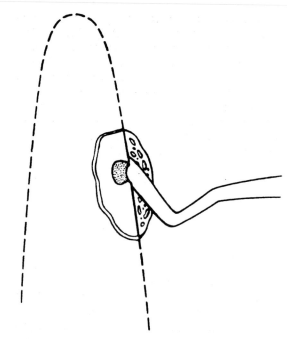

Figure 9.43 Repair of perforation. A flat plastic instrument or the convex side of a small curette is used to apply the filling material to the prepared cavity; it may also serve as a matrix, against which the filling material is condensed.

due to the potential for microbial contamination.

2. Microbial contamination of any perforation will lower its prognosis.
3. The use of any material which is cytotoxic will significantly reduce the prognosis. For example, the placement of phenolic compounds in the root canal after a perforation has occurred and before surgical repair will cause irreparable damage to the periodontium at the perforation site. Likewise, the use of a cytotoxic material to seal the perforation will cause tissue damage.
4. The success of perforation repair is highly dependent on sealing the defect with minimal to no excess material in the surgical site that may cause persistent inflammation and possibly stimulate root resorption. Likewise the seal of the perforation implies that the root canal system coronal to the perforation and the crown of the tooth are properly sealed.
5. The patient must maintain optimal oral hygiene in the area of any perforation repair.

Replantation

Replantation is defined as replacing a tooth in its socket following deliberate or traumatic avulsion. In the case of surgical or deliberate removal of a tooth and its replacement, it is defined as intentional replantation [6].

Few true indications exist for choosing intentional replantation as a primary method of treatment [48]. The presence of calcified canals, separated instruments, non-negotiable root canals, perforations, or anatomical closeness of, for example, the mandibular canal, are not valid indications for choosing intentional replantation. The patient's symptoms and signs, the strategic value of the tooth and the overall dental condition, including arch continuity, occlusion, function, tooth restorability and periodontal status, must be considered along with the patient's understanding and cooperation. Finally, awareness of the potential for adverse sequelae such as bone loss, tooth resorption and tooth fractures during extraction must be considered. When viewed from this perspective the only true indication for intentional replantation is when there is absolutely no other treatment available to maintain a strategic tooth [36,118,139]. Even then it is essential that all phases of this planned procedure be communicated to the patient, providing a realistic appraisal of the treatment plan, sequelae, prognosis and alternatives.

Once a decision has been reached to perform intentional replantation, all efforts should be taken to ensure removal of all tissue debris within the tooth. Root canals must be as clean as possible, canals obturated as far as possible and the access opening closed with a permanent restoration. Occlusal adjustments and teeth cleaning should also be performed.

Ideally a two-person team should perform the procedure, one to remove the tooth and the other to assess and fulfil the endodontic needs of the tooth. The surrounding tissue is disinfected with an antiseptic solution. Elevators should be carefully used to loosen the tooth, minimizing injuries to the soft tissue, bone and root. If necessary the extraction forceps can be wrapped with gauze to minimize damage to the root. Once removed, the tooth is grasped with gauze sponges soaked in sterile saline or it is held in the forceps under a continuous stream of saline. The socket is gently curetted to remove foreign debris. Care is exercised to avoid damage to the socket-retained periodontal fibres; gauze or cotton products should not be placed into the socket.

The extracted tooth is examined for fractures, extra roots or foramina, or any unusual anatomical configurations. Root ends are easily resected with a high-speed fine diamond bur under sterile saline. The nature of the canal system and its orifices are examined and, if necessary, apically prepared and obturated. This is done with a small round bur or inverted cone. Ultrasonic or sonic preparation may also be used. Time is of the essence with these procedures and all members of the team must be fully aware of their responsibilities and skilled in their execution.

When the tooth is ready to be replaced in its socket, the walls should be gently flushed with saline to remove the blood clot. Additionally the tooth is flushed to remove any residual cotton fibres or debris from the root-end filling material. The tooth is carefully and slowly teased into its original position in the socket, allowing for the slow escape of the blood that has built up in the socket. Slight pressure is applied to the buccal and lingual cortical plates to ensure adaptation. The occlusion is rechecked, and a splint is placed if necessary. Often only a periodontal pack is necessary. If a splint is used the tooth must be in physiological function. Convenient splints are made of soft, clear resin or nylon line which is acid-etched and cemented to the buccal surface. Splints are removed after 5–7 days.

The prognosis for intentionally replanted teeth is primarily dictated by the presence or absence of inflammatory and replacement resorption. Long-term studies provide mixed results with this technique: 50–60% success over a 5–10-year period. The reader is referred elsewhere for additional information [7,48].

Success and failure – aetiology and evaluation

Whilst many studies have attempted to determine success–failure rates for periradicular surgery, none have been able to integrate fully all parameters of evaluation with techniques performed, materials used, patient compliance and clinician expertise, variability and interpretative skills. Attempts at multivariate analysis have provided some trends and correlations, but even these findings may only be applicable to specifically controlled cases [112].

Success (complete healing) with periradicular surgery has been reported to range from 25% to 90% using mixed populations, less than ideal percentages of review examinations and minimal evaluation periods [48].

Because of the significant variability in results, comparison of studies is not possible. However, the identification of factors that have contributed to the success or failure of periradicular surgery is essential, and these should be integrated into all phases of case assessment and treatment [69]. Often the aetiology of failure may be difficult to identify and may encompass the integration of multiple factors. For periradicular surgery, most failures can be attributed to specific causes. At the same time, when failure cannot be explained, speculation may lead to uncertain aetiological factors and treatment. Table 9.5 lists aetiological factors often cited as valid or uncertain in the failure of periradicular surgery.

Evaluation of success or failure following root-end surgery is limited to clinical and radiographic examinations. Clinical criteria for success or failure are most commonly used and are integrated with the radiographic findings. Clinically patients are classified into one of three categories at the time of review examinations (Table 9.6). Patient assessment, however, must be made after integrating both clinical and radiographic parameters of evaluation (Table 9.7). If the only goal of periradicular surgery is to retain the tooth in adequate clinical function [119], then many cases can be classified as successful. Many factors, however, such as case selection, evaluator bias and patient factors, can skew

Table 9.5 Factors influencing success or failure of periradicular surgery

Valid causes for surgical failure
Failure to debride the root canal space thoroughly
Failure to seal the root canal space three-dimensionally
Tissue irritation from toxic root canal or root-end fillings
Failure to manage root canal or root-end materials properly
Superimposition of periodontal disease
Vertical root fracture
Recurrent cystic lesions
Improper management of the supporting periodontium

Uncertain causes for surgical failure
Infected dentinal tubules
Infected periradicular lesions
Failure to use antibiotics
Accessory or lateral canals
Loss of alveolar bone
Root resorption
Timing of root canal obturation (before or during surgery)
Type of root-end filling

Table 9.6 Clinical evaluation of success and failure

Clinical success
No tenderness to percussion or palpation
Normal mobility and function
No sinusitis or paraesthesia
No sinus tract or periodontal pocket
No infection or swelling
Adjacent teeth respond normally to stimuli
Minimal to no scarring or discoloration
No subjective discomfort

Clinical uncertainty
Sporadic vague symptoms
Pressure sensation or feeling of fullness
Low-grade discomfort on percussion, palpation or chewing
Discomfort with tongue pressure
Superimposed sinusitis focused on treated tooth
Occasional need to use analgesics

Clinical failure
Persistent subjective symptoms
Discomfort to percussion and/or palpation
Recurrent sinus tract or swelling
Evidence or irreparable tooth fracture
Excessive mobility or progressive periodontal breakdown
Inability to chew on the tooth

levels of success or failure. Likewise, many clinically symptom-free teeth may have histopathological changes at the root apices along with minimal or extensive radiographic changes. Even in the presence of an apparently normal radiographic appearance, a clinically symptom-free tooth may exhibit histopathological changes in the periradicular tissues. This is especially true adjacent to resected root surfaces which are difficult to assess radiographically.

Retreatment of surgical procedures

Not all surgery is successful. With astute case analysis the aetiological factors may be identified and further surgery performed. When this is not the case, some patients undergo multiple operations only to have persistent signs or symptoms of failure. Often these teeth will be extracted, or last-ditch efforts will be made with intentional replantation.

When a case has been identified as failing it is necessary to use all tests and information available to determine the cause before

Table 9.7 Radiographic evaluation of success and failure

Radiographic success
Normal periodontal ligament width or slight increase
Normal lamina dura or elimination of radiolucency
Normal to fine-meshed osseous trabeculae
No resorption evident

Radiographic uncertainty
Slight increase in periodontal ligament width
Slight increase in width of lamina dura
Size of radiolucency static or slight evidence of repair
Radiolucency is circular or asymmetrical
Extension of the periodontal ligament into radiolucency
Evidence of resorption

Radiographic failure
Increased width of the periodontal ligament and lamina
  dura
Circular radiolucency with limited osseous trabeculae
Symmetrical radiolucency with funnel-shaped borders
Evidence of resorption

further surgery is undertaken. Table 9.8 lists some of the more common unsuspected, anatomical and technical causes for failure. Not all of these causes are amenable to further surgery, and often a tooth may require extraction and prosthetic replacement.

Very few studies have evaluated the results of periradicular surgery that was performed

Table 9.8 Causes of surgical failure

Unsuspected
Root fracture not readily visible

Post-hole perforation, especially on the buccal or lingual
  surface

Instrument perforation coronal to the resected root end

Persistent infection in the apically resected tubules

Corrosion of previously placed amalgam root-end filling

Anatomical
Fenestrations or dehiscences – loss of marginal bone

Aberrant root anatomy or canal space

Proximity of root of adjacent teeth

Proximity of maxillary sinus

Technical
Poor canal cleaning and obturation

Inadequate root-end resection

Inadequate root-end preparation and obturation

Toxicity of root-end filling materials

Improper soft-tissue management

subsequent to previous surgical failure [86,111]. Success rates of repeat surgery have been 50% or less with little subsequent alteration in healing after 1 year. Even poorer results have been reported when the periradicular lesion at the time of the first surgery was >5 mm in diameter.

The primary reason for failure following periradicular surgery is the presence of necrotic tissue debris in uncleaned and obturated canal space [112]. The primary cause for failure with non-surgical root canal treatment has been identified as coronal leakage due to poor quality of the coronal restoration [104,116]. Therefore, it is essential to access, clean and obturate as much of the canal space as possible and to seal thoroughly the coronal aspects of the root canal system before resorting to surgical intervention. If this is not adhered to, failure will inevitably result.

References

1. AINAMO J, LÖE H (1966) Anatomical characteristics of gingiva. A clinical and microscopic study of the free and attached gingiva. *Journal of Periodontology* **37**, 5–13.
2. AKTENER BO, PEHLIVAN Y (1993) Sealing ability of cermet ionomer cement as a retrograde filling material. *International Endodontic Journal* **26**, 137–141.
3. AL-AJAM ADK, MCGREGOR AJ (1993) Comparison of the sealing capabilities of Ketac-silver and extra high copper alloy amalgam when used as retrograde root canal filling. *Journal of Endodontics* **19**, 353–356.
4. ALHADAINY HA, ELSAED HY, ELBAGHDADY YM (1993) An electrochemical study of the sealing ability of different retrofilling materials. *Journal of Endodontics* **19**, 508–511.
5. ALTONEN M, MATTILA K (1976) Follow-up study of apicoectomized molars. *International Journal of Oral Surgery* **5**, 33–40.
6. AMERICAN ASSOCIATION OF ENDODONTISTS (1994) *Glossary – Contemporary Terminology for Endodontics*, 5th edn, pp. 1–25. Chicago, IL, USA: American Association of Endodontists.
7. ANDREASEN JO (1992) *Atlas of Replantation and Transplantation of Teeth*, pp. 99–109. Fribourg, Switzerland: Mediglobe.
8. ANDREASEN JO, MUNKSGAARD EC, FREDEBO L, RUD J (1993) Periodontal tissue regeneration including cementogenesis adjacent to dentin-bonded retrograde composite filling in humans. *Journal of Endodontics* **19**, 151–153.

9. ANDREASEN JO, RUD J, MUNKSGAARD EC (1989) Retrograde root obturations using resin and a dentin bonding agent: a preliminary histologic study of tissue reactions in monkeys. *Danish Dental Journal* **93**, 195–197.

10. ARENS DE, ADAMS WR, DECASTRO RA (1981) *Endodontic Surgery*, pp. 31–55. Hagerstown, MD, USA: Harper & Row.

11. BARNES IE (1991) *Surgical Endodontics. A Colour Manual*. Oxford, UK: Butterworth-Heinemann.

12. BARRY GN, HEYMAN RA, ELIAS A (1975) Comparison of apical sealing methods. A preliminary report. *Oral Surgery, Oral Medicine, Oral Pathology* **39**, 806–811.

13. BEATTY R (1986) The effect of reverse filling preparation design on apical leakage. *Journal of Dental Research* **65**, 259 (abstract 805).

14. BELLIZZI R, LOUSHINE R (1991) *A Clinical Atlas of Endodontic Surgery*. pp. 13–15. Chicago, IL, USA: Quintessence.

15. BENENATI FW, ROANE JB, BIGGS JT, SIMON JH (1986) Recall evaluation of iatrogenic root perforations repaired with amalgam and gutta-percha. *Journal of Endodontics* **12**, 161–166.

16. BENNETT CR (1984) *Monheim's Local Anesthesia and Pain Control in Dental Practice*, 7th edn, pp. 181–182. St Louis, MO, USA: Mosby.

17. BIGGS JT, BENENATI FW, SABALA CL (1988) Treatment of iatrogenic root perforations with associated osseous lesions. *Journal of Endodontics* **14**, 620–624.

18. BOSTANCI HS, ARPAK MN, GUNHAN O (1990) New attachment formation following periodontal surgery in a dog. *Journal of Nihon University School of Dentistry* **32**, 159–166.

19. BOYKO GA, BRUNETTE DM, MELCHER AH (1980) Cell attachment to demineralized root surfaces *in vitro*. *Journal of Periodontal Research* **15**, 297–303.

20. BRÄNNSTRÖM M (1984) Smear layer: pathological and treatment considerations. *Operative Dentistry* (suppl 3), 35–42.

21. BRÄNNSTRÖM M, GLANTZ PO, NORDENVALL KJ (1979) The effect of some cleaning solutions on the morphology of dentin prepared in different ways: an *in vivo* study. *Journal of Dentistry for Children* **46**, 19–23.

22. BUCKLEY JA, CIANCIO SG, MCMULLEN JA (1984) Efficacy of epinephrine concentration in local anesthesia during periodontal surgery. *Journal of Periodontology* **55**, 653–657.

23. CALLIS PD, SANTINI A (1987) Tissue response to retrograde root fillings in the ferret canine: a comparison of glass ionomer cement and gutta-percha with sealer. *Oral Surgery, Oral Medicine, Oral Pathology* **64**, 475–479.

24. CAMBRUZZI JV, MARSHALL FJ (1983) Molar endodontic surgery. *Journal of the Canadian Dental Association* **49**, 61–65.

25. CARR GB (1994) Surgical endodontics. In: Cohen S, Burns R (eds) *Pathways of the Pulp*, 6th edn, pp. 531–567. St Louis, MO, USA: Mosby-Year Book.

26. CARRIGAN PJ, MORSE DR, FURST ML, SINAI IH (1984) A scanning electron microscopic evaluation of human dentinal tubules according to age and location. *Journal of Endodontics* **10**, 359–363.

27. CHONG BS, OWADALLY ID, PITT FORD TR, WILSON RF (1994) Antibacterial activity of potential retrograde root filling materials. *Endodontics and Dental Traumatology* **10**, 66–70.

28. CHONG BS, PITT FORD TR, WATSON TF (1993) Light-cured glass ionomer cement as a retrograde root seal. *International Endodontic Journal* **26**, 218–224.

29. CIANCIO SG, BOURGAULT PC (1989) *Clinical Pharmacology for Dental Professionals*, 3rd edn, pp. 146–148. Chicago, IL, USA: Year Book Medical.

30. CODELLI GR, FRY HR, DAVIS JW (1991) Burnished versus nonburnished application of citric acid to human diseased root surfaces: the effect of time and method of application. *Quintessence International* **22**, 277–283.

31. CRAIG KR, HARRISON JW (1993) Wound healing following demineralization of resected root ends in periradicular surgery. *Journal of Endodontics* **19**, 339–347.

32. CRIGGER M, RENVERT S, BOGLE G (1983) The effect of topical citric acid application on surgically exposed periodontal attachment. *Journal of Periodontal Research* **18**, 303–305.

33. CROOKS WG, ANDERSON RW, POWELL BJ, KIMBROUGH WF (1994) Longitudinal evaluation of the seal of IRM root end fillings. *Journal of Endodontics* **20**, 250–252.

34. DEGROOD ME, OGUNTEBI BR, CUNNINGHAM CJ, PINK R (1995) A comparison of tissue reactions to Ketac-Fil and amalgam. *Journal of Endodontics* **21**, 65–69.

35. DORN SO, GARTNER AH (1990) Retrograde filling materials: a retrospective success-failure study of amalgam, EBA, and IRM. *Journal of Endodontics* **16**, 391–393.

36. DUMSHA TC, GUTMANN JL (1985) Clinical guidelines for intentional replantation. *Compendium of Continuing Education in Dentistry* **6**, 604–608.

37. FINN MD, SCHOW RS, SCHNEIDERMAN ED (1992) Osseous regeneration in the presence of four common hemostatic agents. *Journal of Oral and Maxillofacial Surgery* **50**, 608–612.

38. FONG CD (1993) A sonic instrument for retrograde preparation. *Journal of Endodontics* **19**, 374–375.

39. FORSSELL H, TAMMISALO T, FORSSELL K (1988) A follow-up study of apicectomized teeth. *Proceedings of the Finnish Dental Society* **84**, 85–93.

40. GANGAROSA LP, HALIK FJ (1967) A clinical evaluation of local anaesthetic solutions containing graded epinephrine concentrations. *Archives of Oral Biology* **12**, 611–621.

41. GILHEANY PA, FIGDOR D, TYAS MJ (1994) Apical dentin permeability and microleakage associated with root end resection and retrograde filling. *Journal of Endodontics* **20**, 22–26.

42. GOLDBERG M (1984) Structures de l'email et de la dentine: effets d'agents demineralisants et incidences sur le collage de biomateriaux. *Actualites Odonto-Stomatologiques* **147**, 411–434.

43. GUTMANN JL (1984) Principles of endodontic surgery for the general practitioner. *Dental Clinics of North America* **28**, 895–908.

44. GUTMANN JL (1986) Surgical procedures in endodontic practice. In: Levine N (ed.) *Current Treatment in Dental Practice*, pp. 194–201. Philadelphia, PA, USA: Saunders.

45. GUTMANN JL (1992) Clinical, radiographic and histologic perspectives on success and failure in endodontics. *Dental Clinics of North America* **36**, 379–392.

46. GUTMANN JL (1993) Parameters of achieving quality anesthesia and hemostasis in surgical endodontics. *Anesthesia and Pain Control in Dentistry* **2**, 223–226.

47. GUTMANN JL, HARRISON JW (1985) Posterior endodontic surgery: anatomical considerations and clinical techniques. *International Endodontic Journal* **18**, 8–34.

48. GUTMANN JL, HARRISON JW (1994) *Surgical Endodontics*. St Louis, MO, USA: Ishiyaku EuroAmerica.

49. GUTMANN JL, PITT FORD TR (1993) Management of the resected root end: a clinical review. *International Endodontic Journal* **26**, 273–283.

50. GUTMANN JL, SAUNDERS WP, NGUYEN L, GUO IY, SAUNDERS EM (1994) Ultrasonic root-end preparation: part 1. SEM analysis. *International Endodontic Journal* **27**, 318–324.

51. HALSE A, MOLVEN O, GRUNG B (1991) Follow-up after periapical surgery: the value of the one-year control. *Endodontics and Dental Traumatology* **7**, 246–250.

52. HASSE AL, HENG MK, GARRET NR (1986) Blood pressure and electocardiographic response to dental treatment with use of local anesthesia. *Journal of the American Dental Association* **113**, 639–642.

53. HICKEL R (1988) Erste klinische Ergebnisse von retrograden Wurzelfüllungen mit Cermet-Zement. *Deutsche Zahnärztliche Zeitschrift* **43**, 963–965.

54. HIRSCH JM, AHLSTRÖM U, HENRIKSON PÅ, HEYDEN G, PETERSEN LE (1979) Periapical surgery. *International Journal of Oral Surgery* **8**, 173–185.

55. ICHESCO WR, ELLISON RL, CORCORAN JF, KRAUSE DC (1991) A spectrophotometric analysis of dentinal leakage in the resected root. *Journal of Endodontics* **17**, 503–507.

56. INGLE JI, BAKLAND LK. (1994) *Endodontics*, 4th edn, pp. 689–763. Malvern, PA, USA: Williams & Wilkins.

57. JASTAK JT, YAGIELA JA (1983) Vasoconstrictors and local anesthesia: a review and rationale for use. *Journal of the American Dental Association* **107**, 623–630.

58. JEANSONNE BG, BOGGS WS, LEMON RR (1993) Ferric sulfate hemostasis: effect on osseous would healing. II. With curettage and irrigation. *Journal of Endodontics* **19**, 174–176.

59. JESSLÉN P, ZETTERQVIST L, HEIMDAHL A (1995) Long-term results of amalgam versus glass ionomer cement as apical sealant after apicectomy. *Oral Surgery, Oral Medicine, Oral Pathology, Oral Radiology, Endodontics* **79**, 101–103.

60. JOHNSON SA (1991) Periradicular wound healing following the use of IRM as a root-end filling material. Thesis, Baylor University.

61. KADOHIRO G (1984) A comparative study of the sealing quality of zinc-free amalgam and Diaket when used as a retrograde filling material. *Hawaii Dental Journal* **15**, 8–9.

62. KEESLING GR, HINDS EC (1963) Optimal concentration of epinephrine in lidocaine solutions. *Journal of the American Dental Association* **66**, 337–340.

63. KELLERT M, CHALFIN H, SOLOMON C (1994) Guided tissue regeneration: an adjunct to endodontic surgery. *Journal of the American Dental Association* **125**, 1229–1233.

64. KHOURY F, SCHULTE A, BECKER R, HAHN T (1987) Prospektive Vergleichsstudie zwischen prä- und intraoperativer Wurzelfüllung. *Deutsche Zahnärztliche Zeitschrift* **42**, 248–250.

65. KHOURY F, STAEHLE HJ (1987) Retrograde Wurzelfüllungen aus Glasionomerzement. *Deutsche Zeitschrift fur Mund-, Kiefer-, und Gesichts-Chirurgie* **11**, 351–355.

66. KNOLL-KÖHLER E, FÖRTSCH G (1992) Pulpal anesthesia dependent on epinephrine dose in 2% lidocaine. *Oral Surgery, Oral Medicine, Oral Pathology* **73**, 537–540.

67. KNOLL-KÖHLER E, FRIE A, BECKER J, OHLENDORF D (1989) Changes in plasma epinephrine concentration after dental infiltration anesthesia with different doses of epinephrine. *Journal of Dental Research* **68**, 1098–1101.

68. LEMON RR, STEELE PJ, JEANSONNE BG (1993) Ferric sulfate hemostasis: effect on osseous wound healing. I. Left *in situ* for maximum exposure. *Journal of Endodontics* **19**, 170–173.

69. LIN LM, PASCON EA, SKRIBNER J, GÄNGLER P, LANGLELAND K (1991) Clinical, radiographic, and histologic study of endodontic treatment failures. *Oral Surgery, Oral Medicine, Oral Pathology* **71**, 603–611.

70. LLOYD A (1995) The combined effects of angulation of root-end resection using sonic retro-tips or burs on the linear leakage patterns of root-end filling materials. Cardiff: University of Wales College of Medicine, MScD thesis.

71. LUKS S (1956) Root end amalgam technic in the practice of endodontics. *Journal of the American Dental Association* **53**, 424–428.

72. MAALOUF EM, GUTMANN JL (1994) Biological perspectives on the non-surgical management of periradicular pathosis. *International Endodontic Journal* **27**, 154–162.

73. MACDONALD A, MOORE BK, NEWTON CW, BROWN CE (1994) Evaluation of an apatite cement as a root end filling material. *Journal of Endodontics* **20**, 598–604.

74. MALAMED SF (1990) *Handbook of Local Anesthesia*, 3rd edn, pp. 25–35. St Louis, MO, USA: Mosby-Year Book.

75. MÄLMSTROM M, PERKKI K, LUNDQUIST K (1982) Apicectomy: a retrospective study. *Proceedings of the Finnish Dental Society* **78**, 26–31.

76. MATTILA K, ALTONEN M (1968) A clinical and roentgenological study of apicoectomized teeth. *Odontologisk Tidskrift* **76**, 389–408.

77. MEYERS JP, GUTMANN JL (1994) Histological healing following surgical endodontics and its implications in case assessment: a case report. *International Endodontic Journal* **27**, 339–342.

78. MIZUNUMA T (1986) Relationship between bond strength of resin to dentin and structural change of dentin collagen during etching – influence of ferric chloride to structure of the collagen. *Journal of the Japanese Society of Dental Materials* **5**, 54–64.

79. MOLVEN O, HALSE A, GRUNG B (1987) Observer strategy and the radiographic classification of healing after endodontic surgery. *International Journal of Oral and Maxillofacial Surgery* **16**, 432–439.

80. MOLVEN O, HALSE A, GRUNG B (1991) Surgical management of endodontic failures: indications and treatment results. *International Dental Journal* **41**, 33–42.

81. MOOREHEAD FB (1927) Root-end resection. *Dental Cosmos* **69**, 463–467.

82. NEDDERMAN TA, HARTWELL GR, PORTELL FR (1988) A comparison of root surfaces following apical root resection with various burs: scanning electron microscope evaluation. *Journal of Endodontics* **14**, 423–427.

83. NENCKA D, WALIA HD, AUSTIN BP (1995) Histologic evaluation of the biocompability of Diaket. *Journal of Dental Research* **74**, 101 (abstract 716).

84. NERY EB, ESLAMI A, VAN SWOL RL (1990) Biphasic calcium phosphate ceramic combined with fibrillar collagen with and without citric acid conditioning in the treatment of periodontal osseous defects. *Journal of Periodontology* **61**, 166–172.

85. NICHOLLS E (1962) Treatment of traumatic perforations of the pulp cavity. *Oral Surgery, Oral Medicine, Oral Pathology* **15**, 603–612.

86. NORDENRAM Å, SVÄRDSTRÖM G (1970) Results of apicectomy. *Swedish Dental Journal* **63**, 593–604.

87. O'CONNOR RP, HUTTER JW, ROAHEN JO (1995) Leakage of amalgam and super-EBA root-end fillings using two preparation techniques and surgical microscopy. *Journal of Endodontics* **21**, 74–78.

88. OLSEN FK, AUSTIN BP, WALIA H (1994) Osseous reaction to implanted ZOE retrograde filling materials in the tibia of rats. *Journal of Endodontics* **20**, 389–394.

89. OLSON AK, MACPHERSON MG, HARTWELL GR, WELLER N, KULILD JC (1990) An *in vitro* evaluation of injectable thermoplasticized gutta-percha, glass ionomer, and amalgam when used as retrofilling materials. *Journal of Endodontics* **16**, 361–364.

90. OSWALD RJ (1979) Procedural accidents and their repair. *Dental Clinics of North America* **23**, 593–616.

91. OYNICK J, OYNICK T (1978) A study of a new material for retrograde fillings. *Journal of Endodontics* **4**, 203–206.

92. ÖZATA F, ERDILEK N, TEZEL H (1993) A comparative sealability study of different retrofilling materials. *International Endodontic Journal* **26**, 241–245.

93. PASHLEY DH (1984) Smear layer: physiological considerations. *Operative Dentistry* (suppl 3), 13–29.

94. PASSANEZI E, ALVES ME, JANSON WA, RUBEN MP (1979) Periosteal activation and root demineralization associated with horizontal sliding flap. *Journal of Periodontology* **50**, 384–386.

95. PECORA G, KIM S, CELLETTI R, DAVARPANAH M (1995) The guided tissue regeneration principle in endodontic surgery: one-year postoperative results of large periapical lesions. *International Endodontic Journal* **28**, 41–46.

96. PILEGGI R, DERMODY J, MCDONALD NJ, DIANDRETH M, TURNG BF, MINAH GE (1995) Apical leakage of ultrasonically cut retro-preparations: a bacterial evaluation. *Journal of Dental Research* **74**, 101 (abstract 718).

97. PINTO VS, ZUOLO ML, MELLONIG JT (1995) Guided bone regeneration in the treatment of a large periapical lesion: a case report. *Practical Periodontics and Aesthetic Dentistry* **7**, 76–82.

98. PITT FORD TR, ANDREASEN JO, DORN SO, KARIYAWASAM SP (1994) Effect of IRM root end fillings on healing after replantation. *Journal of Endodontics* **20**, 381–385.

99. PITT FORD TR, ANDREASEN JO, DORN SO, KARIYAWASAM SP (1995) Effect of super-EBA as a root end filling on healing after replantation. *Journal of Endodontics* **21**, 13–15.

100. PITT FORD TR, ROBERTS GJ (1990) Tissue response to glass ionomer retrograde root fillings. *International Endodontic Journal* **23**, 233–238.

101. POLSON AM, PROYE GT (1983) Fibrin linkage: a precursor for new attachment. *Journal of Periodontology* **54**, 141–147.

102. POWIS DR, FOLLERAS T, MERSON SA, WILSON AD (1982) Improved adhesion of a glass ionomer cement to dentin and enamel. *Journal of Dental Research* **61**, 1416–1422.

103. PRODGER TE, SYMONDS M (1977) ASPA adhesion study. *British Dental Journal* **143**, 266–270.

104. RAY HA, TROPE M (1995) Periapical status of endodontically treated teeth in relation to the technical quality of the root filling and the coronal restoration. *International Endodontic Journal* **28**, 12–18.

105. REGISTER AA (1973) Bone and cementum induction by dentin, demineralized *in situ*. *Journal of Periodontology* **44**, 49–54.

106. REGISTER AA, BURDICK FA (1975) Accelerated reattachment with cementogenesis to dentin, demi-

neralized *in situ*. I. Optimum range. *Journal of Perio-dontology* **46**, 646–655.

107. REIT C (1987) Decision strategies in endodontics: on the design of a recall program. *Endodontics and Dental Traumatology* **3**, 233–239.

108. RIRIE CM, CRIGGER M, SELVIG KA (1980) Healing of periodontal connective tissues following surgical wounding and application of citric acid in dogs. *Journal of Periodontal Research* **15**, 314–327.

109. ROBERTS DH, SOWRAY JH (1987) *Local Analgesia in Dentistry*, 2nd edn, pp. 84–88. Bristol, UK: Wright.

110. RUD J, ANDREASEN JO (1972) Operative procedures in periapical surgery with contemporaneous root filling. *International Journal of Oral Surgery* **1**, 297–310.

111. RUD J, ANDREASEN JO (1972) A study of failures after endodontic surgery by radiographic, histologic and stereomicroscopic methods. *International Journal of Oral Surgery* **1**, 311–328.

112. RUD J, ANDREASEN JO, MÖLLER JENSEN JE (1972) A multivariate analysis of the influence of various factors upon healing after endodontic surgery. *International Journal of Oral Surgery* **1**, 258–271.

113. RUD J, ANDREASEN JO, RUD V (1989) Retrograde root filling utilizing resin and a dentin bonding agent: frequency of healing when compared to retrograde amalgam. *Danish Dental Journal* **93**, 267–273.

114. RUD J, RUD V, MUNKSGAARD EC (1989) Retrograde root filling utilizing resin and a dentin bonding agent: indication and applications. *Danish Dental Journal* **93**, 223–229.

115. RUSE ND, SMITH DC (1991) Adhesion to bovine dentin – surface characterization. *Journal of Dental Research* **70**, 1002–1008.

116. SAUNDERS WP, SAUNDERS EM (1994) Coronal leakage as a cause of failure in root-canal therapy: a review. *Endodontics and Dental Traumatology* **10**, 105–108.

117. SAUNDERS WP, SAUNDERS EM, GUTMANN JL (1994) Ultrasonic root-end preparation: part 2. Microleakage of EBA root-end fillings. *International Endodontic Journal* **27**, 325–329.

118. SCOTT JN, ZELIKOW R (1980) Replantation – a clinical philosophy. *Journal of the American Dental Association* **101**, 17–19.

119. SELTZER S (1988) *Endodontology: Biologic Considerations in Endodontic Procedures*, 2nd edn, pp. 439–470. Philadelphia, PA, USA: Lea & Febiger.

120. SINAI IH (1977) Endodontic perforations: their prognosis and treatment. *Journal of the American Dental Association* **95**, 90–95.

121. SKOGLUND A, PERSSON G (1985) A follow-up study of apicoectomized teeth with total loss of the buccal bone plate. *Oral Surgery, Oral Medicine, Oral Pathology* **59**, 78–81.

122. SOMMER RF (1946) Essentials for successful root resection. *American Journal of Orthodontics and Oral Surgery* **32**, 76–100.

123. STASHENKO P (1990) Role of immune cytokines in the pathogenesis of periapical lesions. *Endodontics and Dental Traumatology* **6**, 89–96.

124. STERRETT JD, DELANEY B, RIZKALLA A, HAWKINS CH (1991) Optimal citric acid concentration for dentinal demineralization. *Quintessence International* **22**, 371–375.

125. SULTAN M, PITT FORD TR (1995) Ultrasonic preparation and obturation of root-end cavities. *International Endodontic Journal* **28**, 231–238.

126. TETSCH P (1974) Development of raised temperatures after osteotomies. *Journal of Maxillofacial Surgery* **2**, 141–145.

127. TETSCH P (1986) *Wurzelspitzenresektionen*, p. 99. Munchen, Germany: Carl Hanser Verlag.

128. TIDMARSH BG, ARROWSMITH MG (1989) Dentinal tubules at the root ends of apicected teeth: a scanning electron microscopic study. *International Endodontic Journal* **22**, 184–189.

129. TORABINEJAD M (1995) Investigation of mineral trioxide aggregate for root-end filling. PhD thesis. London: University of London.

130. TORABINEJAD M, HIGA RK, MCKENDRY DJ, PITT FORD TR (1994) Dye leakage of four root end filling materials: effects of blood contamination. *Journal of Endodontics* **20**, 159–163.

131. TORABINEJAD M, WATSON TF, PITT FORD TR (1993) Sealing ability of a mineral trioxide aggregate when used as a root end filling material. *Journal of Endodontics* **19**, 591–595.

132. TRICE FB (1959) Periapical surgery. *Dental Clinics of North America* **3**, 735–748.

133. TROPE M, TRONSTAD L (1985) Long-term calcium hydroxide treatment of a tooth with iatrogenic root perforation and lateral periodontitis. *Endodontics and Dental Traumatology* **1**, 35–38.

134. TROULLOS ES, GOLDSTEIN DS, HARGREAVES KM, DIONNE RA (1987) Plasma epinephrine levels and cardiovascular response to high administered doses of epinephrine contained in local anesthesia. *Anesthesia Progress* **34**, 10–13.

135. VERTUCCI FJ, BEATTY RG (1986) Apical leakage associated with retrofilling techniques: a dye study. *Journal of Endodontics* **12**, 331–336.

136. WALIA HD, NEWLIN S, AUSTIN BP (1995) Electrochemical analysis of retrofilling microleakage in extracted human teeth. *Journal of Dental Research* **74**, 101 (abstract 719).

137. WALIA H, STRIEFF J, GERSTEIN H (1988) Use of a hemostatic agent in the repair of procedural errors. *Journal of Endodontics* **14**, 465–468.

138. WANG T, NAKABAYASHI N (1991) Effect of 2-(methacryloxy)ethyl phenyl hydrogen phosphate on adhesion to dentin. *Journal of Dental Research* **70**, 59–66.

139. WEINE FS (1980) The case against intentional replantation. *Journal of the American Dental Association* **100**, 664–668.

140. WILLIAMS SS, GUTMANN JL (1993) Healing response to Diaket-tricalcium phosphate root-end fillings. *Journal of Endodontics* **19**, 199 (abstract 61).

141. WONG WS, ROSENBERG PA, BOYLAND RJ, SCHULMAN A (1994) A comparison of the apical seals

achieved using retrograde amalgam fillings and the Nd:YAG laser. *Journal of Endodontics* **20**, 595–597.

142. WUCHENICH G, MEADOWS D, TORABINEJAD M (1994) A comparison between two root end preparation techniques in human cadavers. *Journal of Endodontics* **20**, 279–282.

143. ZETTERQVIST L, ANNEROTH G, NORDENRAM A (1987) Glass-ionomer cement as retrograde filling material: an experimental investigation in monkeys. *International Journal of Oral and Maxillofacial Surgery* **16**, 459–464.

144. ZETTERQVIST L, HALL G, HOLMLUND A (1991) Apicectomy: a clinical comparison of amalgam and glass ionomer cement as apical sealants. *Oral Surgery, Oral Medicine, Oral Pathology* **71**, 489–491.

10

Endodontics in children

D.C. Rule and S. Patel

Introduction
Treatment of primary teeth
  Indirect pulp capping
  Direct pulp capping
  Coronal pulpotomy
  Formocresol pulpotomy
  Alternative pulpotomy medicaments
  Root canal treatment of non-vital primary
  teeth

Treatment of immature permanent teeth
  Treatment of vital teeth with open apices
  Treatment of non-vital teeth with open apices
  Surgical treatment
References

Introduction

The basic aims of endodontic treatment in children are similar to those for the adult patient: prevention and treatment of apical periodontitis. The relief of pain and the control of sepsis in the pulp and surrounding periradicular tissues are secondary aims. An additional consideration when deciding on a suitable treatment plan for primary teeth is the maintenance of arch length; it is generally accepted that primary molar teeth in particular should be retained until they are shed normally.

The treatment of pulp-involved permanent teeth with immature roots also presents special endodontic problems. Efforts should first be directed to maintaining pulp vitality where possible to allow root formation and maturation. Second, successful obturation of an immature root canal can be complicated.

Treatment of primary teeth

The primary teeth differ morphologically from their permanent successors in both shape and size [14]. Primary molars have fine tapered roots which are flattened mesio-distally to enclose a ribbon-like root canal. Their pulp chambers are relatively larger, and their enamel and dentine are thinner than in permanent teeth. The single root canal may become partially calcified with age [27], to produce several intercommunicating canals, thus making instrumentation of the radicular pulp space difficult. Many lateral canals exist in the furcations of primary molar teeth [61], and these may contribute to the early spread of infection from the pulp chamber to the interradicular area.

The diagnosis of pulp disease is especially difficult in young patients because not infrequently they are unable to give an accurate account of their symptoms. The diagnosis is dependent on the combination of a good history, clinical and radiographic examinations and special tests. The clinical examination should include looking for abnormal tooth mobility, discharging sinus tracts and tenderness to pressure. In primary teeth and newly erupted permanent teeth, assessment of vitality has been shown to be an unreliable guide to the histological status of the pulp [34,43]. Tests carried out with an electric pulp tester involve a gradually increasing current applied to the tooth and rely on conduction along nerve pathways. False-positive results are common, and care must be taken to avoid metal restorations. Extensively necrotic pulps may also still have intact nerve pathways. As with all non-invasive special investigations, the contralateral and adjacent teeth should be tested, preferably before the suspect tooth. This enables the young patient to have some experience of the sensation felt and may help to allay anxiety. Young patients may give a positive response in an attempt to please.

Recent developments in assessing pulp vitality include laser Doppler flowmetry and pulse oximetry. The former concept was originally developed to measure blood flow in skin and other organs [29], and later applied to testing pulp vitality [23]. The present equipment is expensive and the technique of use is time-consuming; specific versions for routine dental use are not yet available. Pulse oximetry originates from the concept of spectrophotometry and gives a reading of pulse rate and oxygen saturation. Both methods are still in experimental stages for vitality testing, but may play an important role for child patients in the future. Advantages include non-invasiveness, no resultant pain and direct assessment of blood flow in the pulp. In addition, no reliance is placed on patients to relate their feelings, and this is especially of benefit in children.

Preoperative radiographic examination is essential to eliminate local contraindications to root canal treatment, such as gross canal destruction, advanced internal or external root resorption and marked alveolar bone loss.

General contraindications to treatment may include poor patient cooperation and lack of parental motivation. A history of a cardiac or renal condition where it is essential to avoid infection may tip a decision towards extraction rather than retaining a pulpless tooth. Patients who have an impaired capacity to respond to infection such as those with a defective immune system will also need careful assessment.

The treatment techniques which have been advocated for use on primary teeth may be grouped as follows:

1. Indirect pulp capping.
2. Direct pulp capping.
3. Coronal pulpotomy (one or two visits).
4. Pulpectomy (one or two visits).

In all cases, the administration of local anaesthesia and adequate tooth isolation, normally with rubber dam, are advised. For maxillary teeth, infiltration anaesthesia is usually satisfactory, whereas a block injection or intraligamentary infiltration is more likely to eliminate pain when pulp treatment is carried out on vital mandibular primary molar teeth.

Indirect pulp capping

This is the term used to describe the placement of a sedative dressing over residual hard carious dentine in an attempt to allow irritation dentine to be formed within the pulp chamber [56]. Thus pulpal exposure is avoided in teeth with deep carious lesions when there is no clinical or radiographic evidence of pulpal degeneration or periradicular disease. Contraindications to this method of treatment include a history of spontaneous pain, associated swelling, tenderness to biting or mobility. Likewise, preoperative radiographs must be examined for root resorption, pulpal calcifications or periradicular radiolucency which, if present, would necessitate more extensive treatment.

At the initial visit, all soft carious dentine is removed with a slow running bur or a hand excavator. The amelodentinal junction must be free from all softened or stained carious dentine. The area of dentine over the site of a potential pulpal exposure is covered with a layer of setting cement containing calcium hydroxide (e.g. Dycal, Caulk, Milford, DE, USA) and sealed with an overlying structural base of a quick-setting reinforced zinc oxide–eugenol preparation (e.g. Kalzinol, Dentsply, Konstanz, Germany). The final restoration can then be placed. A success rate of 92% for indirect pulp capping with calcium hydroxide in primary incisors followed for 42 months has been reported [6]. Hence, for primary teeth, regular review of vitality is preferable to subjecting the patient to subsequent re-entry into the tooth, as was formerly advocated. Some operators prefer to use a zinc oxide–eugenol preparation alone for indirect pulp capping [30].

Direct pulp capping

Direct pulp capping is the application of a material directly on to pulp tissue which has been exposed as a result of cavity preparation or by traumatic injury. This aims to encourage formation of an irritation dentine bridge below the exposure site, and to maintain pulpal vitality. It is recommended that this technique is reserved for treatment of clean traumatic pulpal exposures. The exposure site should be gently irrigated with a non-irritant solution, e.g. saline, to remove any infected debris which may impede healing and also to keep the pulp moist. The capping material should be flowed gently over the exposure and allowed to set. Various capping materials have been employed. Calcium hydroxide, used alone or together with zinc oxide–eugenol, has been most widely investigated [53,59]. Other materials, e.g. antibiotic and steroid preparations, polycarboxylate cement and formocresol, have also been used, without notable success. The final restoration should be a stainless-steel crown to minimize subsequent microleakage and prevent fracture of the tooth.

Coronal pulpotomy

This technique involves removal of the entire coronal pulp which has undergone irreversible inflammatory change or necrosis, leaving remaining vital tissue intact. The cut radicular pulp stumps are covered with a medicament which will result in either healing or fixation of the tissue beyond the interface of dressing and radicular pulp. Pulpotomy provides the most suitable method for treating carious exposures in primary teeth without a history of swelling, sinus tract or any evidence of internal or external root resorption.

Recent literature has implicated the use of lasers [55] and electrosurgery [35] for pulpotomy procedures; the main advantage being

the avoidance of potentially toxic medicaments. When electrosurgery was used to remove the entire coronal pulp and treat the remaining stumps, root resorption occurred [57]. An alternative method may be to remove the coronal pulp mechanically and treat the remaining pulp stumps electrosurgically [50], in order to avoid excessive heat dissipation. Although a clinical and radiographic success rate of 99% has been demonstrated at 2 years [35], the electrosurgical pulpotomy technique is still experimental.

Formocresol pulpotomy

Buckley [5] formulated a solution containing equal parts of formalin and tricresol. A commercial solution containing 19% formaldehyde, 35% cresol in a glycerine/water vehicle (Buckley's formocresol, Cosby Laboratories, Burbank, CA, USA), was later developed as a suitable medicament for the treatment of pulpally exposed primary teeth. The aim of this treatment technique is to fix the coronal portion of the radicular pulp and maintain vitality of the remaining apical portion [58]. Formocresol acts through its aldehyde group and binds to the amino acids of protein and bacteria to prevent autolysis and hydrolysis, so rendering tissue inert [32]. The use of formocresol for pulpotomy has recently been reviewed [60].

Over the years, there has been increasing concern about the toxicity, both local and systemic, of formocresol. Sufficient formocresol has been absorbed systemically from multiple pulpotomy sites in one dog to induce early tissue injury in the kidneys and liver [44–46]. However, with the quantity normally used in humans, the risk is negligible. A definite relationship between formocresol pulpotomies in primary teeth and enamel defects on their permanent successors has been demonstrated [47], but not confirmed in subsequent studies [42,49]. In addition, carcinogenic and mutagenic properties have been recognized which, together with local and systemic effects, have led to extensive investigation of the efficacy of a diluted solution. Clinical studies have confirmed that a 1 : 5 dilution is equally effective and should be used routinely [17,41].

The solution may be prepared by first making up a diluent solution of three parts glycerine with one part distilled water. To this is then added one part concentrated formocresol, and mixed thoroughly.

One-visit formocresol pulpotomy

Originally, a three- to five-stage procedure was described [58,60], but since the 1960s it has become preferable to complete the pulpotomy procedure in a single visit [48], provided adequate analgesia has been achieved. The one-visit formocresol pulpotomy (Figure 10.1) entails the application of a pledget of cotton wool moistened with the medicament to the cut pulp stumps, after removal of the coronal pulp and arrest of haemorrhage. The pledget is left *in situ* for 3–5 min, although a 1-min application has been recommended [31]. Following this, the amputated pulp tissue appears black. A zinc oxide–eugenol dressing is then prepared and pressed into the chamber, before final restoration of the tooth with a stainless-steel crown. It is unnecessary to incorporate formocresol into this zinc oxide–eugenol sub-base [2]. A clinical success rate of 94% in pulpotomized primary teeth using a one-fifth diluted formocresol solution followed-up for 4–36 months has been achieved [17].

Two-visit formocresol pulpotomy

With this technique (Figure 10.1), the formocresol pledget is sealed in the pulp chamber for a period of 1 week, and at the second visit the procedure is completed as for the one-visit pulpotomy. This may be preferable for uncooperative patients as appointment times are reduced, or in cases where a hyperaemic pulp is encountered, or adequate analgesia has not been achieved.

Whichever technique is used, the final restoration of choice is a full-coverage stainless-steel crown, as this minimizes the risks of fracture and microleakage, and hence enhances the prognosis.

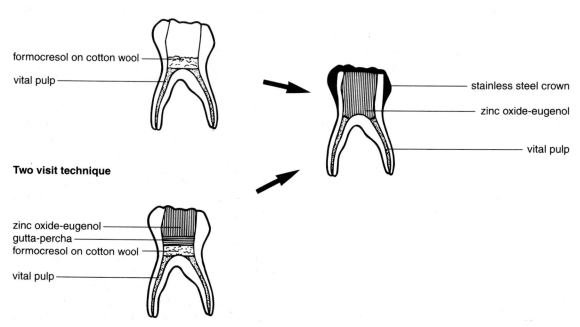

One visit technique

formocresol on cotton wool

vital pulp

stainless steel crown

zinc oxide-eugenol

vital pulp

Two visit technique

zinc oxide-eugenol
gutta-percha
formocresol on cotton wool

vital pulp

Figure 10.1 Formocresol pulpotomy for a primary molar with vital pulp in the root canals. It may be performed as a one-visit or two-visit procedure.

Alternative pulpotomy medicaments

Glutaraldehyde

Glutaraldehyde has been investigated as an alternative fixing medicament to formocresol because of its low toxicity [54]. Glutaraldehyde is a larger molecule than formaldehyde, and as a result diffusion through the tissues is reduced. When 2% unbuffered glutaraldehyde was used, over 96% clinical success was reported after 42 months [21,22]. A 90% clinical success rate was achieved after 1 year, when 2% buffered glutaraldehyde had been applied for 5 min [19]. After 2 years there was a failure rate of 18%, as a result of internal resorption [18].

Although glutaraldehyde is potentially a possible replacement for formocresol, questions are still being raised about its safety [60]. On a weight-for-weight basis there is little difference in toxicity between formocresol and glutaraldehyde [13].

Ferric sulphate

Ferric sulphate is commonly used in dentistry for control of bleeding during surgery or for gingival retraction. When applied directly to pulp tissue, a ferric ion–protein complex is formed which blocks the cut vessels mechanically. Although not a fixative, having only bacteriostatic properties, ferric sulphate is used to control haemorrhage by gentle intermittent application. A zinc oxide–eugenol base is then used to cover the pulp stumps, prior to restoration. A better clinical success rate was reported after 1 year when 15.5% ferric sulphate was used compared with 1 : 5 diluted formocresol [12]. In a more recent study there was no difference between the two medicaments [15]. Despite these promising results, this relatively new technique must be subjected to further clinical investigation with a longer follow-up period.

Calcium hydroxide

Although the application of pure calcium hydroxide to the cut pulp stumps after haemorrhage control was previously favoured for pulpotomy of primary teeth [3], the work of Magnusson [36] cast doubt on the use of this material in primary teeth. However, later studies indicate that if a carefully controlled technique is used then calcium hydroxide may produce long-term results which are comparable with those obtained when formocresol is used [53,59].

Root canal treatment of non-vital primary teeth

Non-vital primary teeth may be retained successfully when this technique is employed. Pulpal necrosis, alveolar swelling, interradicular or periradicular radiolucency are not contraindications to treatment; root canal treatment provides the most satisfactory method of retaining the restorable primary tooth where extraction remains the only other option. The whole procedure can be completed in one visit where there is no abscess, or over two visits when acute discharge is present. In this situation, a pledget of formocresol should be sealed into the pulp chamber for 1 week, after canal preparation, and prior to obturation. There is no consensus as to the preferred filling material, but absorbable materials based on zinc oxide–eugenol, calcium hydroxide and iodoform paste have been used [31].

Once any initial pain or swelling has been relieved, an access cavity is prepared under rubber dam isolation. The use of local anaesthesia is recommended as some vital tissue could still be encountered in one of the root canals. Any pulp tissue in the root canals is removed using fine barbed broaches, or files, and the canals are gently filed to within 2 mm of the apices using Hedstrom files. Dilute sodium hypochlorite solution should be used to irrigate the canals and achieve chemical dissolution of any remaining pulp. Finally, the canals should be flushed thoroughly and dried.

The chosen filling material should be mixed to a creamy consistency and carried into the canals using a pressure syringe, spiral root canal filler or, if mixed to a stiffer consistency, packed into the canal with a plugger. Various filling techniques, including using a spiral filler and the Jiffy tube pressure syringe, have been compared for filling root canals of primary teeth, with the spiral filler performing best [1]. After root canal filling, the pulp chamber should be packed with a suitable cement, and the tooth restored with a stainless-steel crown. A recent study compared pulpectomies using zinc oxide–eugenol and KRI paste in 139 primary molars [28]. Both pastes were introduced into root canals with a Lentulo spiral filler. The follow-up period extended between 6 months and 7 years, with the overall success rate for KRI paste being better than that for zinc oxide–eugenol.

Pulpectomy can also be considered to be an alternative to current pulpotomy techniques when treating vital primary teeth with carious exposure, as it eliminates the need for potentially toxic aldehyde-containing compounds, and can be completed in one visit.

Treatment of immature permanent teeth

Current treatment strategies for immature teeth in which the pulp has been exposed are conservative, and have as their ultimate objective the maintenance of vitality of the radicular pulp to allow root formation to be completed. It is essential to assess the restorability of the tooth and to assess the patient orthodontically.

Treatment of vital teeth with open apices

Traumatic pulp exposure in an immature permanent tooth with a good blood supply leads initially to local haemorrhage in the tissue immediately beneath the exposure site, followed by superficial inflammation. The wound is subsequently covered with fibrin [33]. If the inflamed tissue is removed to a level where healthy pulp is encountered, a dressing of calcium hydroxide placed over the cut pulp will ultimately cause induction of hard tissue and dentine formation by newly differentiated odontoblasts [52].

Pulpotomy

This may be performed at various levels, depending on the size of the exposure and the condition of the pulp observed at the initial exposure site. The classical operation (Figure 10.2) refers to the removal of the coronal pulp to the cervical region with a slowly rotating steel bur [37].

Partial (or Cvek) pulpotomy

A more conservative approach to pulpotomy in those cases where a small exposure is found has been proposed [24]. In this technique (Figure 10.2) the pulp immediately adjacent to the exposure site should be

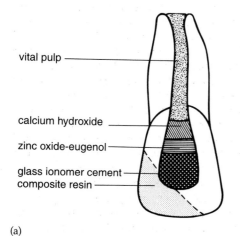

vital pulp

calcium hydroxide

zinc oxide-eugenol

glass ionomer cement
composite resin

(a)

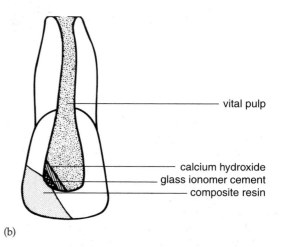

vital pulp

calcium hydroxide
glass ionomer cement
composite resin

(b)

Figure 10.2 (a) Coronal pulpotomy for an immature incisor with extensive damage to the coronal pulp. (b) Partial pulpotomy when pulp damage is superficial.

removed to a depth of 2 mm with an adequately cooled diamond bur in a turbine handpiece. This partial amputation is followed by irrigation with saline and arrest of haemorrhage with cotton-wool pledgets or blunt-ended paper points. If bleeding at the exposure site cannot be controlled, this suggests that inflamed pulp tissue remains; therefore a further deeper cut should be performed. Calcium hydroxide powder mixed with water to form a stiff paste (or a calcium hydroxide base material) is placed against the cut pulp tissue, before restoring the tooth with a fortified zinc oxide–eugenol cement and/or glass ionomer covered by composite resin retained by etched enamel. Within 6–8 weeks, calcific tissue is usually evident adjacent to the site of pulp amputation [4].

The size of the pulpal exposure and the interval between accident and treatment are not critical for healing, hence extensive exposures for long periods of time are no longer a contraindication to pulpotomy in immature permanent incisors [8]. A success rate of over 90% has been reported in other studies [16,20], where permanent teeth were treated by pulpotomy, with the time elapsing between trauma and treatment varying from 1 to 14 days.

The tooth should be kept under review clinically and radiographically at 6 months, and then at annual intervals to assess continued pulp vitality and normal root development. Calcification within the root canal may be observed, but this is no longer an indication for the removal of the remaining pulp tissue followed by root canal treatment.

Partial pulpotomy in carious immature teeth

Treatment of a pulp exposed by caries in a newly erupted permanent tooth is a problem for which extraction is often no longer an appropriate solution. New methods have been developed to maintain pulp vitality allowing continued root development. When calcium hydroxide was used for pulpotomy in immature posterior teeth with carious exposures, a high frequency of pulpal healing was reported [38]. Removal of the superficial layer of the pulp beneath the exposure site, with a diamond bur in a turbine handpiece, is recommended. The wound is then dressed

with calcium hydroxide following haemostasis, and sealed with zinc oxide–eugenol cement before an overlying restoration is placed. Although promising, further studies are required before this treatment can be recommended for routine clinical use [38].

Treatment of non-vital teeth with open apices

The object of endodontic treatment for non-vital teeth with immature roots is essentially the same as that for conventional root canal treatment, namely to produce a filling which seals the canal system by means of laterally or vertically condensed gutta-percha in conjunction with a root canal sealer. However, in immature incisor teeth, the root canal may diverge towards the apex and is oval in cross-section, with a greater labiopalatal than mesiodistal dimension. The apical foramen is patent to varying degrees, from nearly closed to a widely divergent or 'blunderbuss' type. The walls of the root canal are often very thin in the case of a newly erupted immature tooth, and may be further weakened during mechanical preparation of the root canal. In addition, a relatively short root presents an adverse crown : root ratio for the subsequent coronal restoration.

Theoretical considerations suggest that continued root growth with histologically normal dentine and cementum is only possible in those cases where the epithelial root sheath of Hertwig has retained its function. Thus, when a chronically infected immature tooth is treated, the only type of root-end closure that may be anticipated is calcific occlusion. This has been shown to be the result of dystrophic calcifications, formed within apical granulation tissue, which coalesce to form a corporate mass, continuous with the predentine at the root apex [11]. However, some teeth which do not respond to conventional vitality-testing techniques are shown to have vital tissue towards the root apex when instrumentation is carried out within the root canal. For practical purposes, the treatment in each case is virtually identical – to clean the root canal and to deliver calcium hydroxide to within 1–2 mm of the root apex so as to encourage either root growth or apical repair [51]. The tooth is opened on the palatal aspect to give wide access to the root canal, and necrotic tissue removed with barbed broaches or files to within 1 mm of the root apex. The walls of the canal may then be gently cleaned using either hand files or an ultrasonically operated file. It is important at this stage to avoid disruption of the apical tissues, so all instrumentation should be carefully controlled short of the apical foramen.

Various irrigating solutions have been recommended to remove debris and necrotic tissue. While sterile water or saline has been used and has least potential for damage to the periradicular tissues, a 2.5% solution of hypochlorite has been recommended as having a proven antibacterial effect [25,39]. However, when 5% hypochlorite was compared with 0.5% hypochlorite or saline [10], the hypochlorite solutions reduced the bacterial count more effectively than saline, but periapical healing was significantly impaired by use of 5% hypochlorite. A solution of ≤2% hypochlorite is now recommended [40].

After irrigation and drying with paper points, the root canal is filled with a thick aqueous slurry of calcium hydroxide or a commercial product (e.g. Hypocal, Elman, New York, NY, USA). Calcium hydroxide is now widely recommended as the sole root canal dressing (Figure 10.3) [25]. The quality of canal filling with calcium hydroxide should be checked radiographically, before sealing the access cavity with a fortified zinc oxide–eugenol cement. The patient should be reviewed at 1, 3, 6 and 12 months. It has been usual to replace the dressing at these appointments but current practice is to do so only if radiographic evidence of dissolution of the dressing has occurred [25], or the temporary filling has failed. The better condensed the initial dressing, the less likely it is that it will need to be replaced. The time taken for a mechanically detectable calcific barrier to form has been shown to vary between 9 and 18 months [7,62].

When a barrier appears to have formed radiographically, the tooth should be re-isolated and opened and the dressing should be washed out and dried, prior to checking for apical closure by probing with a file. The root canal should be filled with gutta-percha and sealer, using a condensation technique which fills the canal both laterally and apically. The available filling techniques are customized gutta-percha points, lateral condensation, vertical condensation and thermoplastic delivery (Figure 10.3) [25,26].

The prognosis for root-filled immature teeth depends on the degree of immaturity of the root. The thinner the root canal walls, the more likely fracture is to occur [9].

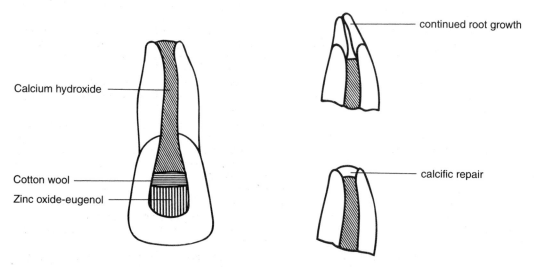

Figure 10.3 Root canal treatment of a non-vital immature tooth. Following canal cleaning, the root canal is filled with calcium hydroxide. Either continued root growth or calcific repair may occur.

Surgical treatment

If attempts to induce root-end closure are ultimately unsuccessful, as for example when a persisting sinus tract is present, then a surgical approach is indicated. In an apprehensive child it may be necessary to carry this out under sedation or general anaesthesia; and consent for all eventualities should be obtained. Surgery may be necessary to look for a vertical root fracture; if present, the tooth would need to be extracted. When surgery is to be undertaken, the root canal is normally filled with gutta-percha beforehand, and the end of the root canal filling trimmed flush with the root end during surgery, or if the thin root walls are sufficiently thick, a root-end filling can be placed. A further alternative is to use a 'through-and-through' technique. Further details of endodontic surgery are given in Chapter 9.

References

1. AYLARD SR, JOHNSON R (1987) Assessment of filling techniques for primary teeth. *Pediatric Dentistry* **9**, 195–198.
2. BEAVER HA, KOPEL HM, SABES WR (1966) The effect of zinc oxide-eugenol on a formocresolized pulp. *Journal of Dentistry for Children* **33**, 381–396.
3. BERK H (1950) Effect of calcium-hydroxide methyl cellulose paste on the dental pulp. *Journal of Dentistry for Children* **17**, 65–68.
4. BRÄNNSTRÖM M, NYBORG H, STRÖMBERG T (1979) Experiments with pulp capping. *Oral Surgery, Oral Medicine, Oral Pathology* **48**, 347–352.
5. BUCKLEY JP (1904) A rational treatment for putrescent pulps. *Dental Review* **18**, 1193–1197.
6. COLL JA, JOSELL S, NASSOF S, SHELTON P, RICHARDS MA (1988) An evaluation of pulpal therapy in primary incisors. *Pediatric Dentistry* **10**, 178–184.
7. CVEK M (1972) Treatment of non-vital permanent incisors with calcium hydroxide. I. Follow-up of periapical repair and apical closure of immature roots. *Odontologisk Revy* **23**, 27–44.
8. CVEK M (1978) A clinical report on partial pulpotomy and capping with calcium hydroxide in permanent incisors with complicated crown fracture. *Journal of Endodontics* **4**, 232–237.
9. CVEK M (1992) Prognosis of luxated non-vital maxillary incisors treated with calcium hydroxide and filled with gutta-percha. A retrospective clinical study. *Endodontics and Dental Traumatology* **8**, 45–55.
10. CVEK M, NORD CE, HOLLENDER L (1976) Antimicrobial effect of root canal debridement in teeth with immature roots. A clinical and microbiologic study. *Odontologisk Revy* **27**, 1–10.
11. DYLEWSKI JJ (1971) Apical closure of nonvital teeth. *Oral Surgery, Oral Medicine, Oral Pathology* **32**, 82–89.
12. FEI AL, UDIN RD, JOHNSON R (1991) A clinical study of ferric sulfate as a pulpotomy agent in primary teeth. *Pediatric Dentistry* **13**, 327–332.
13. FEIGAL RJ, MESSER HH (1990) A critical look at glutaraldehyde. *Pediatric Dentistry* **12**, 69–71.
14. FINN SB (1973) *Clinical Pedodontics*, 4th edn, p. 217. Philadelphia, PA, USA: Saunders.
15. FUKS A, HOLAN G, DAVIS J, EIDELMAN E (1994) Ferric sulfate versus diluted formocresol in pulpotomized primary molars: preliminary report. *Pediatric Dentistry* **16**, 158–159 (abstract).
16. FUKS AB, BIELAK S, CHOSAK A (1982) Clinical and radiographic assessment of direct pulp capping and pulpotomy in young permanent teeth. *Pediatric Dentistry* **4**, 240–244.
17. FUKS AB, BIMSTEIN E (1981) Clinical evaluation of diluted formocresol pulpotomies in primary teeth of school children. *Pediatric Dentistry* **3**, 321–324.
18. FUKS AB, BIMSTEIN E, GUELMANN M, KLEIN H (1990) Assessment of a 2 percent buffered glutaraldehyde solution in pulpotomized primary teeth of schoolchildren. *Journal of Dentistry for Children* **57**, 371–375.
19. FUKS AB, BIMSTEIN E, KLEIN H (1986) Assessment of a 2% buffered glutaraldehyde solution in pulpotomized primary teeth of school children: a preliminary report. *Journal of Pedodontics* **10**, 323–330.
20. FUKS AB, CHOSACK A, KLEIN H, EIDELMAN E (1987) Partial pulpotomy as a treatment alternative for exposed pulps in crown-fractured permanent incisors. *Endodontics and Dental Traumatology* **3**, 100–102.
21. GARCIA-GODOY F (1983) Clinical evaluation of glutaraldehyde pulpotomies in primary teeth. *Acta Odontologica Pediatrica* **4**, 41–44.
22. GARCIA-GODOY F (1986) A 42 month clinical evaluation of glutaraldehyde pulpotomies in primary teeth. *Journal of Pedodontics* **10**, 148–155.
23. GAZELIUS B, OLGART L, EDWALL B, EDWALL L (1986) Non-invasive recording of blood flow in human dental pulp. *Endodontics and Dental Traumatology* **2**, 219–221.
24. GRANATH LE, HAGMAN G (1971) Experimental pulpotomy in human bicuspids with reference to cutting technique. *Acta Odontologica Scandinavica* **29**, 155–163.
25. GUTMANN JL, HEATON JF (1981) Management of the open apex. 2. Non-vital teeth. *International Endodontic Journal* **14**, 173–178.
26. GUTMANN JL, RAKUSIN H (1987) Perspectives on root canal obturation with thermoplasticized injectable gutta-percha. *International Endodontic Journal* **20**, 261–270.
27. HIBBARD ED, IRELAND RL (1957) Morphology of the root canals of the primary molar teeth. *Journal of Dentistry for Children* **24**, 250–257.

28. HOLAN G, FUKS AB (1993) A comparison of pulpectomies using ZOE and KRI paste in primary molars: a retrospective study. *Pediatric Dentistry* **15,** 403–407.

29. HOLLOWAY GA (1983) Laser doppler measurement of cutaneous blood flow. In: Rolfe P (ed.) *Noninvasive Physiological Measurements,* vol 2, pp. 219–249. London, UK: Academic Press.

30. KING JB, CRAWFORD JJ, LINDAHL RL (1965) Indirect pulp capping: a bacteriologic study of deep carious dentine in human teeth. *Oral Surgery, Oral Medicine, Oral Pathology* **20,** 663–671.

31. KOPEL HM (1994) Pediatric endodontics. In: Ingle JI, Bakland LK (eds) *Endodontics,* 4th edn, pp. 835–867. Malvern, PA, USA: Williams and Wilkins.

32. LOOS PJ, HAN SS (1971) An enzyme histochemical study of the effect of various concentrations of formocresol on connective tissues. *Oral Surgery, Oral Medicine, Oral Pathology* **31,** 571–585.

33. LUOSTARINEN V (1971) Dental pulp response to trauma. An experimental study in the rat. *Suomen Hammaslaakariseuran Toimituksia* **67,** (suppl 2), 3–74.

34. MCDONALD RE (1956) Diagnostic aids and vital pulp therapy for deciduous teeth. *Journal of the American Dental Association* **53,** 14–22.

35. MACK RB, DEAN JA (1993) Electrosurgical pulpotomy: a retrospective study. *Journal of Dentistry for Children* **60,** 107–114.

36. MAGNUSSON B (1970) Therapeutic pulpotomy in primary molars – clinical and histological follow up. 1. Calcium hydroxide paste as wound dressing. *Odontologisk Revy* **21,** 415–431.

37. MALONE AJ, MASSLER M (1952) Fractured anterior teeth – diagnosis treatment and prognosis. *Dental Digest* **58,** 442–447.

38. MEJÀRE I, CVEK M (1993) Partial pulpotomy in young permanent teeth with deep carious lesions. *Endodontics and Dental Traumatology* **9,** 238–242.

39. MENTZ TCF (1982) The use of sodium hypochlorite as a general endodontic medicament. *International Endodontic Journal* **15,** 132–136.

40. MOORER WR, WESSELINK PR (1982) Factors promoting the tissue dissolving capability of sodium hypochlorite. *International Endodontic Journal* **15,** 187–196.

41. MORAWA AP, STRAFFON LH, HAN SS, CORPRON RE (1975) Clinical evaluation of pulpotomies using dilute formocresol. *Journal of Dentistry for Children* **42,** 360–363.

42. MULDER GR, VAN AMERONGEN WE, VINGERLING PA (1987) Consequences of endodontic treatment of primary teeth. Part II. A clinical investigation into the influence of formocresol pulpotomy on the permanent successor. *Journal of Dentistry for Children* **54,** 35–39.

43. MUMFORD JM (1967) Pain perception threshold on stimulating teeth and the histological condition of the pulp. *British Dental Journal* **123,** 427–433.

44. MYERS DR, PASHLEY DH, WHITFORD GM, MCKINNEY RV (1983) Tissue changes induced by the absorption of formocresol from pulpotomy sites in dogs. *Pediatric Dentistry* **5,** 6–8.

45. MYERS DR, PASHLEY DH, WHITFORD GM, SOBEL RE, MCKINNEY RV (1981) The acute toxicity of high doses of systemically administered formocresol in dogs. *Pediatric Dentistry* **3,** 37–41.

46. MYERS DR, SHOAF HK, DIRKSEN TR, PASHLEY DH, WHITFORD GM, REYNOLDS KE (1978) Distribution of 14C-formaldehyde after pulpotomy with formocresol. *Journal of the American Dental Association* **96,** 805–813.

47. PRUHS RJ, OLEN GA, SHARMA PS (1977) Relationship between formocresol pulpotomies on primary teeth and enamel defects on their permanent successors. *Journal of the American Dental Association* **94,** 698–700.

48. REDIG DF (1968) A comparison and evaluation of two formocresol pulpotomy techniques using Buckley's Formocresol. *Journal of Dentistry for Children* **35,** 22–30.

49. ROLLING I, POULSEN S (1978) Formocresol pulpotomy of primary teeth and occurrence of enamel defects on the permanent successors. *Acta Odontologica Scandinavica* **36,** 243–247.

50. RUEMPING DR, MORTON TH, ANDERSON MW (1983) Electrosurgical pulpotomy in primates – a comparison with formocresol pulpotomy. *Pediatric Dentistry* **5,** 14–18.

51. RULE DC, WINTER GB (1966) Root growth and apical repair subsequent to pulpal necrosis in children. *British Dental Journal* **120,** 586–590.

52. SCHRODER U, GRANATH LE (1971) On internal dentine resorption in deciduous molars treated by pulpotomy and capped with calcium hydroxide. *Odontologisk Revy* **22,** 179–188.

53. SCHRÖDER U, SZPRINGER-NODZAK M, JANICHA J, WACIŃSKA M, BUDNY J, MLOSEK K (1987) A one-year follow–up of partial pulpotomy and calcium hydroxide capping in primary molars. *Endodontics and Dental Traumatology* **3,** 304–306.

54. 'S-GRAVENMADE EJ (1975) Some biochemical considerations of fixation in endodontics. *Journal of Endodontics* **1,** 233–237.

55. SHOJI S, NAKAMURA M, HORIUCHI H (1985) Histopathological changes in dental pulps irradiated by CO_2 laser: a preliminary report on laser pulpotomy. *Journal of Endodontics* **11,** 379–384.

56. SHOVELTON DS (1972) The maintenance of pulp vitality. *British Dental Journal* **133,** 95–101.

57. SHULMAN ER, MCIVER FT, BURKES EJ (1987) Comparison of electrosurgery and formocresol as pulpotomy techniques in monkey primary teeth. *Pediatric Dentistry* **9,** 189–194.

58. SWEET CA (1930) Procedure for treatment of exposed and pulpless deciduous teeth. *Journal of the American Dental Association* **17,** 1150–1153.

59. TURNER C, COURTS FJ, STANLEY HR (1987) A histological comparison of direct pulp capping agents in

primary canines. *Journal of Dentistry for Children* **54,** 423–428.

60. WATERHOUSE PJ (1995) Formocresol and alternative primary molar pulpotomy medicaments: a review. *Endodontics and Dental Traumatology* **11,** 157–162.

61. WINTER GB (1962) Abscess formation in connexion with deciduous molar teeth. *Archives of Oral Biology* **7,** 373–379.

62. YATES JA (1988) Barrier formation time in non-vital teeth with open apices. *International Endodontic Journal* **21,** 313–319.

11

Endodontic aspects of traumatic injuries

T.R. Pitt Ford amd T.M. Odor

Introduction

This chapter is principally concerned with the endodontic aspects of traumatic injuries to the teeth, and does not set out to cover traumatology comprehensively. Injuries may occur for many different reasons. In infancy and the preschool group, falls are the most common cause. This continues in the early school years, but in the teenage years many injuries are due to sports. Boys are affected twice as often as girls, and there are peak incidences of injuries at 2–4 years and at 8–10 years [8]. A good history and thorough examination are essential if dental injuries are to be properly managed. The management of patients following a traumatic injury can be classified as:

1. Immediate.
2. Short-term.
3. Long-term.

History, examination and immediate management

A dental injury should always be treated as an emergency. Immediate treatment will help to relieve pain, allowing repositioning of displaced teeth and for treatment priorities to be determined.

A full account of when, where and how the injury occurred must be recorded [30]. Knowing how the injury occurred gives some indication of the type and extent of injury. The place of injury can indicate possible contamination of the wounds and the need for tetanus prophylaxis; it may also have legal implications.

The time interval between injury and presentation can influence choice of treatment, and is critical to the success of replantation of avulsed teeth.

Any period of unconsciousness, amnesia, headache, nausea or vomiting may indicate cerebral involvement, and the patient should therefore be immediately referred for medical examination and appropriate care [30].

At examination, any previous treatment as well as previous injuries must be recorded. Disturbances to the occlusion should be investigated, as these may indicate jaw fracture or condylar displacement. Thermal sensitivity of the teeth may be a consequence of exposed dentine or pulp. The medical history must be reviewed in case antibiotic prophylaxis is required, or there may be bleeding or other problems.

The clinical examination should include assessment of the soft tissues and facial skeleton. Any soft-tissue injury should be noted and the possible presence of a foreign body considered; radiographic examination may be necessary to locate this. Injuries to the oral mucosa should be investigated, especially bleeding from the gingival sulcus; lacerations may occur with displaced teeth, whereas bleeding from a non-lacerated gingival margin may indicate periodontal damage. The teeth should next be examined for infractions or fractures. Pulpal exposures should be noted along with any colour changes. Lost pieces of fractured teeth should be accounted for, in case they are embedded in soft tissue or have been swallowed or inhaled. Mobility and percussion testing should be carried out as they can indicate damage to the periodontal ligament. Reactions to pulp testing of permanent teeth should be recorded; immediately after trauma teeth may not respond, but the results of tests provide a baseline for later comparison. A negative response to vitality testing *per se* does not indicate a need for root canal treatment, as some pulps may recover. Research using laser Doppler flowmetry has shown blood flow in traumatized teeth some time ahead of pulps responding to electric pulp testing [33]. At present laser Doppler flowmetry is not a technique suitable for routine use in general dental practice.

Radiographic examination of permanent teeth should include a paralleling-technique periapical film of each affected tooth using a film-holder to standardize projections for later comparison. For luxation injuries a further film with the tube rotated mesially

(or distally) is often helpful [3]. In addition, if the maxillary incisor region is involved, an occlusal film may also be used, as two views at different vertical angles are better able to demonstrate a root fracture. For primary teeth an occlusal film alone is usually sufficient.

A systematic approach to examination is important; however, if there is severe bleeding, respiratory problems or unconsciousness, their management becomes the first priority. The replantation of avulsed permanent teeth is also a high priority in the period immediately after trauma.

Any inconsistencies between the history and the injuries sustained, particularly if accompanied by late presentation, should alert one to the possibility of non-accidental injury.

Following a thorough examination, a diagnosis should be made for each tooth injured. If one tooth has been avulsed, it is likely that the adjacent ones will also have sustained some trauma.

Soft-tissue injuries may need to be sutured after careful cleaning, and in the case of the lips, possible removal of tooth fragments could be required. Avulsed permanent teeth should be replanted into sockets which have been irrigated of blood clot, and should then be splinted. Luxated teeth should be repositioned and splinted. These injuries are covered in more detail later.

As the patient and parent are frequently very upset, it is often prudent to delay non-urgent treatment to another visit. However, if the patient is not very distressed and the dental injuries are not severe, then pulpotomy or covering exposed dentine could be carried out at the initial appointment.

Short-term management

This is carried out some days after injury, when the swelling and soreness have subsided. It consists of covering exposed dentine or pulpotomy where appropriate, if these have not already been done, removal of sutures and pulpal extirpation in the case of avulsion or intrusion of mature teeth with fully formed apices. Splints may be removed 1–2 weeks after placement following luxation or avulsion. Further details on procedures and timings are given in the respective sections later.

Long-term management

The pulps of traumatized teeth, particularly those with mature roots at the time of injury, are at risk of dying, or in some cases not revascularizing following infarction. It is therefore necessary to monitor pulpal status in the weeks and months after injury by systematic testing for signs of pulp survival, revascularization or death. Where there has been damage to the clinical crown, a potential route for infection of the pulp exists. Thus it is important to provide a satisfactory long-term restoration to prevent late pulp death. Teeth with immature roots which have been intruded or replanted following avulsion are at risk of replacement or inflammatory resorption, and therefore need careful and regular monitoring, with prompt intervention if inflammatory resorption becomes evident.

Types of injury

Anterior teeth are usually damaged by direct blows that may result in fractures which are horizontal or oblique [8]. Often more than one tooth is affected, and the types of injury which they have suffered are likely to differ. In children, trauma to anterior teeth commonly affects sound teeth, which frequently have large pulps and wide dentinal tubules, so any injury which exposes dentine can potentially damage the pulp; therefore early treatment is necessary. Direct trauma may cause the following damage:

1. Infraction of enamel.
2. Fracture of enamel.
3. Fracture of dentine.
4. Fracture exposing the pulp.
5. Crown-root fracture.
6. Intra-alveolar root fracture.
7. Subluxation or luxation.
8. Intrusion.
9. Avulsion.

A blow to the mandible may cause vertical fracture of the cusps of posterior teeth, ranging from minimal loss of hard tissue to crown-root fracture.

Tissues damaged

Trauma to the teeth may cause damage to the dental hard tissues, the pulp, the supporting tissues or to any combination; there are specific consequences to damage to each of these. First, loss of enamel creates potential routes for infection of the pulp, as well as any cosmetic disfigurement. Second, the pulp may lose its blood supply and hence vitality as a result of concussion, luxation or intrusion; in the case of avulsion it may also become infected. Third, the cementum on the tooth surface may be damaged by luxation, intrusion or avulsion; the natural repair mechanism involves limited resorption, which ought not to be of serious consequence. However, where there is extensive damage to the cementum, ankylosis (replacement resorption) is a frequent complication, and is virtually untreatable. If infection complicates damage to cementum, then inflammatory resorption of dentine may rapidly occur, particularly with immature teeth. With replanted immature teeth the pulp is often the site of infection, and the inflammatory resorption can be effectively halted by thorough canal cleaning followed by obturation with calcium hydroxide [23].

Management of primary teeth

Infractions and coronal fractures

Young children may not be very cooperative, particularly after a traumatic injury in which the soft tissues are sore, swollen and bruised; therefore immediate treatment may need to be limited to doing the minimum, such as smoothing sharp edges. If the pulp has been exposed, a partial pulpotomy and restoration should be carried out if there is sufficient cooperation; if there is not, extraction of the tooth is indicated. The technique of pulpotomy is covered in the section on permanent teeth.

Intra-alveolar root fracture

This may occur in primary teeth, but is much less common than in permanent teeth. Management is generally observation. If the coronal fragment is very loose and at risk of being inhaled, or pulpal infection occurs, extraction is indicated; however the apical fragment is normally left *in situ* to resorb naturally and to avoid surgical damage to the developing permanent tooth.

Luxation or intrusion

In general a conservative approach to management is adopted with primary teeth. Intruded teeth will usually re-erupt spontaneously. If there is concern that a displaced primary tooth has damaged the developing permanent tooth then it should be extracted atraumatically. If a luxated tooth interferes with the occlusion, it should be repositioned or extracted; where there is a danger of inhalation, immediate extraction is indicated. Pulpal damage is a frequent complication of luxation injuries, and as a result primary teeth may discolour. Immediate discoloration indicates bleeding in the pulp and the possibility of repair. Later-developing discoloration that is generally a darkening of the tooth signifies pulp necrosis, while later discoloration that is a yellowing of the tooth indicates pulp canal obliteration. Where discoloration is caused by pulp canal obliteration, no intervention is required. However, where discoloration is caused by pulp necrosis, and there is an associated abscess, root canal treatment or extraction should be carried out; root canal treatment of primary teeth has been covered in Chapter 10.

Avulsion

Replantation of avulsed primary teeth is not normally carried out because of the potential risk of damage to the developing permanent

tooth from infection of the pulp of the primary tooth.

Management of permanent teeth

Infractions and fracture of enamel

Infraction of enamel rarely requires operative treatment, but the pulpal status should be monitored for several years in case the pulp which might have suffered as a result of concussion or subluxation does not recover, and subsequently shows evidence of necrosis. Where there is clear evidence of pulp necrosis, confirmed by more than one test, root canal treatment is indicated. A lack of a positive response to electric pulp testing or discoloration on their own provides insufficient evidence to remove a pulp.

Loss of a small amount of enamel does not normally require restorative treatment; any sharp edge may be smoothed for comfort or appearance. Loss of a larger amount of enamel requires its replacement by composite resin retained by etched enamel either because dentine is exposed or to improve appearance.

The likelihood of pulp canal obliteration or pulp necrosis occurring is low for both enamel infractions and enamel fractures [36]. The chance of pulp damage is increased if there is associated subluxation of the tooth [34].

Fracture of dentine

Fractures involving dentine open up numerous dentinal tubules, which frequently become very sensitive. If left untreated, bacterial plaque will grow on the exposed surface and cause pulpal inflammation, which may in time lead to pulp necrosis. The early placement of a restoration prevents permanent pulp damage and relieves sensitivity. The use of composite resin retained by etched enamel restores the appearance and does not hinder subsequent monitoring of pulp vitality (Figure 11.1). In recent years fractured fragments have been reattached with composite resin retained by etched enamel; the longevity of

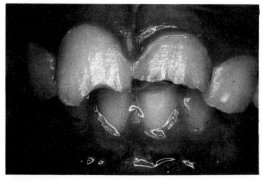

(a)

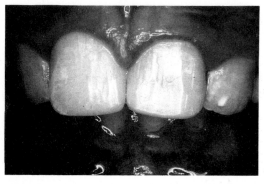

(b)

Figure 11.1 (a) Fractured incisal edges of maxillary central incisors exposing dentine. (b) Restoration of incisal edges using composite resin retained by etched enamel.

such restorations is acceptable [8]. Immediately after trauma the exposed dentine may be covered with glass ionomer cement as a temporary measure, especially if there is no piece of tooth to put back in place, or there is insufficient time or cooperation to place a permanent restoration in composite resin.

The likelihood of pulp canal obliteration or pulp necrosis occurring is also low following fractures involving dentine [36,40]. The chance of pulp damage is increased if there is associated subluxation of the tooth [34].

Fracture exposing the pulp

Immature tooth

If this type of injury occurs in a young patient whose tooth has an immature root, then treatment is directed at maintaining pulp vitality to allow continued root formation; this considerably improves the long-term prognosis of the tooth by reducing the risk of subsequent root fracture [13]. The pulp can usually be treated conservatively as it has a good blood supply and rarely becomes necrotic [12,25]. Although pulp capping may be suitable treatment, partial pulpotomy is the treatment of choice, particularly when there is any delay [12,20,21,24]. The advantages of partial pulpotomy over pulp capping are that inflamed pulp tissue is removed, the pulp dressing is placed in a cavity and can be covered by a protective base, and adjacent infected dentine is removed.

It is necessary to give a local anaesthetic in order to carry out pulpotomy. The tooth must be isolated with rubber dam to exclude salivary contamination; retention of rubber dam on an immature tooth is facilitated by a suitable clamp (e.g. Ash EW, Dentsply, Weybridge, UK). Pulp removal is confined to the superficial 2 mm since removal of deeper pulp tissue is normally unnecessary. The pulp is best removed with a bur in the turbine handpiece using copious waterspray [24]; it creates less damage than a bur at low speed or use of an excavator. A 2-mm deep cavity is created in the fractured dentine surface, with the periphery of the cavity floor on dentine (Figure 11.2). After arrest of haemorrhage, the wound is covered by calcium hydroxide (either a slurry which is subsequently compressed and dried with cotton wool or a hard-setting base material may be used). A lining of fortified zinc oxide–eugenol should be placed over the calcium hydroxide material to prevent subsequent bacterial contamination, which has been shown to cause pulpal inflammation and necrosis. The tooth is restored with composite resin retained by etched enamel; glass ionomer cement may be placed over the zinc oxide–eugenol cement to prevent any adverse effect of the eugenol on the resin. The tooth should be reviewed at least annually for several years to ensure continued pulp vitality by regular pulp testing and continued root formation by examination of radiographs. Should the restoration fail, it must be replaced immediately to stop infection of the pulp via the pulpotomy site, since the hard tissue barrier is frequently porous [24]. This treatment has a high rate of success

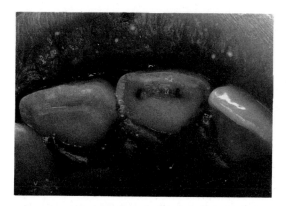

(a)

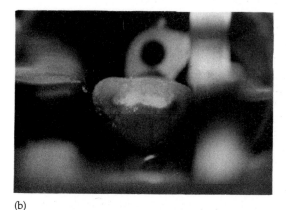

(b)

Figure 11.2 (a) Maxillary right central incisor with a fracture involving the pulp. (b) After placement of a hard-setting calcium hydroxide material in the partial pulpotomy preparation.

when it is correctly performed; the pulp remains alive and healthy [12,20,24]. There is no need for root canal treatment subsequent to partial pulpotomy, unless the pulp becomes infected [14].

At one time coronal pulpotomy, involving removal of the entire coronal pulp, was recommended [32]; however it is difficult to perform, causes the tooth to be weak at its neck, and can result in pulp canal obliteration or necrosis [12,24]. It has largely been superseded by partial pulpotomy. In circumstances where the entire clinical crown of an immature tooth has been lost, coronal pulpotomy is indicated to allow root formation to continue and to provide sufficient tooth structure on which to place a restoration.

Mature teeth

In the case of a mature tooth where tooth fracture extends into the pulp, conservative treatment by partial pulpotomy should still be considered as the first treatment option. However, where the entire clinical crown has been lost or the tooth has had an associated luxation injury, more radical treatment consisting of pulpal extirpation, root canal filling and construction of a post crown is indicated.

Crown-root fracture

In this type of extensive tooth fracture, the coronal fragment is usually retained by a limited amount of periodontal ligament, and the pulp is frequently exposed. Crown-root fractures can be very difficult to treat, particularly if the fracture line is a long way subgingival on the palatal aspect. When the patient first presents, the coronal fragment is often loose and painful to bite on. It is usually necessary to give local anaesthesia to allow removal of the fragment and to assess the extent of the fracture.

In the case of an immature tooth with a minimal amount of root loss, coronal pulpotomy may be carried out (as described above). Where loss of the root is more extensive, the tooth will be difficult to restore long term and is likely to have a poor prognosis. In some cases it may be possible to extrude the tooth orthodontically, otherwise extraction will need to be considered.

In a mature tooth where the fracture is superficial, it will be possible to carry out root canal treatment and restore the tooth by a post crown. If the fracture is deeper, it will be difficult to isolate the tooth for root canal treatment, and orthodontic extrusion of the root will need to be considered to improve the periodontal condition before restoration by a post crown [8,26]. When the fracture is very deep, there may be too little root remaining to support a restoration even after orthodontic extrusion; such teeth are also more likely to fail subsequently [18]. Where the prognosis is very poor, extraction of the remaining root should be considered along with appropriate immediate replacement and long-term prostheses (denture, bridge or implant).

Intra-alveolar root fracture

Intra-alveolar root fractures are relatively uncommon, and fortunately often occur without the complication of contamination by bacteria from the mouth. Immediately post-trauma, teeth with root fractures may be mobile and slightly extruded. The teeth should be examined carefully for periodontal injuries which communicate between the mouth and the fracture; these substantially reduce the prognosis.

Diagnosis of intra-alveolar root fracture is frequently made by exclusion of clinical signs of other traumatic injury, and by radiographic examination with films taken at different tube angulations. This type of root fracture is more easily observed on an occlusal film rather than a paralleling technique film (Figure 11.3), because the X-ray beam passes through rather than across the fracture. Treatment consists of repositioning the tooth in its correct position, checking the position with a radiograph, and then splinting for 2–3 months. Splinting is easily achieved by using a polymeric material with wire reinforcement, retained by etched enamel [8]. The purpose of the splint is to prevent excessive movement of the coronal fragment and to improve the long-term prognosis for the pulp.

The tooth should be reviewed clinically and radiographically at the time of intended splint removal; in the absence of periodontal breakdown, the splint should be removed. Pulp vitality should be checked. Where a vital response is obtained, the tooth should be reviewed again at 1 year. Where no vital response is obtained, and there is no radiographic evidence of periradicular inflammation, no tenderness to palpation or a sinus tract, pulp testing should be carried out at 3-monthly intervals either until a response

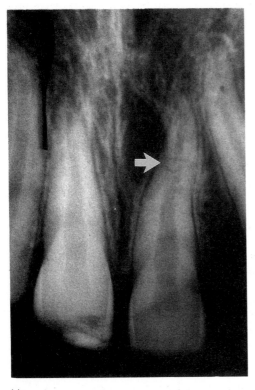

(a)

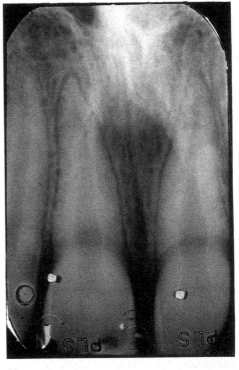

(b)

Figure 11.3 (a) Part of an occlusal radiograph more easily demonstrates an intra-alveolar root fracture (arrow) of the left maxillary central incisor than (b) a paralleling technique radiograph of the same tooth, on which the fracture is very difficult to observe.

occurs or until other evidence of pulp necrosis appears. Teeth that have fractures remote from the gingival sulcus have the best long-term prognosis (Figure 11.4).

The most favourable response is uniting of the two fragments by hard tissue laid down both in the root canal and on the root surface. A less favourable but still satisfactory outcome may occur when the coronal fragment has not been adequately repositioned; there is continued pulp vitality in the coronal fragment but no union of the fragments. The sharp end of the tooth is rounded by remodelling, and bone is formed between the fragments. Often the pulp in the coronal fragment calcifies and radiographically gives an appearance of an obliterated pulp space [4], however the pulp responds to vitality testing [2,9,39]. Pulp canal obliteration is not an indication for root canal treatment [8,28].

Pulp necrosis occurs in a minority of intra-alveolar root-fractured teeth and is related to initial coronal displacement, coronal position of the fracture, lack of splinting and maturity of the root [4,9,39]. Pulp necrosis is invariably confined to the coronal fragment [9]. As well as the loss of response to thermal and electrical stimuli, there is frequently a radiolucency of the bone around the tooth at the fracture line (Figure 11.5). Root canal treatment should be carried out in the coronal fragment alone unless there is definite evidence to implicate the apical fragment. Following cleaning and shaping of the canal in the coronal fragment, a well-packed dressing of calcium hydroxide is placed to allow healing at the fracture site. After 1 year, when there should be radiographic evidence of repair, the root canal can be filled with gutta-percha (Figure 11.5). If there is an inadequate apical stop at the end of the coronal fragment, the top millimetre may first be packed with calcium hydroxide to avoid gutta-percha being extruded at the fracture site. This treatment has a high rate of success [11,29]. It is most unusual to need to treat the apical fragment, and its removal is rarely indicated; in most instances the pulp in the apical fragment remains vital.

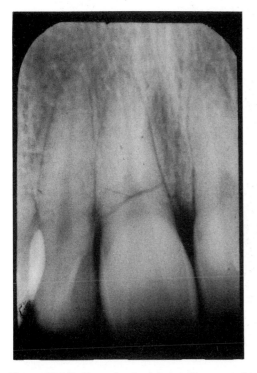

Figure 11.4 Radiograph of a right maxillary central incisor with a horizontal root fracture close to the gingival margin. The pulp responds to electric pulp testing 1 year after trauma; however, the long-term prognosis is poor.

Subluxation or luxation

Subluxation of a tooth is simply loosening without displacement. Luxation of a tooth implies its displacement rather than completely coming out of its socket (avulsion). Luxation injuries are the most common type of dental trauma [7]. With subluxation there is unlikely to be severance of the blood vessels supplying the pulp, giving the possibility of pulp survival. However, with other luxation injuries pulpal blood vessels will have been severed at the apex; the pulp may revascularize with prompt repositioning, if infection is avoided, and the root is immature with a large apex. A luxated tooth may need to be disimpacted from its new position to allow correct repositioning.

Mature teeth

Mature teeth, which have been luxated, are unlikely to undergo pulpal revascularization. Therefore the pulp should be extirpated 2 weeks after repositioning and a root canal filling subsequently placed; obturation with

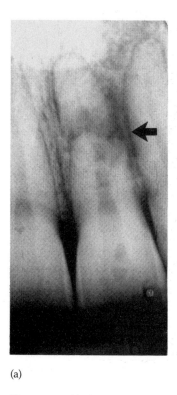
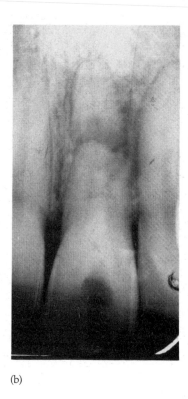
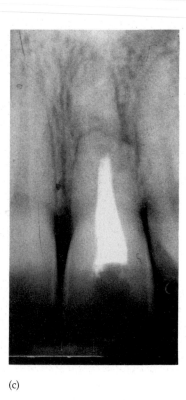

(a)   (b)   (c)

Figure 11.5 (a) The left maxillary central incisor has a root fracture in the mid-third, and there is periradicular radiolucency at the fracture line (arrow). (b) The root canal of the coronal fragment has been cleaned, shaped and filled with calcium hydroxide. (c) One year later the root canal has been filled by lateral condensation of gutta-percha.

gutta-percha soon after pulp extirpation is recommended, and there is no benefit in placing calcium hydroxide dressings for prolonged periods [16].

Immature teeth

In the case of immature teeth, there is a good chance of pulp revascularization [5], and therefore root canal treatment is not undertaken until there is evidence of pulpal infection. Revascularization of pulps in immature teeth may take some weeks but return of functioning nerve fibres may take up to 1 year [33]. Initial treatment is to reposition the tooth using local anaesthesia if necessary, and splint for 2–3 weeks; in the case of lateral luxation, the period may need to be increased if the tooth is mobile. The patient is reviewed at 2–3 weeks when the patient is carefully re-examined and the splint is normally removed. Radiographs are taken to check for continued root formation (Figure 11.6) or signs of dis-

ease, i.e. periapical radiolucency, and inflammatory resorption on the sides of the roots. If there are signs of inflammatory root resorption, the pulp should be removed and root canal treatment carried out (see later). If no signs of disease are observed, the patient is reviewed again after 2, 3, 6 months and 1 year. Pulp vitality is assessed at each period using thermal and electric tests; electric pulp testing often does not produce a response in the early period after luxation injury.

Concurrent with return of vitality, as assessed by pulp testing, may be evidence of pulp canal obliteration (Figure 11.7), which is very common in luxated teeth but less so in subluxated teeth [6]. Discoloration caused by pulp canal obliteration is not an indication for intervention, and should be differentiated from that caused by pulp necrosis. Pulp necrosis only occurs in a minority of teeth, and therefore only when several tests clearly point to this diagnosis is it appropriate to undertake root canal treatment. In some

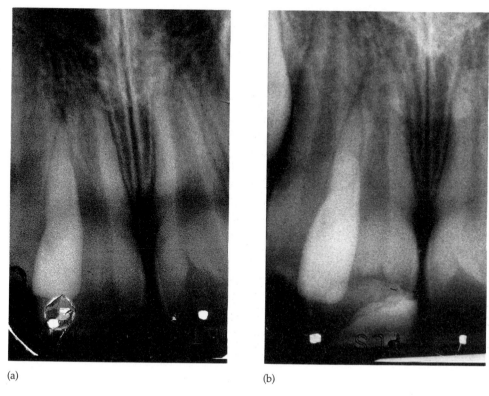

Figure 11.6 (a) The immature right central incisor was luxated. (b) One year later the root has continued to form.

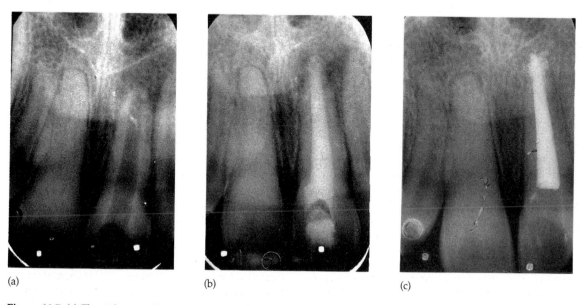

Figure 11.7 (a) The right central incisor displays pulp canal obliteration following a luxation injury. The pulp in the left central incisor was necrotic, necessitating root canal treatment. (b) Following cleaning and shaping, the root canal was filled with calcium hydroxide mixed with barium sulphate to give enhanced radiopacity. (c) One year later the root canal was filled by laterally condensed gutta-percha.

luxated teeth radiolucency is a temporary phenomenon and disappears as healing progresses [1].

Intrusion

Intrusion is when a tooth is forced into its socket, so crushing the blood vessels that supply the pulp. The tooth is likely to be stuck in the supporting bone, therefore displaying a lack of mobility and a ringing note on percussion. Many of these teeth will re-erupt spontaneously, but if this has not occurred after 3 weeks, orthodontic repositioning should be undertaken. Pulp necrosis is a very frequent complication of intrusion, and even affects 60% of teeth with immature roots [6]. Treatment of mature teeth consists of pulp extirpation, dressing with calcium hydroxide for a short period and subsequent root canal filling. Immature teeth should be observed for signs of pulp vitality returning or complications developing. If evidence of pulp necrosis or infection appears, root canal treatment should be undertaken. Another complication of intrusion is a high incidence of replacement resorption [5], as a result of damage to the periodontal ligament. The regime for reviewing intrusions is similar to that for other luxations; however, these teeth must be regularly assessed for replacement resorption by percussion, recording mobility and by radiography.

Avulsion

This is where a tooth has been completely displaced from its socket. Many avulsed teeth can be replanted with a good long-term prognosis, therefore the lost tooth should be found, preserved until it can be replanted and then followed up. The avulsed tooth needs careful handling while it is out of the mouth to prevent damage to the periodontal ligament. It should not be allowed to dry out, and should be kept in isotonic saline; since that is rarely available at the site of the accident, milk is an acceptable alternative, or the tooth could be kept moist in the buccal sulcus of the patient (or possibly a relative). The patient should be taken to an experienced practitioner as soon as possible. The tooth should be examined for missing parts, and rinsed of dirt with saline; under no circumstances should it be scrubbed or severe periodontal ligament damage will occur. Where doubt remains, the jaw may need to be radiographed to check that no part of the root remains. The socket is then syringed with saline to remove any clot, and the tooth gently repositioned into its socket; the position should be confirmed radiographically. The tooth is then splinted for 1–2 weeks. It is usually unnecessary to give local anaesthesia to achieve this. For optimal healing it is essential to avoid infection, therefore in the days following replantation the mouth should be rinsed with a chlorhexidine mouthwash. Splinting for longer periods should be avoided to reduce the risk of replacement resorption.

With mature teeth the chances of pulp revascularization are so low that the necrotic pulp is extirpated through a conventional access cavity at the time of splint removal. The cleaned and shaped root canal is initially filled with a dressing of calcium hydroxide prior to root canal filling with gutta-percha. There appears to be no benefit in leaving calcium hydroxide in the tooth for a prolonged period [16].

With immature teeth there is a good chance of pulp revascularization, so the pulp is not electively removed; this is to allow root formation and maturation to continue, and reduce the risk of subsequent fracture of the tooth [13]. However, there is a risk that infection present on the root surface or on the apical surface of the pulp at the time of replantation may initiate, or perpetuate, inflammatory resorption, which can rapidly destroy the thin wall of the immature root. Therefore, regular clinical and radiographic reviews should be undertaken at 1, 2, 3, 6 months and 1 year. The patient should be asked to return immediately any problems develop.

Inflammatory resorption

If inflammatory resorption is observed (Figure 11.8), the necrotic pulp should be removed at once, since inflammatory resorption can progress very rapidly in a few weeks in an immature root. The root canal must be cleaned with sodium hypochlorite to kill bacteria, and

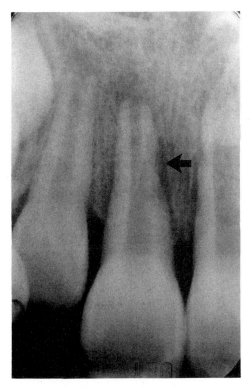

Figure 11.8 The right central incisor displays inflammatory resorption on the mesial aspect (arrow); there is a radiolucency of the bone adjacent to that in the tooth. The pulp of the tooth was necrotic as a consequence of a luxation injury.

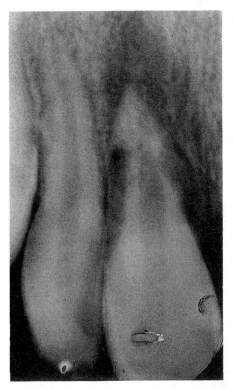

Figure 11.9 The right central incisor displays replacement resorption on the mesial and distal root surfaces; there is a moth-eaten appearance. The tooth had been replanted 2 h after avulsion 1 year previously.

it is then filled with calcium hydroxide. The most important attribute of the calcium hydroxide is to create an unsuitable environment for the continued survival of bacteria in the pulp space or dentinal tubules; less importantly, it raises the pH to halt osteoclastic activity [23]. Should the seal of the coronal access cavity subsequently fail, bacteria may re-enter the root canal with serious consequences.

Replacement resorption

If the root surface is allowed to dry out before replantation, replacement resorption (ankylosis) is likely to occur. This can be detected at follow-up appointments as the tooth gives a ringing note to percussion testing and lacks mobility. The condition can often only be observed on radiographs much later (Figure 11.9). In replacement resorption the body treats the tooth as bone, and the tooth is gradually resorbed and replaced by bone. In a healthy tooth, the cementum resists osteoclastic activity. Being a natural process, replacement resorption cannot be treated, therefore carrying out root canal treatment to stop the process or replacing gutta-percha in a root-filled tooth by calcium hydroxide is not indicated. Ultimately the tooth will be lost, but how long the process will take is variable and depends on bone turnover. In some young patients it can progress rapidly, and during the growth phase can cause the ankylosed tooth to appear to sink into the jaw as the surrounding alveolar bone grows, causing further eruption of the adjacent teeth. Under such circumstances, it may be necessary to extract the tooth surgically; however, in most instances the tooth can be left until symptoms arise from later infection. It may be appropriate to restore the incisal edge of an ankylosed tooth to improve its appearance.

Root canal treatment of immature teeth

When it is necessary to carry out root canal treatment of a replanted immature tooth, local anaesthesia is given so that a rubber dam clamp can be placed securely on the tooth and in case the apical pulp stump is still vital. The access cavity on the palatal surface of the crown should be sufficiently large to allow adequate removal of the entire remaining pulp (Figure 11.7). Instrumentation should be carried out 1–2 mm short of the radiographic apex, unless necrotic tissue is encountered at this level, when instruments should be taken further. It is necessary to measure the length of the root canal by taking a radiograph of a file of known length. Aggressive filing of root canal walls must be avoided as the canal walls are thin; instead the pulp space should be cleaned by irrigation with sodium hypochlorite [22]. After thorough cleaning a stiff paste of calcium hydroxide (mixed with some barium sulphate to increase radiopacity) should be packed into the canal with root canal pluggers. The quality of the calcium hydroxide filling should be checked radiographically (Figure 11.7) before closure of the access cavity with an effective temporary filling (e.g. intermediate restorative material (IRM) or Kalzinol, Dentsply). It is essential that the temporary filling does not break down during the course of treatment, or the canal space will become recontaminated.

The patient's tooth should be reviewed after 1 month, and a radiograph taken to ascertain whether any calcium hydroxide has disappeared from the apical part of the root canal. If none has, the tooth should be reviewed after a further 2 months. On the other hand, if it has disappeared, the entire calcium hydroxide dressing should be removed, the canal irrigated and the calcium hydroxide replaced; this should be reviewed again after 1 month. Where a dressing repeatedly disappears or a large periapical radiolucency fails to heal, a cause such as a discharging sinus tract or a vertical root fracture needs to be considered.

With most teeth further reviews after the second at 3 months are carried out at 6 and 12 months, provided that there are no problems. After 1 year a hard-tissue barrier should have formed, and be visible radiographically [10,19,38]. The type of barrier formed is dependent on the state of the apical pulp stump at the time of root canal treatment. Where the apical pulp stump and Hertwig's root sheath are undamaged, continuing root formation can be expected, but if it has been destroyed a calcific barrier is expected [17,19,27]. Histological examination of barriers shows that they resemble cellular cementum and appear to be continuous with cementum [15]. When there is radiographic evidence of barrier formation, the tooth should be isolated and the dressing removed so that the presence of a barrier can be verified with a file (e.g. International Organization for Standardization (ISO) size 40). If there is an apical stop, the root canal should be filled by a suitable gutta-percha technique (Figure 11.7; this has been covered in Chapter 10).

Late presentation

There are occasions when the patient first presents a long time after the original injury, and has a poor recollection of events. It is essential to conduct a thorough examination. Sometimes the patient presents with a new injury to an already traumatized tooth. Therefore if the history of the presenting injury fails to correlate with the findings of the clinical and radiographic examinations and special tests, the patient should be questioned specifically about a previous injury.

If a patient presents with signs or symptoms related to a root-filled immature tooth and there are technical deficiencies in the previous treatment, root canal retreatment is indicated, and is more successful than surgery, which is often complicated by a short root with thin walls. Root canal retreatment is covered in Chapters 6 and 13. If the technical quality of the previous treatment is very good, the possibility of recent root fracture must be considered.

Sometimes a late complication of trauma, particularly luxation, is inflammatory resorption close to the neck of the tooth (Figure 11.10). It may occur in vital as well as root-filled teeth and is often unrelated to the pulpal status, as infection has come from the

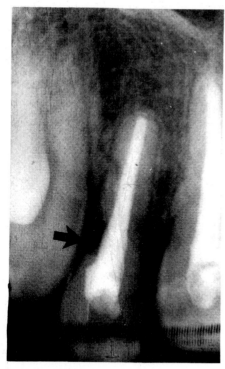

Figure 11.10 Cervical inflammatory resorption (arrow) has occurred on the distal surface of the right lateral incisor approximately 3 years after trauma. If surgical access is good, the defect may be repaired, or the tooth may need to be extracted, as in this example.

damaged root surface [37]. Root canal treatment, or retreatment, is not the appropriate method of dealing with the problem. Where the condition is limited and surgical access is good, surgical repair of the defect may be undertaken; if it is considered that surgical repair will expose the pulp, then root canal treatment should be undertaken first. However, if the condition is extensive or surgical access is poor, extraction is usually indicated.

Conclusions

Orthodontists are very concerned about causing resorption of root-filled previously traumatized teeth during tooth movement. However, there is no scientific evidence to show that these teeth are more at risk than vital ones [31,35]. It is essential that the root canal treatment has been carried out properly prior to orthodontic movement and that

infection has been eliminated; where there is any concern about the technical quality of the root canal filling, the root canal treatment should be redone first. However, it is illogical to replace a perfectly good gutta-percha root canal filling with calcium hydroxide in order to move the tooth. There is no hard evidence to support the clinical practice of delaying permanent filling of root canals of teeth containing calcium hydroxide until the completion of orthodontic treatment; it is essential to ensure that the temporary coronal restoration does not fail and so allow the introduction of infection into the canal space.

Because most general practitioners only see a small number of patients with traumatic injuries, it may be appropriate to refer these patients to a colleague with a special interest. These injuries and their management are further considered in an appropriate textbook [8].

References

1. ANDREASEN FM (1986) Transient apical breakdown and its relation to color and sensibility changes after luxation injuries to teeth. *Endodontics and Dental Traumatology* **2,** 9–19.
2. ANDREASEN FM (1989) Pulpal healing after luxation injuries and root fracture in the permanent dentition. *Endodontics and Dental Traumatology* **5,** 111–131.
3. ANDREASEN FM, ANDREASEN JO (1985) Diagnosis of luxation injuries: the importance of standardized clinical, radiographic and photographic techniques in clinical investigations. *Endodontics and Dental Traumatology* **1,** 160–169.
4. ANDREASEN FM, ANDREASEN JO, BAYER T (1989) Prognosis of root-fractured permanent incisors – prediction of healing modalities. *Endodontics and Dental Traumatology* **5,** 11–22.
5. ANDREASEN FM, VESTERGAARD PEDERSEN B (1985) Prognosis of luxated permanent teeth – the development of pulp necrosis. *Endodontics and Dental Traumatology* **1,** 207–220.
6. ANDREASEN FM, YU Z, THOMSEN BL, ANDERSEN PK (1987) Occurrence of pulp canal obliteration after luxation injuries in the permanent dentition. *Endodontics and Dental Traumatology* **3,** 103–115.
7. ANDREASEN JO (1970) Etiology and pathogenesis of traumatic dental injuries. A clinical study of 1,298 cases. *Scandinavian Journal of Dental Research* **78,** 329–342.
8. ANDREASEN JO, ANDREASEN FM (1994) *Textbook and Color Atlas of Traumatic Injuries to the Teeth*, 3rd edn. Copenhagen: Munksgaard.

9. ANDREASEN JO, HJORTING-HANSEN E (1967) Intra-alveolar root fractures: radiographic and histologic study of 50 cases. *Journal of Oral Surgery* **25**, 414–426.

10. CVEK M (1972) Treatment of non-vital permanent incisors with calcium hydroxide. I. Follow-up of peri-apical repair and apical closure of immature roots. *Odontologisk Revy* **23**, 27–44.

11. CVEK M (1974) Treatment of non-vital permanent incisors with calcium hydroxide. IV. Periodontal healing and closure of the root canal in the coronal fragment of teeth with intra-alveolar fracture and vital apical fragment. A follow-up. *Odontologisk Revy* **25**, 239–246.

12. CVEK M (1978) A clinical report on partial pulpotomy and capping with calcium hydroxide in permanent incisors with complicated crown fracture. *Journal of Endodontics* **4**, 232–237.

13. CVEK M (1992) Prognosis of luxated non-vital maxillary incisors treated with calcium hydroxide and filled with gutta-percha. A retrospective clinical study. *Endodontics and Dental Traumatology* **8**, 45–55.

14. CVEK M, LUNDBERG M (1983) Histological appearance of pulps after exposure by a crown fracture, partial pulpotomy, and clinical diagnosis of healing. *Journal of Endodontics* **9**, 8–11.

15. CVEK M, SUNDSTRÖM B (1974) Treatment of non-vital permanent incisors with calcium hydroxide. V. Histologic appearance of roentgenographically demonstrable apical closure of immature roots. *Odontologisk Revy* **25**, 379–392.

16. DUMSHA T, HOVLAND EJ (1995) Evaluation of long-term calcium hydroxide treatment in avulsed teeth – an *in vivo* study. *International Endodontic Journal* **28**, 7–11.

17. FEIGLIN B (1985) Differences in apex formation during apexification with calcium hydroxide paste. *Endodontics and Dental Traumatology* **1**, 195–199.

18. FEIGLIN B (1986) Problems with the endodontic-orthodontic management of fractured teeth. *International Endodontic Journal* **19**, 57–63.

19. FRANK AL (1966) Therapy for the divergent pulpless tooth by continued apical formation. *Journal of the American Dental Association* **72**, 87–93.

20. FUKS AB, CHOSACK A, KLEIN H, EIDELMAN E (1987) Partial pulpotomy as a treatment alternative for exposed pulps in crown-fractured permanent incisors. *Endodontics and Dental Traumatology* **3**, 100–102.

21. GRANATH LE, HAGMAN G (1971) Experimental pulpotomy in human bicuspids with reference to cutting technique. *Acta Odontologica Scandinavica* **29**, 155–163.

22. GUTMANN JL, HEATON JF (1981) Management of the open apex. 2. Non–vital teeth. *International Endodontic Journal* **14**, 173–178.

23. HAMMARSTRÖM LE, BLOMLÖF LB, FEIGLIN B, LINDSKOG SF (1986) Effect of calcium hydroxide treatment on periodontal repair and root resorption. *Endodontics and Dental Traumatology* **2**, 184–189.

24. HEIDE S, KEREKES K (1986) Delayed partial pulpotomy in permanent incisors of monkeys. *International Endodontic Journal* **19**, 78–89.

25. HEIDE S, MJÖR I (1983) Pulp reactions to experimental exposures in young permanent monkey teeth. *International Endodontic Journal* **16**, 11–19.

26. HEITHERSAY GS (1973) Combined endodontic–orthodontic treatment of transverse root fractures in the region of the alveolar crest. *Oral Surgery, Oral Medicine, Oral Pathology* **36**, 404–415.

27. HEITHERSAY GS (1975) Calcium hydroxide in the treatment of pulpless teeth with associated pathology. *Journal of the British Endodontic Society* **8**, 74–93.

28. JACOBSEN I, KEREKES K (1977) Long-term prognosis of traumatized permanent anterior teeth showing calcifying processes in the pulp cavity. *Scandinavian Journal of Dental Research* **85**, 588–598.

29. JACOBSEN I, KEREKES K (1980) Diagnosis and treatment of pulp necrosis in permanent anterior teeth with root fracture. *Scandinavian Journal of Dental Research* **88**, 370–376.

30. KOPEL HM, JOHNSON R (1985) Examination and neurologic assessment of children with oro-facial trauma. *Endodontics and Dental Traumatology* **1**, 155–159.

31. LEVANDER E, MALMGREN O (1988) Evaluation of the risk of root resorption during orthodontic treatment: a study of upper incisors. *European Journal of Orthodontics* **10**, 30–38.

32. MALONE AJ, MASSLER M (1952) Fractured anterior teeth – diagnosis, treatment and prognosis. *Dental Digest* **58**, 442–447.

33. OLGART L, GAZELIUS B, LINDH-STRÖMBERG U (1988) Laser Doppler flowmetry in assessing vitality in luxated permanent teeth. *International Endodontic Journal* **21**, 300–306.

34. RAVN JJ (1981) Follow-up study of permanent incisors with enamel-dentin fractures after acute trauma. *Scandinavian Journal of Dental Research* **89**, 355–365.

35. SPURRIER SW, HALL SH, JOONDEPH DR, SHAPIRO PA, RIEDEL RA (1990) A comparison of apical root resorption during orthodontic treatment in endodontically treated and vital teeth. *American Journal of Orthodontics and Dentofacial Orthopedics* **97**, 130–134.

36. STALHANE I, HEDEGARD B (1975) Traumatized permanent teeth in children aged 7–15 years. Part II. *Swedish Dental Journal* **68**, 157–169.

37. TRONSTAD L (1988) Root resorption – etiology, terminology and clinical manifestations. *Endodontics and Dental Traumatology* **4**, 241–252.

38. YATES JA (1988) Barrier formation time in non-vital teeth with open apices. *International Endodontic Journal* **21**, 313–319.

39. ZACHRISSON BU, JACOBSEN I (1975) Long-term prognosis of 66 permanent anterior teeth with root fracture. *Scandinavian Journal of Dental Research* **83**, 345–354.

40. ZADIK D, CHOSACK A, EIDELMAN E (1979) The prognosis of traumatized permanent anterior teeth with fracture of the enamel and dentin. *Oral Surgery, Oral Medicine, Oral Pathology* **47**, 173–175.

12

Periodontal disease and the dental pulp

A.L. Frank

Introduction

An important publication [17] was presented in the 'original' *Journal of Endodontia* in 1948 by two of the early giants in Endodontics and Periodontics, Drs Harry Johnston and Balint Orban. This publication remains the classic introduction of the endodontic–periodontal relationship. Clinicians noted at the time that success could be obtained following root canal treatment. Radicular bone healing would be expected if the disease was due to pulpal necrosis as opposed to periodontal disease, in which case the prognosis would be guarded. Unfortunately, in some clinical situations, it was often impossible to differentiate predictably the origin as endodontic or periodontal. For this reason, a combination of endodontic and periodontal treatment was performed. This double approach resulted in healing in a substantial number of cases; and it was often accompanied by unnecessary hemisections and root amputations [34]. These redesigning techniques, although introduced in the 1880s [5,14], enjoyed a rebirth of interest and usage. However, when indicated, they still remain an important and useful form of treatment. The purpose of this chapter is to discuss the relationship between pulpal and periodontal disease, and especially the diagnosis and treatment of these problems.

Pulpo-periodontal communications

Pulpal and periodontal tissues have a close relationship, both anatomically and functionally. Their communications can be divided into two groups: vascular and tubular.

Vascular

The possibility that periodontal disease might be related to or cause pulpal disease was reported by Colyer [9] and Cahn [7], who described structures that are termed lateral canals. Cahn [7] stated: 'it does not require a wide stretch of the imagination to see how easily an infective process might spread from without inwards, rapidly involving the pulp, especially in teeth having these side canals'. By means of Indian ink perfusion studies, a vascular communication via these channels has been demonstrated [8,20]. They represent an original communication between the developing dental sac and the dental papilla. The majority of lateral canals are found in the apical part of the root. Accessory root canals have been reported to occur in 27% of teeth, with 2% occurring in the coronal third of the root, 9% in the middle third and 17% in the apical third [11]. The observations were made after the teeth had been rendered transparent and their root canal systems filled with China ink. Lateral canals in the furcation have been found in 59–76% of molars [6,23]. The vessels running in lateral canals do not provide a major source of collateral circulation, although they contribute to nutrition of the pulp. However, they do provide a major communication between the pulp and the periodontal ligament and vice versa [21]. Although anastomoses of this type usually become sealed by continuous deposition of dentine and cementum, some still remain patent in adults.

Tubular

Exposed dentinal tubules may serve as a pathway between the pulp and the periodontal ligament [30,32]. No evidence has yet been presented which indicates that the non-vital pulp can cause inflammation of the periodontal tissues through 'normal' walls of dentine and cementum [36]. Injuries of the root cementum, such as traumatic fractures or cemental tears, may establish tubular communication between the pulp and periodontal ligament. The same would occur with extensive horizontal or vertical fractures involving the crown of the tooth (Figure 12.1). Developmental grooves on the crown and root are most often found in maxillary lateral incisors and, when exposed to plaque bacteria, may initiate inflammatory alterations in the pulp. Advanced periodontal disease may also be associated with root surface resorption.

The nature and frequency of tissue changes in the dental pulps of monkeys with moderately advanced periodontitis have been studied [4]; 30% of roots showed inflammation of the pulp adjacent to areas of attachment loss, especially where root-surface resorption had occurred. A more recent study has suggested that the presence of pathogenic microorganisms in the dentinal tubules and pulp may be related to the failure of periodontal treatment [2].

Classification of endodontic–periodontal lesions

It is helpful to classify lesions according to their primary source of origin (Figure 12.2) [33]:

1. Primary endodontic lesion.
2. Primary endodontic lesion with secondary periodontal involvement.
3. Primary periodontal lesion.
4. Primary periodontal lesion with secondary endodontic involvement.
5. Combined lesions.

Effort should be made to determine the diagnosis in order to establish the correct treatment plan and achieve an accurate prognosis [24].

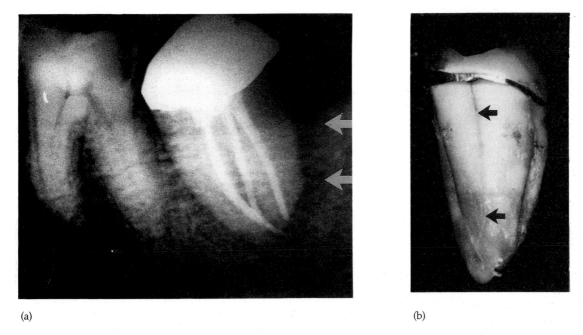

(a)   (b)

Figure 12.1 Vertical fracture. (a) A distal vertical pocket (arrows), probable to the apex on a mandibular left second molar, persisted following root canal treatment and necessitated extraction. (b) Following extraction, a vertical fracture on the distal root surface (arrows) was evident, extending the length of the tooth. Fused roots prevented 'anatomical redesigning'.

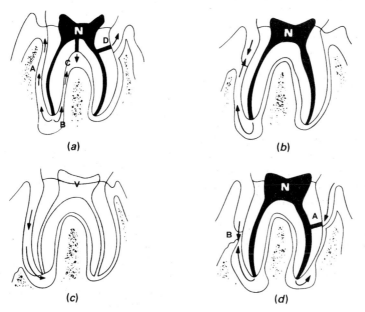

Figure 12.2 Classification of endodontic–periodontal lesions. (a) Primary endodontic lesions: pathway extending from apex to gingival sulcus via periodontium (A); apex to furcation (B); lateral canal to furcation (C); lateral canal to pocket (D). (b) Primary endodontic lesion with secondary periodontal involvement. (c) Primary periodontal lesion extending to the apex. (d) Primary periodontal lesion with secondary endodontic involvement via a lateral canal (A). Combined lesion from coalescence of separate lesions (B). N = Necrotic pulp; V = Vital pulp.

Primary endodontic lesion

An acute exacerbation of a chronic apical lesion on a tooth with a necrotic pulp may drain coronally through the periodontal ligament into the gingival sulcus area (Figure 12.2a). This situation may mimic a periodontal abscess. However, it is only periodontal in that it passes through the periodontal ligament area (Figures 12.3–12.6). In reality, it is a sinus tract resulting from pulpal disease.

Thus it is essential that a gutta-percha cone is inserted into the sinus tract and one or more radiographs taken to determine the origin of the lesion. When the pocket is probed, it is narrow and lacks width. A similar situation occurs where drainage from the apex of a molar tooth extends coronally into the furcation area (Figure 12.7). Direct extension of inflammation from the pulp may also occur into the furcation area of a non-vital tooth when a lateral canal is present (Figure 12.8).

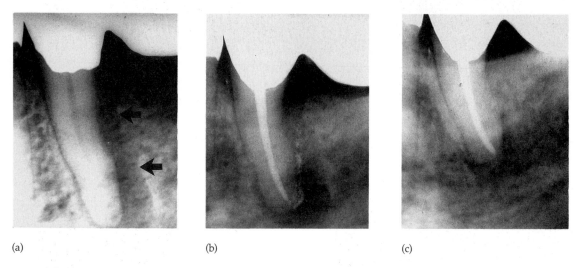

(a)   (b)   (c)

Figure 12.3 Primary endodontic lesion. Mandibular premolar with a radiolucency along the distal surface of the root. (a) Pretreatment, the lesion (arrows) drained through the gingival sulcus. (b) Immediately after treatment, root canal sealer can be observed in the sinus tract. (c) Six months later, there is evidence of considerable healing and bone filling.

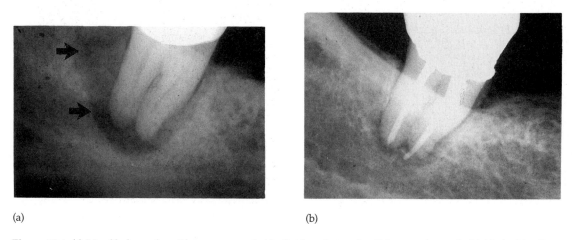

(a)   (b)

Figure 12.4 (a) Mandibular molar with a narrow probable distal pocket and radiolucency (arrows). (b) Marked healing apparent at 1-year recall, confirming that the original 'pocket' was of endodontic origin.

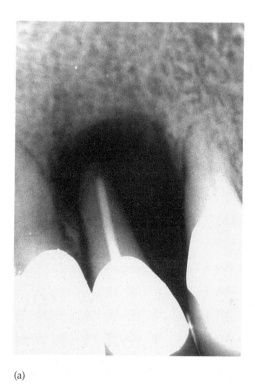

(a)

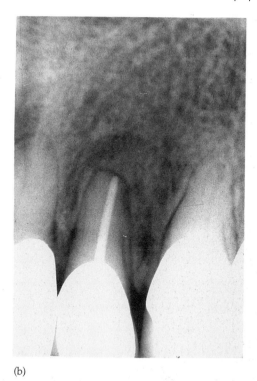

(b)

Figure 12.5 (a) Immediately after root canal filling a non-vital lateral incisor with extensive loss of surrounding bone. (b) Radiograph taken 1 year later showing healing, and confirming that the lesion was of endodontic origin.

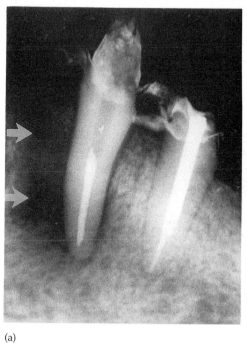

(a)

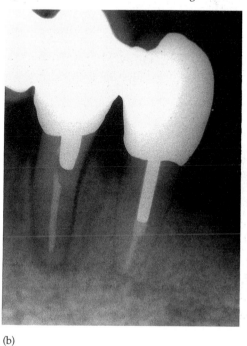

(b)

Figure 12.6 Success following treatment of a primary endodontic lesion. (a) Immediate post-treatment radiograph of a mandibular canine showing mesial radiolucency (arrows). (b) Radiograph at 15 months showing healing.

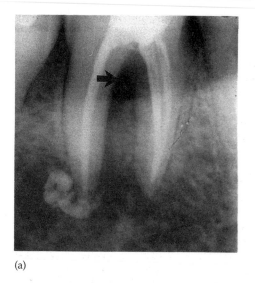
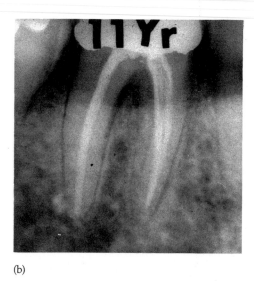

(a)　　　　　　　　　　　　　　　　　　　　(b)

Figure 12.7 Mandibular molar where apical involvement extends into the furcation (arrow). (a) Immediately following root canal treatment, excess sealer is present at the apex of the distal root. (b) Radiograph 11 years later, showing healing apically and in the furcation.

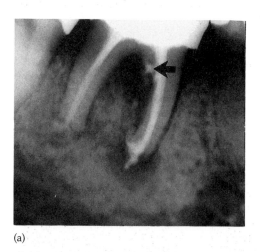
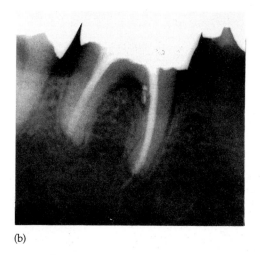

(a)　　　　　　　　　　　　　　　　　　　　(b)

Figure 12.8 Primary endodontic lesion with a lateral canal in the furcation. (a) Post-treatment radiograph demonstrates a filled lateral canal opening into the furcation (arrow). (b) After 18 months, total healing of lesions at the apex and adjacent to the lateral canal is demonstrated.

Primary endodontic lesions usually heal following root canal treatment; the sinus tract extending into the gingival sulcus or furcation area disappears at an early stage once the necrotic pulp has been treated. It is important to recognize that failure of any periodontal treatment will occur when the presence of a necrotic pulp has not been diagnosed, and therefore not treated.

Primary endodontic lesion with secondary periodontal involvement

If after a period of time a suppurating primary endodontic lesion remains untreated, it may then become secondarily involved with marginal periodontal breakdown (Figure 12.2b). Plaque forms at the gingival margin of the sinus tract and leads to marginal periodontitis. When plaque or calculus is encountered with a probe, the treatment and prognosis of the tooth are altered; the tooth now requires both endodontic and periodontal treatment. If the endodontic treatment is adequate, the prognosis depends on the severity of the marginal periodontal damage and the efficacy of periodontal treatment. With endodontic treatment alone, only part of the lesion can heal to the level of the secondary periodontal lesion. In general, healing of the tissues damaged by suppuration from the pulp space can be anticipated.

Primary endodontic lesions with secondary periodontal involvement may also occur as a result of root perforation during root canal treatment, or where pins or posts have been misplaced during coronal restoration (Figure 12.9). Symptoms may be acute, with periodontal abscess formation associated with pain, swelling, exudation of pus, pocket formation and tooth mobility. A more chronic response may sometimes occur without pain, and involves the sudden appearance of a pocket with bleeding on probing or exudation of pus.

When the root perforation is situated close to the alveolar crest, it may be possible to raise a flap and repair the defect with an appropriate filling material, and then to replace the flap apically, so exteriorizing the repaired perforation. In deeper perforations, or in the roof of the furcation, immediate repair of the perforation has a better prognosis than management of an infected one [26,27]. Amalgam has been widely used but the long-term results have been disappointing [12,26,27]. Recent experimental work with mineral trioxide aggregate has demonstrated cemental healing following immediate repair [27]; delayed repair was not as good but indicates potential for further investigation.

Root fractures may also present as primary endodontic lesions with secondary periodontal involvement. These typically occur on root-treated teeth (Figure 12.1), often with post crowns *in situ*. The signs may range from a local deepening of a periodontal pocket to more acute periodontal abscess formation. Root fractures have also become an increasing problem with molar teeth that have been treated by root resection. In a study of 100 patients, a total of 38 teeth failed during the 10-year period of observation [22]; 47% of the failures were due to root fractures, the vast majority being in mandibular molar teeth.

Primary periodontal lesion

These lesions (Figure 12.2c) are caused by periodontal disease; the process of chronic marginal periodontitis progressing apically along the root surface until the apical region

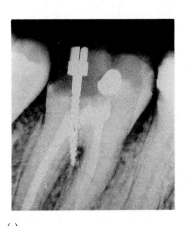
(a)

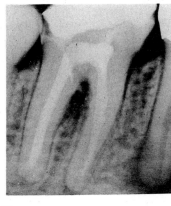
(b)

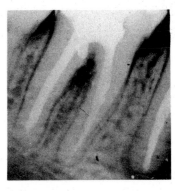
(c)

Figure 12.9 Primary endodontic lesion with secondary periodontal involvement. (a) A Dentatus screw has perforated the furcation of a mandibular second molar. (b) After 6 months, bone loss is evident in the furcation and a pocket has formed. (c) The perforation has been treated with calcium hydroxide and curettage of the pocket. Some new bone has formed in the furcation; however, no pocket is probable clinically.

is approximated. In primarily periodontally involved teeth, pulp-testing procedures reveal a clinically normal pulpal response (Figure 12.10). In addition one would anticipate a probable pocket of some depth and width; as the probe is moved around the tooth, the V-shaped pocket progressively deepens then becomes progressively shallower. There is frequently an accumulation of plaque and calculus [24].

The prognosis in this situation depends wholly upon the stage of periodontal disease and the efficacy of periodontal treatment. The clinician must also be aware of the radiographic appearance of periodontal disease associated with developmental radicular anomalies (see later).

Primary periodontal lesion with secondary endodontic involvement

The apical progression of a periodontal pocket can continue until the apex is reached; the vital pulp may become necrotic as a result of infection entering via a lateral canal or the apical foramen (Figure 12.2d). In single-rooted teeth the prognosis is usually hopeless, which is totally the opposite of the primary endodontic lesion. In molar teeth not all the roots may suffer the same loss of supporting tissues to the apex, in which case

the possibility of root resection should be considered.

The treatment of periodontal disease can lead to secondary endodontic involvement. Lateral canals and dentinal tubules may be opened to the oral environment by curettage, scaling or surgical flap procedures (Figure 12.11). In addition, it is possible for a blood vessel within a lateral canal to be severed by a curette during treatment. Controversy exists as to whether progressive periodontitis has any effect on the vitality of the pulp. Pulpal changes resulting from periodontal disease have been reported [2,4,19,29,31,37]. Terminal breakdown of the pulp does not seem to occur until periodontal disease involves the main apical foramen [21]. Provided that the blood supply through the apex is intact, the pulp has a strong capacity for survival (Figure 12.10). A strong relationship between the cultivable microorganisms from the root canals of human caries-free teeth with advanced periodontitis and from their periodontal pockets has been shown [19], with the microorganisms in the pocket being a possible source of root canal infection. Support for this concept has come from research in which cultured samples obtained from the pulp tissue and radicular dentine of human periodontally involved teeth showed bacterial growth in 87% of the teeth [2]. It was suggested that the reservoir of bacteria in the dentine and pulp tissue might contribute to the failure of periodontal treatment. The possibility might also exist that these teeth would develop pulpal necrosis.

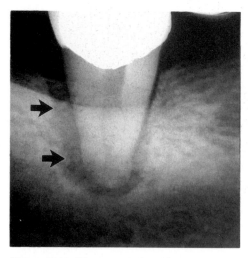

Figure 12.10 Primary periodontal lesion. A mandibular molar presented with a probable pocket distally (arrows). Pulp testing gave a vital response indicating a lesion of periodontal origin; the tooth was extracted.

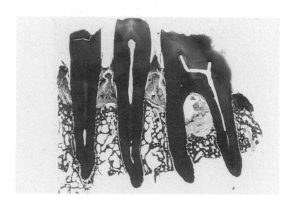

Figure 12.11 Histological examination shows that in advanced marginal periodontitis, furcation involvement can be severe. The pulp might become affected through a lateral canal.

There is often a lack of relationship between periodontal disease and pulpal involvement [10]; the histological status of the pulps of 100 periodontally involved teeth was the same as 22 control teeth with a normal periodontium [25]. Normal pulp tissue in the roots of molar teeth amputated for periodontal reasons has been reported [35]. The results of retrospective studies of periodontal treatment indicated that 'retrograde pulpitis' was not a causative factor in the loss of 460 out of a total of 1464 molar teeth with furcation involvement observed over a period of 22 years [16], or in the loss of 46 out of a total of 387 maxillary molar teeth with furcation lesions maintained from 5 to 24 years [28].

Despite the conflict of opinion from various research studies [4,37], it would seem that, on a clinical basis at least, plaque-associated periodontal disease rarely causes 'significant' pathological changes in the pulp, and this remains true until the periodontal pocket reaches the apical foramen.

Combined lesions

Combined lesions (Figure 12.2d) occur where an endodontic lesion progressing coronally becomes continuous with a plaque-infected periodontal pocket progressing apically [32]. The degree of attachment loss in this type of lesion is invariably large and the prognosis guarded. This is particularly true in single-rooted teeth, but the situation may be salvaged in molars by sectioning where not all the roots are as severely involved. Periapical healing may be anticipated following successful endodontic treatment (Figure 12.12). The periodontal aspects then may (or may not) respond to periodontal treatment, depending on the severity of involvement. A similar radiographic appearance may result from a vertically fractured tooth. If a sinus tract is present, it may be necessary to raise a flap to help determine the exact cause of the lesion. A fracture that has penetrated to the pulp space, with resultant necrosis, may also be labelled a 'true' combined lesion and yet not be amenable to successful treatment (Figure 12.1).

Retrospective classification

The classifying of primary endodontic and primary periodontal lesions presents no clinical difficulty. In a primarily endodontically involved tooth the pulp is infected and

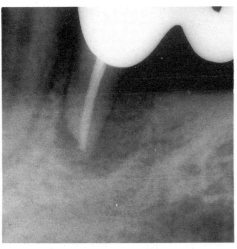

(a)

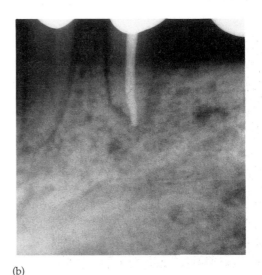

(b)

Figure 12.12 Combined endodontic–periodontal lesion, in which healing will occur to the level of the marginal periodontal breakdown. (a) Immediate postoperative radiograph after root canal treatment of a non-vital premolar, which received periodontal curettage. (b) Recall radiograph at 2 years demonstrated stable healing.

non-vital; however, in a tooth with a primary periodontal defect the pulp is vital and responsive to testing [24]. This is not true in the differential classification of primary endodontic lesions with secondary periodontal involvement, or primary periodontal lesions with secondary endodontic involvement, or the combined lesions. All of these three entities are clinically and radiographically very similar, with probable pockets to the apex of a non-vital root in each of them. If it is diagnosed and treated as primarily endodontic because of lack of evidence of marginal periodontitis, and there is soft-tissue healing on clinical probing and bony healing on a recall radiograph, a valid retrospective diagnosis can then be made. The degree of healing that has taken place following root canal treatment will determine the retrospective classification. At that stage, in the absence of adequate healing, further periodontal treatment would be indicated.

Prognosis

The prognosis of each classification has been discussed along with aetiology. To assist in their comparative understanding, each will be repeated in this summary:

Primary endodontic lesion

Treatment – Root canal treatment.
Prognosis – Good.

Primary periodontal lesion

Treatment – Periodontal treatment.
Prognosis – Depends on periodontal treatment and patient response.

Primary endodontic lesion with secondary periodontal involvement

Primary periodontal lesion with secondary endodontic involvement

Combined lesions

Treatment – Endodontic and periodontal treatment.
Prognosis – Dependent on periodontal treatment and patient response.

Differential diagnosis

Sinus tracts

Where a sinus tract opens into the gingival sulcus or at the mucogingival junction, the origin of the lesion can be determined by the insertion of a gutta-percha point. The gutta-percha point has the advantage that, being pliable, it can follow the soft-tissue tract around the root of the tooth. There are instances where the sinus tract emerges through the periodontium of the adjacent tooth which has a healthy pulp [18]. Sinus tracts of endodontic origin are usually narrow, while periodontal lesions tend to be more broad-based [3,24].

Pulp testing

An acute lesion that is of endodontic origin may often mimic periodontal abscess formation, especially in the furcation areas of molar teeth. Establishing that the tooth is non-vital, with either electric or thermal pulp testing, is essential to prevent failure if periodontal treatment alone is provided. The problem with vitality testing is that it can be imprecise, especially with very heavily restored teeth. Occasionally, false-positive responses may be obtained due to the transmission of electric current to the periodontal ligament. Confusion may also occur where the different roots of a molar tooth are not all vital. Heavily restored teeth may sometimes necessitate a test cavity where a small hole is drilled through the restoration into the dentine without anaesthesia to test for pulpal response. This subject has been covered in Chapter 4.

Radiographic examination

Paralleling technique radiographs are essential for good diagnosis of the crest of the bone interdentally and the furcation area of molar teeth. Vertical bitewing radiographs omit the apices of teeth, but give an undistorted representation of the interdental and furcation areas. Sinus tracts are not visible on radiographs, therefore a radiopaque marker, such as a gutta-percha point, can be used to establish the origin of the lesion. It is also important to look at the radiographic evidence from other parts of the mouth. Severe bone loss on one aspect of a tooth in a mouth where bone levels around all other teeth are normal should point to a suspicion of an endodontic lesion; this would particularly apply to a heavily restored tooth. Root fractures present a severe problem in radiographic diagnosis, since these hairline defects are not visible unless the fractured parts of the root or restorations are displaced; however, if the fracture space is infected, bone loss will be observed around the root on the radiograph.

Surgical exploration

Where a root fracture is suspected it may be impossible to establish a diagnosis, either clinically or radiographically. In this case a mucoperiosteal flap is raised to expose the root and look for the presence of a fracture.

Lighting and magnification

The use of a fibreoptic light source, together with magnifying binocular loops, will often provide valuable information when examining and treating furcation areas and in searching for root fractures and perforations.

Furcation involvement

Progressive marginal periodontal disease may lead to exposure of the furcation region of posterior teeth, usually from more than one aspect. Destruction of the furcation attachment may also occur following the spread of pulpal infection, as a result of tooth fracture, the consequence of poor restorations or via lateral canals in the furcation [6,23]. The lesion of endodontic origin is likely to be probable from only one aspect.

Dimension of the root trunk

Multirooted teeth have a common root trunk which is that part of the root extending from the cervix to the furcation. Teeth with a short root trunk have the highest incidence of furcation involvement because of the close proximity to marginal periodontal breakdown. However, they are the easiest teeth on

which to perform root resection procedures. Teeth with long root trunks will only show periodontally involved furcation areas when the disease is more advanced, and are often difficult to section.

Diagnostic complications due to radicular anomalies

Observation of extracted teeth and clinical cases has disclosed a particular group that fails to respond to treatment. These are directly associated with an invagination or a vertical developmental radicular groove, which can lead to an untreatable periodontal condition (Figures 12.13 and 12.14). These grooves usually begin in the central fossa of maxillary central and lateral incisors crossing over the cingulum, and continuing apically down the root for varying distances. Such a groove is apparently the result of an attempt of the tooth germ to form another root. This fissure-like channel provides a nidus for plaque and an avenue for the progression of periodontal disease.

Aetiology

From the time the tooth develops with this anomalous root defect, the potential for isolated periodontal involvement exists. As long as the epithelial attachment remains intact, the periodontium remains healthy. However, once this attachment is breached and the groove becomes involved, a self-sustaining infrabony pocket can be formed along its length. This condition often does not respond to periodontal treatment. Radiographically, this may appear as a coronal extension of a periapical radiolucency. The area of bone destruction follows the course of the groove.

Diagnosis

The clinical diagnosis of this condition is all important. The patient may have the symptoms of a periodontal abscess or a variety of symptomless endodontic conditions. If the condition is purely periodontal, it can be diagnosed by visually following the groove to

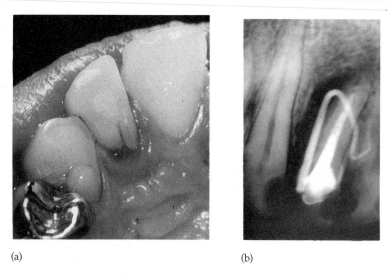

(a)   (b)

Figure 12.13 Radicular anomaly. (a) A lingual groove on the lateral incisor was probable to the apex. (b) Root canal treatment did not improve the situation and the defect remained probable to a gutta-percha point.

the gingival margin and by probing the depth of the pocket, which is usually tubular in form and localized to this one area, as opposed to a more generalized periodontal problem. The tooth will be responsive to pulp-testing procedures. Bone destruction that vertically follows the groove may be apparent radiographically. If this entity is also associated with an endodontic problem, the patient may present clinically with any of the spectrum of endodontic symptoms.

The prognosis of root canal treatment will be guarded, depending upon the apical extent of the groove. The dentist must look for the groove because it may have been altered by a previous access opening or restoration in the access cavity. The appearance of a teardrop-shaped area on the radiograph should immediately arouse suspicion. The developmental groove may actually be visible on the radiograph; if so, it will appear as a dark vertical line. This condition must be

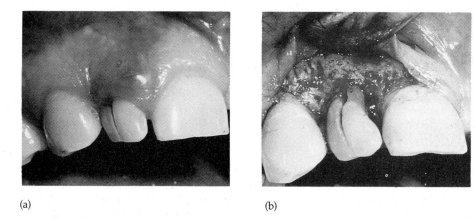

(a)   (b)

Figure 12.14 (a) A developmental groove in the labial surface of a maxillary incisor presenting with an acute abscess. (b) Subsequent surgical exploration shows the groove extending on to the root.

differentiated from a vertical fracture, which may give the same radiographic appearance.

Treatment

In essence, since this is a self-sustaining infrabony pocket, scaling and root planing may be inadequate. Although the acute nature of the problem may be alleviated initially, the source of the chronic or acute inflammation must be eradicated by burring out the groove and surgical management of the soft tissues and underlying bone, or by extraction.

Anatomical redesigning

To assist in periodontal treatment and in certain endodontic situations, anatomical redesigning may become necessary. Such redesigning, which includes root amputation, resection and bicuspidization techniques, develops a periodontally maintainable environment for the remaining root or roots.

Definition of terms

1. *Root amputation* is the removal of one or more roots from a multirooted tooth, leaving the majority of the crown and any existing restoration intact.
2. *Tooth resection* involves the removal of one or more roots of a tooth along with their coronal portion; it is sometimes referred to as hemisection.
3. *Bicuspidization* is the separation of a multirooted tooth by a vertical cut through the furcation.

Indications for root amputation or tooth resection

1. Advanced periodontal disease. The pattern of alveolar and supporting bone loss in periodontal disease may be unequal on the different roots of a molar tooth. If left untreated, the adjacent healthier root support would eventually become involved by direct extension of the periodontal lesion and the prognosis of the tooth would then become hopeless. Removal of the offending root or roots would allow the well-supported part of the tooth to be retained as a functional tooth with a normal clinical and radiographic appearance.
2. Close root proximity. The distobuccal root of the maxillary first molar and the mesiobuccal root of the second molar often tend to flare towards each other. Periodontal disease in these areas may lead to angular bone loss, which is difficult to treat and also provides the patient with a difficult problem of plaque control management. Selective root removal will allow the re-establishment of a proper embrasure area.
3. Furcation involvement.
4. Extensive root caries or external or internal root resorption.
5. Root fracture or perforation.
6. Inability to perform root canal treatment. The canal may be calcified, a broken instrument present, or there may be ledging as a result of procedural errors.

Indications for bicuspidization

1. Gross perforation in the furcation. The uninvolved root lengths must be favourable.
2. Close root proximity. This prevents periodontal treatment or patient home maintenance; it can be improved by root separation.

Contraindications for anatomical redesigning

1. Poor patient motivation and plaque control. This is particularly so if there has been inadequate improvement following initial periodontal treatment.
2. Unfavourable bony support. This relates to all remaining roots of the involved tooth, particularly if it is an abutment for a fixed prosthesis.
3. Fused roots. These prevent root removal. A special clinical situation with a more favourable prognosis exists when there is apical fusion only and adequate interradicular bone, allowing for root removal.

4. Short thin roots.
5. A long root trunk. The furcation area is situated so far apically that considerable supporting bone would need to be sacrificed.
6. Surrounding anatomy. This may preclude the formation of a functional band of attached gingiva around the remaining roots.
7. Non-negotiable canals. The canals are sclerosed or blocked by broken instruments in the remaining roots, and root-end surgery is impossible.
8. Non-restorable tooth.

Root amputation of maxillary molar teeth

This form of treatment relates primarily to maxillary molar teeth and the most common root to be removed by amputation is the distobuccal of the first molar. Whenever possible, root canal treatment and sealing of the pulp chamber with a permanent restorative material extending into the coronal part of the root to be resected should be carried out, prior to root removal (Figure 12.15). Coronal reshaping and buccolingual narrowing should also be completed to bring occlusal forces over the solid roots that remain (Figure 12.16).

The need for root removal may become apparent during diagnosis and treatment planning of the case, as a solution to treating roots with extensive periodontal breakdown. Root canal treatment is completed on the tooth in question with amalgam placed in the pulp chamber and coronal part of the root to be amputated, as soon as the patient's plaque control has reached a satisfactory level and the inflammatory phase has been resolved. Full-thickness mucoperiosteal flaps are reflected to expose the furcation area. Careful exploration with a Nabers probe is required to make sure that the furcation has not been exposed on all three surfaces. If so, tooth resection would be required, leaving one root *in situ*, or the tooth would need to be extracted. The cut in the root is made with an International Organization for Standardization (ISO) 012L bur, or pencil diamond, which is long enough to reach from one side of the root to the other. Care is taken to

maintain the correct angulation of the bur, so as not to damage the remaining root(s) or the crown. The fissure bur is held at a 45° angle to the tooth at the level of the furcation. Removal of some of the buccal cortical plate of bone may be required so that the separated root can be gently elevated out of its socket, without undue pressure being applied to the adjacent tooth or bone.

Once the root has been removed, the area of the stump should be reshaped with diamond burs, so that it blends imperceptibly into the remaining tooth structure. Enough clearance should also be left between the undersurface of the crown and the gingival tissue to allow for adequate plaque control. The tooth surface should finally be finished with fine diamond burs and then polished.

A re-evaluation of the periodontal situation is carried out some 3 months after root removal. If mucogingival and osseous deformities are present in this quadrant of the mouth, definitive periodontal surgery is now carried out.

An alternative method of treatment allows for root amputation to be carried out at the time of periodontal surgery; this has the advantage of allowing for only one surgical procedure. The disadvantage is that the bony healing has yet to occur, and the extent to which this will progress cannot always be predicted; this may result in more radical reshaping in the area than might otherwise be required. In this approach, a cavity is cut over the pulp stump with an inverted cone bur and a dressing of calcium hydroxide placed over the exposed pulp. Definitive root canal treatment is carried out at a later stage after the periodontal dressings have been removed [35], but it is more difficult to control root canal irrigants, prevent pulp space contamination, and fill the orifice of the resected root.

Root amputation of mandibular molar teeth

Situations may present where it is reasonable to amputate the root of a mandibular molar. If such a tooth presents with a periodontally involved mesial root and it is part of a multiunit bridge or splinted crowns, its amputation should be considered. The buccolingual

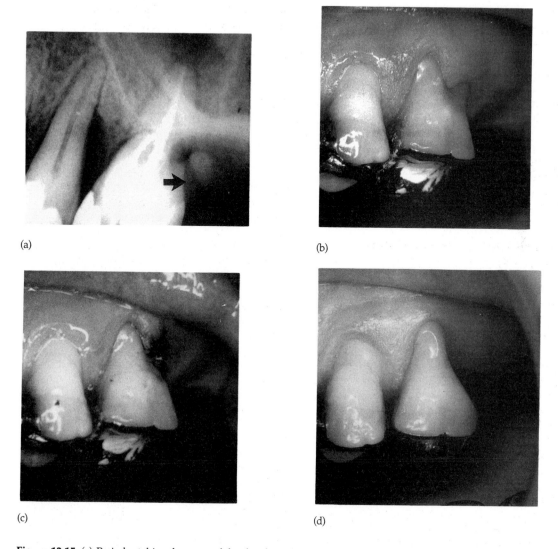

(a)

(b)

(c)

(d)

Figure 12.15 (a) Periodontal involvement of the distobuccal root (arrow) of the maxillary first molar necessitated its amputation. (b) Prior to amputation. (c) Following amputation. (d) The remaining tooth after being smoothed and polished.

dimension of the occlusal aspect of the tooth and pontics should be reduced to minimize and redirect the occlusal forces if possible (Figure 12.17).

Another situation where an amputation could be considered is when the periodontally involved root of a crowned tooth is adjacent to another crowned tooth and they could be firmly splinted to each other to avoid vertical fracture of the remaining root (Figure 12.18); broad interproximal contact without splinting is not sufficient (Figure

12.19). Maxillary molars do not normally present a similar problem because of the support provided by the two remaining roots. The remaining coronal portion of the amputated root should be physiologically contoured to allow for maintenance of periodontal health.

The canal at the amputation site should be prepared and filled with a suitable restorative material to prevent the accumulation of plaque and caries. It is best to place the filling internally prior to root removal. If this is not feasible, a filling should be placed into the

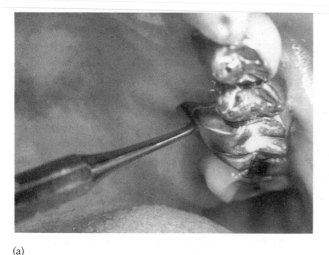

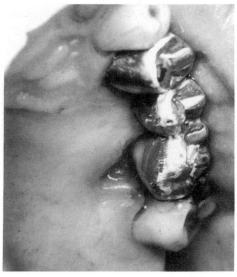

(a)

Figure 12.16 (a) The pocket on the palatal root of the first molar was probable to the apex. (b) Following amputation of the palatal root, the remaining crown was reshaped and polished. The buccolingual width of the clinical crown was reduced.

(b)

resected root end during the surgical procedure. Root-filling materials such as gutta-percha and cements do not provide adequate long-term restorations of such cavities exposed to the oral environment.

Tooth resection

Tooth resection is often the treatment of choice in deep furcation involvements. It is also the treatment of choice where teeth are

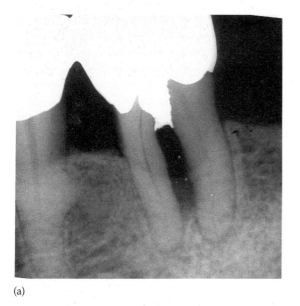

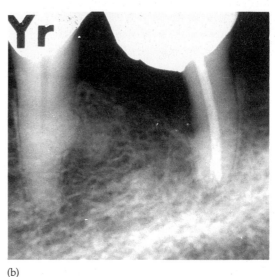

(a)

(b)

Figure 12.17 (a) A perforation with periodontal breakdown in the furcation of a mandibular molar; the tooth was part of a 4-unit splint. The mesial root was amputated and the coronal restoration recontoured and reduced buccolingually. (b) Recall at 13 years demonstrates long-term success.

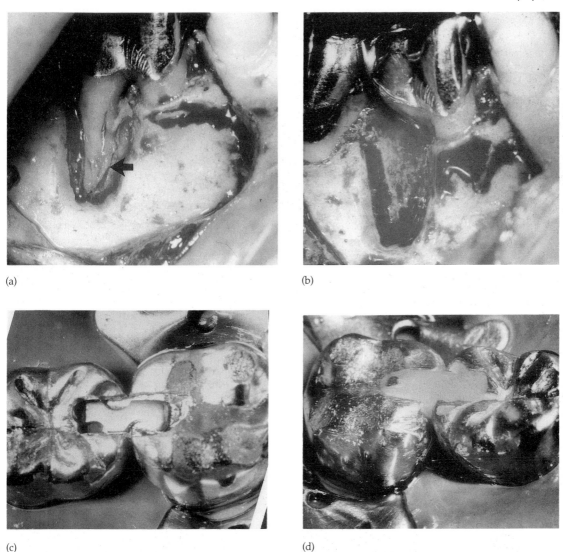

Figure 12.18 Splinting of lower molars. (a) The distal root of a mandibular first molar had a vertical fracture (arrow) necessitating removal. (b) Following amputation of the root and contouring of the remaining structure. (c) An occlusal preparation was fitted with a metal splint. (d) A restorative filling material has been used to keep the splint in place.

to be included in a fixed prosthesis [1]. A considerable advantage is achieved if the initial crown preparation is completed first. This then serves as a guide to entering the furcation.

Full-thickness mucoperiosteal flaps are reflected and the tooth is sectioned using an ISO 016L bur. In maxillary molars, depending on the degree of furcation involvement, it may be possible to retain two roots, providing the furcation is not open between them, such

as mesial and palatal, or distal and palatal, or the two buccal roots. If the furcation proves to be open mesially, buccally and distally, only the best supported root is retained. Sometimes this can only be judged by sectioning all three roots and assessing them individually [15]. The fissure bur is positioned in the long axis of the tooth at the most coronal level of the involved furcation. Initial cuts are made in the crown in the direction of the adjacent furcation. The same step is then

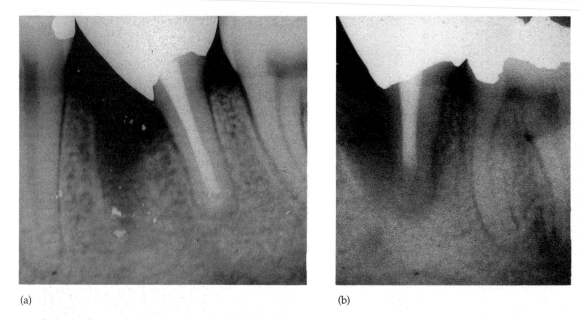

(a)

(b)

Figure 12.19 Broad interproximal contact is not sufficient support following amputation. (a) A crown was prepared on the distal root of the first molar to provide broad interproximal contact with the adjacent tooth. (b) Although successful for 4 years, a vertical fracture then occurred; a diffuse radiolucency is present around the root.

followed from the adjacent furcation towards the initial cut. The bur is then alternated between the two cuts until they are joined. The mandibular molars are sectioned bucco-lingually into two halves. As a general rule it is important to make the cut at the expense of the portion which is to be removed (Figure 12.20a). This minimizes the risk of over-cutting the retained section. When sectioning has been completed, the involved part of the tooth is extracted with forceps.

In finishing the preparation it is important to remove the overhang of the crown that may be left at the roof of the furcation and to blend the cut surface into the retained portion of the tooth. This should be checked radiographically. When the vertical cut to the furcation ends in close proximity to or at the level of bone, it is necessary to remove approximately 1 mm of the bone with a sharp scalpel in order to expose some intact cementum beyond the cut surface (Figure 12.20b). It is not advisable to end the restoration within the cut, leaving raw-cut dentine exposed because of the potential for later marginal caries (Figure 12.21). This will facilitate the preparation for the restoration to follow

(Figure 12.22). There may be situations where it is necessary to consider occlusal factors, as in amputations, and reduce the size of the occlusal table (Figure 12.23). Root fracture is a common cause of failure [13].

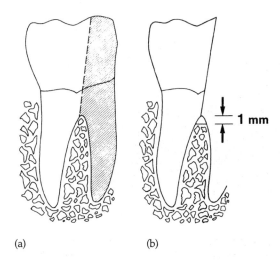

(a)

(b)

Figure 12.20 Resection. (a) The cut should be made at the expense of the part to be removed. (b) The restoration should not leave the raw cut exposed; 1 mm of the bone should be removed to facilitate preparation.

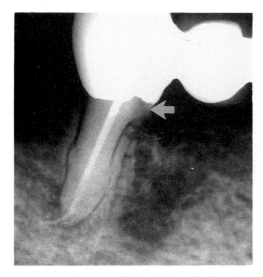

Figure 12.21 The lack of the 1-mm space in bone led the restoration to end on the raw-cut dentine, with the long-term adverse consequence of marginal caries (arrow).

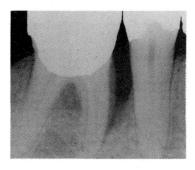

(a)

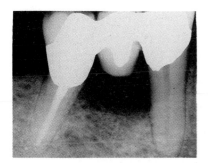

(b)

Figure 12.22 (a) Angular bone loss extending close to the apex of the mesial root of the mandibular first molar. The widely displayed roots made hemisection suitable. (b) The mesial root has been removed, and the distal root after root canal treatment and surgery has been used as a bridge abutment.

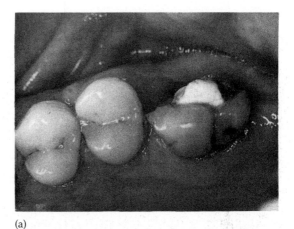

(a)

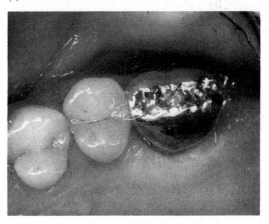

(b)

Figure 12.23 Reduction of masticatory pressure following resection. (a) A mesiodistal fracture of the maxillary first molar necessitated loss of the buccal roots; the thick palatal root was retained. (b) It was necessary to reduce the occlusal table.

Bicuspidization

Bicuspidization, when indicated, is the separation of the roots of a multirooted tooth. This procedure is primarily used in mandibular molars (Figure 12.24). Adequate length and width of the root and clinical crown are primary considerations in case selection. The cut should be vertically directed to the middle of the furcation. It is necessary to expose the margin of the cut surface to facilitate later crown preparation. When there is close root proximity, it is necessary to separate the roots by orthodontic techniques (Figure 12.25). Both roots are then restored as single units to simulate two premolars.

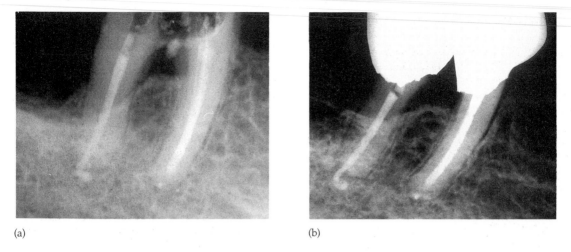

(a)   (b)

Figure 12.24 (a) Perforation into the furcation of the lower molar necessitated bicuspidization. (b) Recall examination after 6 years; the enlarged furcation space permitted effective oral hygiene.

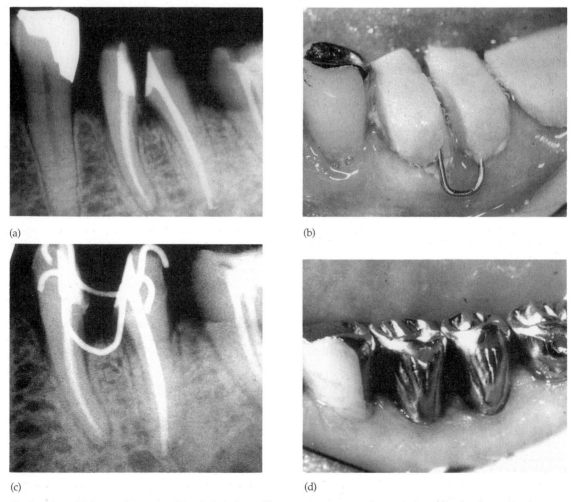

(a)   (b)

(c)   (d)

Figure 12.25 (a) Bicuspidization could only be achieved by root separation; radiograph immediately after sectioning. (b) The roots were separated orthodontically. (c) Radiograph after separation. (d) After cementation of the separate crowns.

Summary

Research findings are somewhat ambiguous about the effects of periodontal disease on the dental pulp [10,25,35]; however the adverse effects of pulp disease on the perio-dontium are well-documented [24,26,27, 33]. Clinical management of endodontic-periodontal lesions is firmly based on careful diagnosis and treatment planning [24,33], and may well involve a team approach.

References

1. ABRAMS L, TRACHTENBERG DI (1974) Hemisection – technique and restoration. *Dental Clinics of North America* **18**, 415–444.
2. ADRIAENS PA, DEBOEVER JA, LOESCHE WJ (1988) Bacterial invasion in root cementum and radicular dentin of periodontally diseased teeth in humans. A reservoir of periodontopathic bacteria. *Journal of Periodontology* **59**, 222–230.
3. BENDER IB, SELTZER S (1972) The effect of periodontal disease on the pulp. *Oral Surgery, Oral Medicine, Oral Pathology* **33**, 458–474.
4. BERGENHOLTZ G, LINDHE J (1978) Effect of experimentally induced marginal periodontitis and periodontal scaling on the dental pulp. *Journal of Clinical Periodontology* **5**, 59–73.
5. BLACK GV (1886) In: Litch W (ed.) *The American System of Dentistry*, pp. 990–992. Philadelphia, PA, USA: Lea Brothers.
6. BURCH JG, HULEN S (1974) A study of the presence of accessory foramina and the topography of molar furcations. *Oral Surgery, Oral Medicine, Oral Pathology* **38**, 451–455.
7. CAHN LR (1927) The pathology of pulps found in pyorrhetic teeth. *Dental Items of Interest* **49**, 598–617.
8. COHEN DW, KELLER G, FEDER M, LIVINGSTON E (1960) Effects of excessive occlusal forces in the gingival blood supply. *Journal of Dental Research* **39**, 677 (abstract 71).
9. COLYER F (1924) Infection of the pulp in pyorrhoeic teeth. *British Dental Journal* **45**, 558–559.
10. CZARNECKI RT, SCHILDER H (1979) A histological evaluation of the human pulp in teeth with varying degrees of periodontal disease. *Journal of Endodontics* **5**, 242–253.
11. DE DEUS QD (1975) Frequency, location and direction of the lateral, secondary, and accessory canals. *Journal of Endodontics* **1**, 361–366.
12. ELDEEB ME, ELDEEB M, TABIBI A, JENSEN JR (1982) An evaluation of the use of amalgam, Cavit, and calcium hydroxide in the repair of furcation perforations. *Journal of Endodontics* **8**, 459–466.
13. ERPENSTEIN H (1983) A 3-year study of hemisected molars. *Journal of Clinical Periodontology* **10**, 1–10.
14. FARRAR J (1884) Radical and heroic treatment of alveolar abscess by amputation of roots of teeth. *Dental Cosmos* **26**, 135–139.
15. HAMP SE, NYMAN S, LINDHE J (1975) Periodontal treatment of multirooted teeth. Results after 5 years. *Journal of Clinical Periodontology* **2**, 126–135.
16. HIRSCHFELD L, WASSERMAN B (1978) A long-term survey of tooth loss in 600 treated periodontal patients. *Journal of Periodontology* **49**, 225–237.
17. JOHNSTON HB, ORBAN B (1948) Interradicular pathology as related to accessory root canals. *Journal of Endodontia* **3**, 21–25.
18. KELLY WH, ELLINGER RF (1988) Pulpal-periradicular pathosis causing sinus tract formation through the periodontal ligament of adjacent teeth. *Journal of Endodontics* **14**, 251–257.
19. KIPIOTI A, NAKOU M, LEGAKIS N, MITSIS F (1984) Microbiological findings of infected root canals and adjacent periodontal pockets in teeth with advanced periodontitis. *Oral Surgery, Oral Medicine, Oral Pathology* **58**, 213–220.
20. KRAMER IRH (1960) The vascular architecture of the human dental pulp. *Archives of Oral Biology* **2**, 177–189.
21. LANGELAND K, RODRIGUES H, DOWDEN W (1974) Periodontal disease, bacteria and pulpal histo-pathology. *Oral Surgery, Oral Medicine, Oral Pathology* **37**, 257–270.
22. LANGER B, STEIN SD, WAGENBERG B (1981) An evaluation of root resections. A ten-year study. *Journal of Periodontology* **52**, 719–722.
23. LOWMAN JV, BURKE RS, PELLEU GB (1973) Patent accessory canals: incidence in molar furcation region. *Oral Surgery, Oral Medicine, Oral Pathology* **36**, 580–584.
24. MANDEL E, MACHTOU P, TORABINEJAD M (1993) Clinical diagnosis and treatment of endodontic and periodontal lesions. *Quintessence International* **24**, 135–139.
25. MAZUR B, MASSLER M (1964) Influence of periodontal disease on the dental pulp. *Oral Surgery, Oral Medicine, Oral Pathology* **17**, 592–603.
26. NICHOLLS E (1962) Treatment of traumatic perforations of the pulp cavity. *Oral Surgery, Oral Medicine, Oral Pathology* **15**, 603–612.
27. PITT FORD TR, TORABINEJAD M, MCKENDRY D, HONG CU, KARIYAWASAM SP (1995) Use of mineral trioxide aggregate for repair of furcal perforations. *Oral Surgery, Oral Medicine, Oral Pathology, Oral Radiology, Endodontics* **79**, 756–763.
28. ROSS IF, THOMPSON RH (1978) A long term study of root retention in the treatment of maxillary molars with furcation involvement. *Journal of Periodontology* **49**, 238–244.
29. RUBACH WC, MITCHELL DF (1965) Periodontal disease, accessory canals and pulp pathosis. *Journal of Periodontology* **36**, 34–38.

30. SELTZER S, BENDER IB (1984) *The Dental Pulp. Biologic Considerations in Dental Procedures*, pp. 303–323. Philadelphia, PA, USA: Lippincott.

31. SELTZER S, BENDER IB, ZIONTZ M (1963) The interrelationship of pulp and periodontal disease. *Oral Surgery, Oral Medicine, Oral Pathology* **16**, 1474–1490.

32. SIMON JHS, DE DEUS QD (1991) Periodontal/endodontic treatment. In: Cohen S, Burns RC (eds) *Pathways of the Pulp*, 5th edn, pp. 548–573. St Louis, MO, USA: Mosby-Year Book.

33. SIMON JH, GLICK DH, FRANK AL (1972) The relationship of endodontic–periodontic lesions. *Journal of Periodontology* **43**, 202–208.

34. SIMON P, JACOBS P (1969) The so-called combined periodontal-pulpal problem. *Dental Clinics of North America* **13**, 45–52.

35. SMUKLER H, TAGGER M (1976) Vital root amputation. A clinical and histological study. *Journal of Periodontology* **47**, 324–330.

36. STALLARD RE (1972) Periodontic–endodontic relationships. *Oral Surgery, Oral Medicine, Oral Pathology* **34**, 314–326.

37. WONG R, HIRSCH RS, CLARKE NG (1989) Endodontic effects of root planing in humans. *Endodontics and Dental Traumatology* **5**, 193–196.

13

Problems in endodontic treatment

T.R. Pitt Ford

Emergency treatment

It is axiomatic that a patient in pain must be rendered comfortable as soon as possible. Treating the patient with antibiotics and analgesics without attempting to discover and treat the cause of the pain is bad practice.

Even in the emergency situation, where the cause of the problem appears obvious, an accurate diagnosis must be established before any treatment is provided. This can only be achieved by taking a careful history and conducting a thorough clinical examination, followed by appropriate radiographic examination and special tests. If one has no idea precisely what the cause of the pain is at the end of this initial examination, active treatment should be delayed because it might be incorrect and could cause the patient harm [16]. This should be explained to the patient, and analgesics prescribed until symptoms change and the diagnosis becomes clearer.

Although the following three conditions – acute pulpitis, acute apical periodontitis and acute periradicular abscess – cause patients to present as an emergency, it must be remem-

bered that other non-endodontic conditions can cause pain, such as food packing, sinusitis and temporomandibular joint syndrome.

Where the diagnosis is clear, the emergency treatment consists of applying one or more of the basic surgical principles, which are:

1. Remove the cause of pain.
2. Provide drainage if fluid exudate is present.
3. Prescribe analgesics if required.
4. Adjust the occlusion if indicated.

Acute pulpitis

The causes of pulp injury, its prevention and treatment have been discussed in Chapter 4. The question is often asked: at what stage should palliative treatment cease and be replaced by pulp extirpation? Ideally the treatment should be related to the state of the pulp, but this can only be determined indirectly. The clinician thus relies on the history given by the patient and a thorough examination. As a rule of thumb, if the pulp of a mature permanent tooth causes severe and prolonged pain after an exciting factor such as thermal stimuli, or the patient is woken at night, then it is likely that the pulp has been irreversibly injured and pulp extirpation is indicated. Emergency pulpotomy can usually achieve relief of pain, if the clinician does not have time to extirpate the entire pulp [19]. It may be difficult to anaesthetize an acutely inflamed pulp and this problem is covered later in this chapter (page 241).

Acute apical periodontitis

This may be defined as acute inflammation of the periodontium. It is often a direct result of irritation through infection of the root canal [18], and may be associated with acute pulpitis.

A purulent exudate is not present periapically, and treatment consists of removing any pulp remnants, irrigation of the canal system with sodium hypochlorite, drying the canal, possibly sealing in a dressing, and closure of the access cavity. The importance of cleaning the canal system thoroughly cannot be overemphasized, and the use of ultrasonic instruments that have an internal irrigating facility helps considerably. This approach to treatment has been widely adopted by practising endodontists [8,9].

Care must be taken not to injure the periapical tissues by instrumenting past the apex or by over-medicating the canal with an irritant drug which may diffuse periapically and cause irritation. Indeed, the necessity of using a potent medicament within the canal has been questioned if the irrigating solution used to clean the canal is antiseptic, such as sodium hypochlorite (see Chapter 7). When a medicament is used, the corticosteroid preparations have been found to be very effective at relieving the acute phase of pain.

The tooth may be slightly extruded and the occlusion can be relieved by grinding either the tooth itself or, in exceptional circumstances, the opposing tooth. Clinically, heavily worn or restored teeth that require root canal treatment should be protected against fracture, therefore the occlusion should be adjusted and a well-adapted band cemented around the tooth. The importance of preventing a tooth from fracturing by placing a band cannot be overemphasized.

Acute periradicular abscess

This condition may develop as a sequel to acute apical periodontitis or present as an acute phase of chronic apical periodontitis. Diagnosis may sometimes be difficult. It is essential to pulp-test adjacent teeth so that the correct tooth is treated. Radiography may not be helpful as lesions do not become radiographically visible until bone, including the cortical plates, has been resorbed.

Where a soft-tissue swelling exists, the diagnosis is generally easier, but it is important to verify to which tooth the swelling relates. Relief of pain can be obtained speedily by adjusting slightly the occlusion of the causative tooth and obtaining drainage. The practice of prescribing an antibiotic without obtaining drainage is incorrect and unnecessarily prolongs the patient's misery. Opening into the pulp chamber may cause considerable discomfort because of vibration, but this can be minimized by stabilizing the tooth with fingers, and obtaining access with a small round bur in the turbine handpiece.

Ideally, the tooth should be allowed to drain until the discharge stops and then the canals irrigated gently with sodium hypochlorite, cleaned of debris and prepared fully, dressed and sealed as normal. Such a regime rarely leads to complications [2]. However, this is not always possible either because of lack of time or because the tooth is exceedingly tender and there is copious discharge of exudate. In this case it is permissible to leave the tooth on open drainage for no longer than 24 h. At the end of this period the patient should be seen again and, if comfortable, the canal instrumented, irrigated and cleaned conventionally before closure [48]. It is important that the root canal is cleaned and sealed as soon as possible so that food does not pack into the canal and microorganisms cause an acute flare-up. The practice of leaving the canal open for weeks, if not months, has nothing to commend it and usually leads to periodic flare-ups due to reinfection from the oral cavity, and even to dentinal caries of the pulp chamber and root canal; this latter makes subsequent restoration of the tooth very difficult, if not impossible.

If a tooth so treated is symptomless while on open drainage but flares up as soon as it is sealed, then the thoroughness of debridement must be questioned. This is probably the commonest cause of postoperative flare-up for no tooth will settle until the canal is thoroughly cleaned. The coronal seal must be effective, so if the clinical crown contains caries or inadequate restorations, these must be removed. It is also remotely possible that a tooth adjacent to the one being treated has a periradicular abscess, which communicates with that on the first tooth. As a precaution, two teeth on either side of any obviously non-vital tooth should be routinely tested for vitality prior to root canal treatment. Sometimes, because of anatomical difficulties or because there is an immovable obstruction in the root canal, it may not be possible to obtain drainage through the canal. In such instances emergency treatment will depend on the presence or absence of swelling. If the swelling is fluctuant, incision and drainage, or aspiration through a large-bore needle into a syringe, are advisable and generally relieve acute pain. If there is no swelling, supportive antibiotic therapy is essential, followed by post removal or surgical treatment when the acute symptoms have subsided (see Chapter 9).

Acute flare-up

Following instrumentation of a symptomless tooth, the patient can expect little pain; however, if the patient has severe pain prior to treatment, the likelihood of severe postoperative pain is higher [13,45]. The intensity of pain will reduce with time and is substantially helped by prescribing analgesics such that pain is of a low order after 24 h. Patients who present with pain and swelling are best managed by prescribing analgesics and antibiotics [45]. Flare-ups are more likely to occur in teeth with necrotic pulps [25,46,47], and in those patients who suffer from allergies. The low incidence of flare-ups reported in clinical studies is a reflection of the high standards of

treatment, but a much higher incidence of pain could be expected where treatment is inadequate.

Inadequate analgesia

Profound analgesia is essential for pulpotomy or vital pulp extirpation, yet there are occasions where, in spite of normally adequate dosage and technique, inadequate analgesia is obtained. Such occasions are distressing to the patient and embarrassing to the dentist. The main reasons for failure are enumerated below, but the subject is covered further in reviews [34,37,53].

Failure of analgesia in acute inflammation

Such a tooth may be excessively stimulated by heat or cold, and may be tender to bite on; it may be difficult, if not impossible, to achieve analgesia of sufficient depth despite repeated injections. The reason for this failure is not entirely clear, although various theories have been propounded:

1. Pulpal inflammation in the affected tooth produces hyperexcitability of the nerve fibres, particularly C fibres, such that the local anaesthetic solution is unable to block the conduction of all these impulses [1].
2. There is usually increased vascularity of the tissues in the region of the inflamed tooth and hence the local anaesthetic may be more rapidly removed by the blood stream, shortening its period of duration.
3. It has been postulated that there is a tendency for pain to increase neural transmission in the spinal cord, so countering effects of analgesics in the central nervous system; there may be a similar explanation when poor results are achieved with local anaesthetics.
4. There is a possible spread of inflammatory mediators along the myelin sheaths of nerves which restrict the absorption of the local anaesthetic; this is likely to contribute only a small part.

5. The pH of inflammatory products in the region of the tooth may be more acidic, thus making the local anaesthetic solution potentially less effective; however, this is considered unlikely [37].

Failure of analgesia

This may be due to one or a combination of the following.

1. Deposition of anaesthetic solution in the wrong place. For infiltrations, the solution should always be placed supraperiosteally and as close to the apex of the tooth as possible. For mandibular blocks, the solution must be injected close to the mandibular foramen. Common errors are:
   (a) Injecting too far posteriorly because the barrel of the syringe is not far enough back over the opposite premolars.
   (b) Injecting too low down: this is often because the lower lip is allowed to lie between the barrel of the syringe and the teeth, thus giving it downward angulation.
2. Wrong amount. The amount of anaesthetic solution required must be assessed correctly, the dosage depending on the thickness and density of the bone through which it has to pass. Most local anaesthetics have a wide safety margin so dosage can be generous. Lignocaine with adrenaline provides longer anaesthesia than plain lignocaine, or solutions of prilocaine with or without vasoconstrictor [5,31]. When a mandibular block is given the duration of anaesthesia is shorter for molars than for teeth further forward [28]. Dosage varies with:
   (a) *The patient.* If the patient is well-built and has a heavy bone structure, a larger dosage will be required than if he or she is small and frail. As a generalization, men tend to need more anaesthetic than women.
   (b) *Local anatomy.* A larger dose may be required where the root lies comparatively deeply in relatively dense bone. For example, some maxillary canines will require more anaesthetic than

upper second molars whose roots are more superficial and lie in less dense bone.
3. Incorrect technique. Analgesia which may be fully adequate for an extraction may be insufficient for pulp extirpation. Surgical procedures also require a deep level of analgesia, possibly because of the presence of inflammatory mediators around the apex of the tooth. Where deep prolonged analgesia is required, regional anaesthesia will often prove more satisfactory than an infiltration technique.
4. Intravascular injection. An aspirating syringe should be used to prevent intravascular injection. Although this complication may occur during any injection, it is more likely to happen when injecting in the maxillary molar region or when giving a mandibular block. If this occurs the patient may feel palpitations or there may be sudden pallor of the face. As soon as the patient shows any sign of intravascular injection, the needle should be withdrawn to remove it from the blood vessel. It is very important to reassure the patient to prevent endogenous adrenaline from compounding the problem, which should resolve in a few minutes. It is frequently necessary to repeat the injection of local anaesthetic to achieve analgesia, as the solution did not go where it was intended.
5. Variation in individual response. Individuals vary considerably in their response to local anaesthetics. For some patients, not more than 1 ml is needed for an infiltration injection, whereas some others may invariably require 3 ml. Similarly, the duration of analgesia may vary between individuals from 60 to 150 min with the same amount of anaesthetic [29]. Therefore it is desirable to record in the patient's notes the type and quantity of anaesthetic used, particularly when the patient's response is abnormal.
6. Variation in pain threshold of individuals. The degree of pain tolerance varies widely with different individuals, and the sensation that one person may interpret as pain another would merely consider discomfort. Therefore in the former patient a far deeper level of analgesia is required through a greater dosage, and by reassurance. In a few very nervous individuals

premedication may be indicated. The tolerance of an individual may vary from time to time as a result of such factors as systemic disease, lack of sleep, hunger or domestic worries.

Alternative techniques

In endodontic practice, failure to obtain analgesia ultimately is an infrequent occurrence, and when it does occur is likely to be in a mandibular molar tooth [6]. One must accept that an acutely inflamed pulp can remain exquisitely painful in spite of what appears to be an otherwise satisfactory mandibular block. In such infrequent instances several alternative techniques are available:

1. Sedation of the pulp.
2. Intrapulpal anaesthesia.
3. Periodontal ligament injection.
4. Sedation or general anaesthesia.

Sedation of the pulp

The kindest treatment to the patient is to accept failure of local analgesia, dress the tooth to reduce the pulpal inflammation and attempt pulpal extirpation on a subsequent occasion. The pulp may be sedated with a zinc oxide–eugenol dressing [21], or with a corticosteroid antibiotic dressing [10,38].

If the pulp has been exposed and it is hyperaemic, it bleeds copiously and should be allowed to do so for 2–3 min to wash out inflammatory mediators. The exposure is then covered with a pledget of cotton wool damped by a medicament. The cotton wool is covered by a fortified zinc oxide–eugenol cement. On the subsequent visit a local anaesthetic should again be given, and when it appears effective attempts should be made to extirpate the pulp. It is usually possible to achieve effective anaesthesia when it was not possible on a previous occasion.

Intrapulpal anaesthesia

This may be used to supplement existing inadequate anaesthesia. The technique consists of injecting local anaesthetic solution into the pulp. The needle is advanced into the pulp chamber and a few drops of solution are injected. This is initially painful but usually effective in allowing sufficient analgesia for pulp extirpation.

Periodontal ligament injection

This may be used to supplement existing inadequate anaesthesia [6]. This technique has superseded the intraosseous injection because it is easier to perform and as effective in augmenting incomplete dental analgesia. Special syringes allow small preset increments of anaesthetic solution to be injected intraosseously through the periodontal ligament. The anaesthetic carpule is inserted into an autoclavable protective sleeve to guard against breakage and a 30-gauge ultrashort needle used to inject the solution into the ligament. Prior to injection, the gingival sulcus must be disinfected and topical anaesthetic used to reduce discomfort during injection. The primary injection is given on the distal of the tooth, and the needle with the bevel towards the root face is slid into the periodontal ligament space until it is stopped by alveolar bone. The lever is squeezed extremely slowly and 0.2 ml of anaesthetic deposited. The procedure may be repeated on the mesial of the tooth, and in the case of molars on other surfaces. Anaesthesia is almost instantaneous and lasts up to 30 min if a solution containing adrenaline is used.

This technique has some disadvantages:

1. Infection can be introduced into the tissues unless the soft tissues have been disinfected.
2. The injection is painful unless a surface anaesthetic has been used.
3. In medically compromised patients, injections of adrenaline that are in effect intravascular may be contraindicated.
4. The injection alters the occlusion of the tooth very slightly by raising it out of its socket, and a careful check of the occlusion of the temporary restoration must be made.

Sedation or general anaesthesia

There are rare and exceptional cases where the use of relative analgesia, intravenous sedation or general anaesthesia is the only way that a vital pulp can be extirpated, or an abscess drained. Generally the reasons are not related to the effectiveness of local anaesthesia but to the attitude of the patient. In such instances, before embarking on such a course, the clinician must be satisfied that the patient is fit enough, the tooth is of sufficient importance to the patient's well-being, and that the patient will accept subsequent treatment without recourse to further intravenous sedation or general anaesthesia. For further information on this subject the reader is referred elsewhere [35,36,39,40].

Radiography

Radiography is an invaluable and essential aid to endodontic treatment and without its use treatment cannot be considered satisfactory. However, radiographs can be misleading, particularly if badly taken, poorly processed and examined in a cursory manner under poor viewing conditions, so that essential diagnostic features are overlooked.

Quality control

Radiographs must be as clear and undistorted as possible and this is best achieved using the paralleling technique [42,51]. This eliminates foreshortening or elongation of tooth images [12] and in the maxillary molar region avoids superimposition of the zygoma on the root apices; the technique also avoids coning off. Film-holder and beam-aiming devices are available not only for preoperative radiographs but also for the length-measurement radiograph. Good-quality dental X-ray film is necessary, and E-speed film is now considered the standard. The E-speed film requires approximately half the X-ray exposure of D-speed film, and yields as good an image [32]. Films must be carefully processed to ensure that they have good contrast and do not fade; well-maintained automatic processors achieve consistent results. Films should be examined, preferably under magnification, on a viewer with extraneous light blocked out. If the image on the film is not satisfactory, the radiograph should be retaken.

Radiographic image

It should be remembered that the radiograph gives limited information because it displays a shadow of the object under investigation and for shadows of different objects to be discernible there must be adequate contrast between them. Further, a radiograph is a two-dimensional picture of a three-dimensional object, and so superimposition and loss of detail are to be expected.

Before considering what can be seen on a radiograph it is as well to recall what *cannot* be seen. A pulp with acute pulpitis looks identical, on the radiograph, to a normal healthy pulp. Similarly, there is no difference in the radiographic appearance of a vital from a necrotic pulp within a tooth, but the latter will ultimately cause periradicular changes which are visible on the radiograph. These take the form of an initial widening of the periodontal ligament space, which may ultimately develop into a visible periradicular radiolucency.

A tooth with an acute periradicular abscess will initially show no periradicular bone changes on the radiograph. Some experimental studies have shown that a lesion does not become radiographically visible until cortical bone becomes resorbed [3,4,33,49].

Detection of extra roots and canals

Abnormalities in root anatomy may occur in any tooth, although it is more common in some teeth. Generally, if the external shape deviates from normal, the root canal system is also likely to be abnormal. For this reason preoperative radiographs should be examined very carefully. Any variation of the outline or contour of the root should raise suspicion of an extra root. Sharp differences in density of the radiographic image of roots are often indicative of the presence of an extra root.

Extra canals cannot be distinguished easily on the preoperative radiograph, but the length radiograph is more useful. In such instances it is possible to follow the file within the root canal and if an extra canal is present, it will show as a dark line adjacent to the file. This line may not be parallel to the file but may leave the main canal, curve and rejoin further along [41]. If the image of a file is not central in the root in an angled film, e.g. in the distal root of a mandibular molar, an additional canal should be suspected.

The coronal part of the root should be examined carefully because the root canal is generally widest in this area. A sharp change in density along the canal may be due to divergence of the main canal into finer branches, e.g. in a mandibular first premolar. In some teeth divergent canals may rejoin a short distance from the apical foramen and this can be confirmed by placing a file to within 1 mm of the foramen and then attempting to negotiate the second canal to the same point. If the second file binds short of the calculated length, then it may be assumed that the canals join at that point. Rubber dam clamps may obscure the image of the coronal part of the root canal, particularly if there is excessive angulation of the X-ray tube.

Certain teeth, such as maxillary first premolars and mandibular incisors, may have two canals in a buccolingual direction, one behind the other. These canals are usually superimposed on the preoperative radiograph and it may help diagnosis if such teeth are routinely radiographed from a different angle as well [23]. In this way the extra canal may be demonstrated and it is also possible to determine the buccolingual position of each canal.

Alternative imaging systems

Xeroradiography

This is a process whereby images are recorded on electrostatically charged plates without the use of chemicals or the need for a darkroom. The process has been used for a number of years in dental radiography. However, its use has never become widespread because of its high cost. It allows paper prints to be viewed rapidly without the need for processing chemicals [14,52]. It has the advantage of edge enhancement of structures such as the pulp space.

Radiovisiography

More recently a new system of radiography has been introduced – radiovisiography (RVG; Trophy Radiologie, Paris, France) [26].

In this system, an intraoral electronic sensor is used instead of an X-ray film. The image produced on the sensor is converted into an electronic signal that is transmitted to a processing and display unit where it is instantly displayed on a small screen. The processing unit can enhance the image to make it clearer. Permanent copies of the image may be stored on computer disk, or paper printouts made.

The advantage of this technique is that instant viewing is possible and the exposure required is low. The size of the sensor allows an image of a molar tooth to be viewed. Its full potential will depend on further development, refinement of the rather bulky intraoral sensor and reduction in cost. Clinical evaluation has shown that RVG is a viable technique for alternatives to the conventional-length radiographic film [30].

Obstructions in the root canal

The preoperative radiograph must be examined carefully prior to beginning root canal treatment. From the radiograph the course, length and approximate size of the root canals should be assessed, together with the presence of any obstructions that might prevent instrumentation. Whether it is necessary or possible to remove an obstruction will depend on its composition, size and position within the root canal system. Obstructions can be naturally occurring or iatrogenic.

Natural obstructions

Natural obstructions include pulp chamber obliteration, pulp stones, calcified canals or anatomical anomalies which make instrumentation difficult or impossible. It is essential to prepare a sufficiently large access cavity so that visual and physical access are not restricted. If the tooth has been crowned, the access is considerably improved by removal of the crown. This is an easy decision if the crown is technically deficient, but less so if it is very well-made; endodontic treatment must not be compromised to conserve the crown. The presence of a rubber dam clamp fitting squarely on the tooth helps to define the buccal and lingual surfaces clearly so that the access cavity is not misplaced.

Pulp chamber obliteration

Careful examination of the pulp space on the preoperative radiograph will show its size and to what extent it has been filled with irritation dentine. The mesiodistal angulation of the tooth should also be assessed on the radiograph. It is helpful to gauge the depth of the pulp space on the radiograph with a bur in a handpiece; this should help prevent damage to the floor of the pulp chamber. Irritation dentine in the original pulp space must be carefully removed with a long-shanked bur in the low-speed handpiece; periodically, the operator should stop and assess whether the cavity is in the correct position. Irritation dentine is darker than normal dentine, and may feel slightly softer on probing with an endodontic probe (DG 16). Where the pulp chamber is only partially obliterated, the patent canal orifices are useful landmarks for orientation. If a canal orifice remains elusive, a radiograph can be taken to check that the cavity is not deviating off course in a mesiodistal direction; the jaws of the rubber dam clamp help in the bucco-lingual direction. Once the probe will stick in the canal orifice it is usually possible to negotiate the canal with a fine file (International Organization for Standardization (ISO) size 06).

Pulp stones

Provided pulp stones can be identified from the preoperative radiograph and occur within the pulp chamber, they present little difficulty in removal. However, it is more difficult to remove a stone from a root canal, particularly if it is attached to the wall. In such an instance, if a file can be passed alongside the stone, it may be removed by careful filing. The introduction of ultrasonic instrumentation has considerably facilitated the removal of pulp stones from root canals.

Calcified canals

Canals that are completely calcified from the pulp chamber to the apical foramen are very rare. Calcification normally begins in the pulp chamber and continues in an apical direction as a result of mild pulpal inflammation. Sometimes canals that look completely calcified on a radiograph can be instrumented because a very fine pathway remains within the calcified material. This may not be visible on the radiograph because of inadequate contrast. For this reason, where endodontic treatment is indicated, an attempt should always be made to negotiate this fine canal using a fine file (ISO size 06), rather than opting for surgery. Once this file has negotiated the canal, its enlargement is relatively simple. The use of ethylenediaminetetraacetic acid (EDTA) alone, or as RC Prep, will help canal enlargement, but is of no use in finding an obstructed canal.

It should be made quite clear that a symptomless tooth with a calcified canal and no periradicular radiolucency does not require root canal treatment [22].

Iatrogenic obstructions

Iatrogenic obstructions include posts, old gutta-percha, silver or cement root fillings and broken root canal instruments.

Posts

Where root canal retreatment is indicated, it is usually possible to remove all but the largest cast posts by ultrasonic vibration, use of special post removers, or the Masserann trepan [24]. Ultrasonic vibration of posts is achieved with a scaler tip placed on the post, or its cement lute, and operated at high power with waterspray cooling; in many instances the post will be worked loose. Special post removers need to have a sufficient collar of dentine against which to apply force, and they are not suitable for screw posts. The Masserann trepan, which is available in different diameters, fits over the post and aims to cut away the cement lute; it works best on parallel-sided posts, and least satisfactorily on oval tapered cast posts. One advantage of the Masserann trepan is that it will work on a post fractured within the root. If cement remains after post removal in the bottom of the hole, it may be removed by an ultrasonic scaler tip.

Gutta-percha

If the existing gutta-percha points have been poorly condensed, it is often possible to negotiate a file alongside and use it to withdraw the gutta-percha points. Sometimes a Hedstrom file will achieve this when other files have failed. Well-condensed gutta-percha resists file penetration, therefore that in the coronal part of the canal should be removed with Gates-Glidden burs of appropriate size that remove gutta-percha but not dentine. The burs should be rotated sufficiently fast to soften the gutta-percha without waterspray. Remaining gutta-percha should then be removed with solvent, e.g. chloroform, methyl chloroform or xylol [50]. This is introduced into the pulp chamber in a syringe; only a small amount is necessary to achieve softening, limit environmental effects and avoid damaging the rubber dam. A file will then pass easily into the mass of gutta-percha, which clings to the file as it is withdrawn. After all the gutta-percha has been removed, canal preparation proceeds as for an initial treatment (see Chapter 6).

Silver points

Although these are not placed in root canals any more, there are still a number of patients who present with symptoms associated with teeth filled with silver points. These points can usually be removed provided that it is possible to grab hold of the coronal end. It is therefore most important not to cut off the coronal ends during preparation of the access cavity. The cement in the pulp chamber around the heads of the silver points is best removed with an ultrasonic scaler. If space exists alongside the silver point in the coronal part of the root canal, an ultrasonic file may be used to break up the sealer cement. Then the silver point may be gripped with fine forceps if access permits, or alternatively the silver point should be elevated with a blunt excavator [20]. If this fails, it is necessary to return to more ultrasonic loosening. The great majority of silver points can be removed [20], but those that will resist removal may have been inserted with a resin-based sealer, e.g. AH 26.

Cement root fillings

Cements based on zinc oxide can usually be removed with ultrasonic files, as can non-setting pastes. Hard-setting materials, e.g. AH 26 and SPAD, are almost impossible to remove; in a straight canal it may be possible to drill out such a material, but in a curved canal the bur is very likely to deviate.

Broken root canal instruments

Management of these may be considered according to their presence in the various thirds of a root canal [11]; if the instrument is superficial, it is normally possible to remove it; deeper down it may be possible to bypass it and incorporate it into the new filling; apically it may only be possible to clean, shape and fill the canal to the fractured end of the instrument [16].

Within the coronal third. If an instrument is present in the pulp chamber, it may be possible, provided access is sufficiently large, to grab hold of it with fine forceps and withdraw it. If the instrument is present in the coronal third of the canal, the access should be enlarged and files worked around the instrument to create more room. It may be possible to create space around the instrument using a Masserann trepan before using the special extractor (Figure 13.1). This is essentially a tube which fits over the instrument, and into the back end of the tube a small stylet is then inserted to trap the instrument against a constriction in the tube. Once the instrument is gripped in the extractor, it can be pulled out.

Within the middle third. When the broken file is not present in the coronal third, it is much more difficult to remove it from the middle third, particularly in a curved root canal. Attempts to use the Masserann trepan frequently fail to get the tube over the head of the instrument. In addition, the furcal wall of a mesial root of a mandibular molar may easily be over-thinned in the attempt; this reduces the long-term prognosis of the tooth. Instead, it may be better to accept being able to negotiate files past the broken instrument to the apical constriction, and then to fill the canal alongside the instrument, thereby

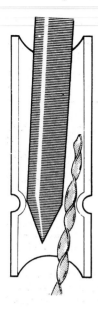

Figure 13.1 Diagram of a Masserann extractor, which consists of a tube with a constriction; into this a stylet is inserted to trap the broken instrument against the constriction.

incorporating it into the new filling. There is no evidence that such an action adversely affects the prognosis.

Within the apical third. It is rarely feasible to use a Masserann trepan in this part of a curved root canal. However, it may be possible to work an ultrasonic file alongside and possibly loosen the broken instrument [27]. If the instrument cannot be removed, then it may be possible to bypass it and incorporate it into the root canal filling. Should it be neither possible to remove the instrument nor to bypass it, then the canal should be cleaned, shaped and filled to the broken end of the instrument; in teeth without periradicular radiolucencies this does not adversely affect the prognosis [7,15].

Through the apical foramen. If a broken file which protrudes through the apical foramen is long enough to have part in the coronal third of the canal, then it is usually possible to remove it as described above. On the other hand, if there is only a small part of the file in the apical part of the canal, then its removal via the coronal access cavity is likely to be impossible. It should normally be managed in the same way as a piece confined to the apical third of the canal, that is, by cleaning, shaping and filling the canal to the broken end of the instrument. Should the patient continue to experience pain, swelling or a discharging sinus tract after this, then assessment for endodontic surgery is needed. It is worth pointing out that the instrument is very likely to be made from a non-corrodible alloy (e.g. stainless steel), therefore it is not the instrument which causes any continued inflammation, but the associated infection.

Prevention of instrument fracture

Generally instruments break because of abuse – either because they have been used too many times, or they have been twisted excessively within the root canal. Fine files (ISO size 06–20) should preferably be used for only one tooth and then discarded. Larger sizes may be autoclaved and used again provided that they are examined carefully and discarded if the blades show any irregularity, this being an indication of overuse. Rotatory use of files is more damaging than vertical filing, so if fine files are used in a rotation technique, they must be discarded after use on one tooth. If the tip of a fine file becomes bent at a sharp angle during use, it should not be straightened but discarded. The breaking of an instrument in a root canal is distressing to the operator and may alarm the patient; its retrieval is very time-consuming. For these reasons, the use of damaged instruments is a false economy.

Prevention and management of fractured root-filled teeth

Patients with tooth wear are at risk of cusp fracture, and preparation of an access cavity to the pulp chamber weakens the tooth further. Where there is a high risk of tooth fracture occurring during root canal treatment, particularly in a molar with a large mesio-occluso-distal restoration, the clinical crown should first be protected by cementing a band (e.g. an orthodontic band) around the tooth. If this precaution is not taken, a cusp or the side of a tooth may fracture during treatment. The gingival extent of fracture may be supragingival, supracrestal or below bone level. The vertical fracture may even extend sufficiently far into the root that the tooth becomes non-restorable and needs to be extracted. If the tooth fractures between visits, the temporary filling in the access cavity is lost, the canal space becomes contaminated and the tooth may be tender to bite on if a loose cusp still has some periodontal attachment. Subsequent isolation of the tooth by rubber dam becomes more difficult as clamps may be far less retentive.

Single-rooted teeth with vertical root fractures have a hopeless prognosis, and therefore need to be extracted [44]. Vertical fractures of root-filled posterior teeth may present with a variety of symptoms [43]. The fate of vertically fractured multirooted teeth will depend on the site of the fracture. Sometimes it is possible to resect part of the tooth, and retain the remaining part, which must be restorable. This treatment has been covered in Chapter 12. After root canal treatment it is generally advised that molar and maxillary premolar teeth should be crowned, as leaving MOD amalgam restorations leads to a high incidence of long-term tooth fracture [17]. The restoration of root-filled teeth is covered in Chapter 14.

References

1. AHLBERG KF (1978) Influence of local noxious heat stimulation on sensory nerve activity in the feline dental pulp. *Acta Physiologica Scandinavica* **103**, 71–80.
2. AUGUST DS (1977) Managing the abscessed tooth: instrument or close? *Journal of Endodontics* **3**, 316–318.
3. BENDER IB, SELTZER S (1961) Roentgenographic and direct observation of experimental lesions in bone. Part I. *Journal of the American Dental Association* **62**, 152–160.
4. BENDER IB, SELTZER S (1961) Roentgenographic and direct observation of experimental lesions in bone. Part II. *Journal of the American Dental Association* **62**, 708–716.
5. CHONG BS, PITT FORD TR, MCDONALD F (1996) Effects of prilocaine local anaesthesic solutions on pulpal blood flow in maxillary canines. *Endodontics and Dental Traumatology* **12**, 89–95.
6. COHEN HP, CHA BY, SPANGBERG LSW (1993) Endodontic anesthesia in mandibular molars: a clinical study. *Journal of Endodontics* **19**, 370–373.
7. CRUMP MC, NATKIN E (1970) Relationship of broken root canal instruments to endodontic case prognosis: a clinical investigation. *Journal of the American Dental Association* **80**, 1341–1347.
8. DORN SO, MOODNIK RM, FELDMAN MJ, BORDEN BG (1977) Treatment of the endodontic emergency: a report based on a questionnaire – part I. *Journal of Endodontics* **3**, 94–100.
9. DORN SO, MOODNIK RM, FELDMAN MJ, BORDEN BG (1977) Treatment of the endodontic emergency: a report based' on a questionnaire – part II. *Journal of Endodontics* **3**, 153–156.
10. EHRMANN EH (1965) The effect of triamcinolone with tetracycline on the dental pulp and apical periodontium. *Journal of Prosthetic Dentistry* **15**, 144–152.
11. FORS UGH, BERG JO (1986) Endodontic treatment of root canals obstructed by foreign objects. *International Endodontic Journal* **19**, 2–10.
12. FORSBERG J (1987) A comparison of the paralleling and bisecting–angle radiographic techniques in endodontics. *International Endodontic Journal* **20**, 177–182.
13. GENET JM, WESSELINK PR, THODEN VAN VELZEN SK (1986) The incidence of preoperative and postoperative pain in endodontic therapy. *International Endodontic Journal* **19**, 221–229.
14. GRATT BM (1979) Xeroradiography of dental structures. III. Pilot clinical studies. *Oral Surgery, Oral Medicine, Oral Pathology* **48**, 276–280.
15. GROSSMAN LI (1968) Fate of endodontically treated teeth with fractured root canal instruments. *Journal of the British Endodontic Society* **2**, 35–37.
16. GUTMANN JL, DUMSHA TC, LOVDAHL PE (1992) *Problem Solving in Endodontics; Prevention, Identification, and Management.* St Louis, MO, USA: Mosby-Year Book.
17. HANSEN EK, ASMUSSEN E, CHRISTIANSEN NC (1990) *In vivo* fractures of endodontically treated posterior teeth restored with amalgam. *Endodontics and Dental Traumatology* **6**, 49–55.
18. HASHIOKA K, YAMASAKI M, NAKANE A, HORIBA N, NAKAMURA H (1992) The relationship between clinical symptoms and anaerobic bacteria from infected root canals. *Journal of Endodontics* **18**, 558–561.
19. HASSELGREN G, REIT C (1989) Emergency pulpotomy: pain relieving effect with and without the use of sedative dressings. *Journal of Endodontics* **15**, 254–256.
20. HÜLSMANN M (1990) The retrieval of silver cones using different techniques. *International Endodontic Journal* **23**, 298–303.
21. HUME WR (1988) *In vitro* studies on the local pharmacodynamics, pharmacology and toxicology of eugenol and zinc oxide–eugenol. *International Endodontic Journal* **21**, 130–134.
22. JACOBSEN I, KEREKES K (1977) Long-term prognosis of traumatized permanent anterior teeth showing calcifying processes in the pulp cavity. *Scandinavian Journal of Dental Research* **85**, 588–598.
23. KAFFE I, KAUFMAN A, LITTNER MM, LAZARSON A (1985) Radiographic study of the root canal system of mandibular anterior teeth. *International Endodontic Journal* **18**, 253–259.

24. MASSERANN J (1971) Entfernen metallischer Fragmente aus Wurzelkanälen. *Journal of the British Endodontic Society* **5**, 55–59.

25. MOR C, ROTSTEIN I, FRIEDMAN S (1992) Incidence of interappointment emergency associated with endodontic therapy. *Journal of Endodontics* **18**, 509–511.

26. MOUYEN F, BENZ C, SONNABEND E, LODTER JP (1989) Presentation and physical evaluation of Radio-VisioGraphy. *Oral Surgery, Oral Medicine, Oral Pathology* **68**, 238–242.

27. NAGAI O, TAGI N, KAYABA Y, KODAMA S, OSADA T (1986) Ultrasonic removal of broken instruments in root canals. *International Endodontic Journal* **19**, 298–304.

28. ODOR TM, PITT FORD TR, MCDONALD F (1994) Effect of inferior alveolar nerve block anaesthesia on the lower teeth. *Endodontics and Dental Traumatology* **10**, 144–148.

29. ODOR TM, PITT FORD TR, MCDONALD F (1994) Adrenaline in local anaesthesia: the effect of concentration on dental pulpal circulation and anaesthesia. *Endodontics and Dental Traumatology* **10**, 167–173.

30. ONG EY, PITT FORD TR (1995) Comparison of Radio-visiography with radiographic film in root length determination. *International Endodontic Journal* **28**, 25–29.

31. PITT FORD TR, SEARE MA, MCDONALD F (1993) Action of adrenaline on the effect of dental local anaesthetic solutions. *Endodontics and Dental Traumatology* **9**, 31–35.

32. POWELL-CULLINGFORD AW, PITT FORD TR (1993) The use of E-speed film for root canal length determination. *International Endodontic Journal* **26**, 268–272.

33. REGAN JE, MITCHELL DF (1963) Evaluation of periapical radiolucencies found in cadavers. *Journal of the American Dental Association* **66**, 529–533.

34. ROBERTS DH, SOWRAY JH (1987) *Local Analgesia in Dentistry*, 3rd edn. Oxford, UK: Wright.

35. ROBERTS GJ (1990) Inhalation sedation (relative analgesia) with oxygen/nitrous oxide gas mixtures: 1. Principles. *Dental Update* **17**, 139–146.

36. ROBERTS GJ (1990) Inhalation sedation (relative analgesia) with oxygen/nitrous oxide gas mixtures: 2. Practical techniques. *Dental Update* **17**, 190–196.

37. ROOD JP (1977) Some anatomical and physiological causes of failure to achieve mandibular analgesia. *British Journal of Oral Surgery* **15**, 75–82.

38. SCHROEDER A (1962) Cortisone in dental surgery. *International Dental Journal* **12**, 356–373.

39. SCULLY C, CAWSON RA (1993) *Medical Problems in Dentistry*, 3rd edn. Oxford, UK: Butterworth-Heinemann.

40. SKELLY AM (1992) Sedation in dental practice. *Dental Update* **19**, 61–67.

41. SLOWEY RR (1974) Radiographic aids in the detection of extra root canals. *Oral Surgery, Oral Medicine, Oral Pathology* **37**, 762–772.

42. SMITH NJD (1988) *Dental Radiography*, 2nd edn. Oxford, UK: Blackwell Scientific Publications.

43. TAMSE A (1988) Iatrogenic vertical root fractures in endodontically treated teeth. *Endodontics and Dental Traumatology* **4**, 190–196.

44. TESTORI T, BADINO M, CASTAGNOLA M (1993) Vertical root fractures in endodontically treated teeth: a clinical survey of 36 cases. *Journal of Endodontics* **19**, 87–90.

45. TORABINEJAD M, CYMERMAN JJ, FRANKSON M, LEMON RR, MAGGIO JD, SCHILDER H (1994) Effectiveness of various medications on postoperative pain following complete instrumentation. *Journal of Endodontics* **20**, 345–354.

46. TROPE M (1990) Relationship of intracanal medicaments to endodontic flare-ups. *Endodontics and Dental Traumatology* **6**, 226–229.

47. TROPE M (1991) Flare-up rate of single-visit endodontics. *International Endodontic Journal* **24**, 24–27.

48. WALKER RT (1984) Emergency treatment – a review. *International Endodontic Journal* **17**, 29–35.

49. WENGRAF A (1964) Radiologically occult bone cavities. An experimental study and review. *British Dental Journal* **117**, 532–536.

50. WENNBERG A, ØRSTAVIK D (1989) Evaluation of alternatives to chloroform in endodontic practice. *Endodontics and Dental Traumatology* **5**, 234–237.

51. WHAITES EJ (1992) *Essentials of Dental Radiography and Radiology*. Edinburgh, UK: Churchill Livingstone.

52. WHITE SC, STAFFORD ML, BEENINGA LR (1978) Intraoral xeroradiography. *Oral Surgery, Oral Medicine and Oral Pathology* **46**, 862–870.

53. WONG MKS, JACOBSEN PL (1992) Reasons for local anesthesia failures. *Journal of the American Dental Association* **123(1)**, 69–73.

14

Restoration of endodontically treated teeth

R. Ibbetson

Introduction

Modern root canal treatment has a high rate of success: teeth with vital pulps have a successful outcome >90% [31]. The same study also showed that if the endodontic condition of the tooth was poor at the beginning of treatment, e.g. with an inadequate root canal filling already present and a periapical radiolucency, the success rate was approximately 60%. Such information is of considerable importance to the restorative dentist in timing when to restore the root-treated tooth. It is unfortunate that there is little information about how successful restorative procedures are for root-treated teeth when compared with their vital counterparts. It is however apparent that there are many methods available. Some of these are traditional, but in this, as in many other areas of dentistry, the availability of modern adhesive techniques is expanding the options for treatment.

Effects of endodontic treatment on the tooth

It is known that the failure rate of restored root-treated teeth can be higher than for vital teeth [28]. There has always been the belief that the removal of a pulp from a tooth changes the physical properties of the tooth structure. Terms such as brittle are used to describe root-treated teeth and this is often given as the major reason why fractures are common. There is certainly a reduction in moisture content in dentine following loss of the pulp. However, apart from perhaps a very small increase in the modulus of elasticity [12], which could be interpreted to be consistent with making the tooth more brittle, most other research has failed to show any change in the physical properties of dentine [30]. This does not necessarily mean that there is none; it may be more a reflection of the difficulties in carrying out tests on very small samples of tooth structure. Alternatively, it is known that teeth undergo very rapid postmortem changes after extraction and it may be that by the time tests of extracted teeth take place, significant changes in the physical properties of the teeth have already occurred.

In practical terms, whether the tooth structure undergoes some fundamental alteration is probably of little consequence. The major effect of root canal treatment is the removal of tooth structure. Many teeth that undergo root canal treatment have previously been extensively restored. Modern root canal treatment requires access cavities that are not only correctly positioned but are large enough to allow straight-line access into the root canal system. This produces a further loss of tooth structure, to which is added canal preparation that removes yet more dentine. Stresses generated in restorative and endodontic procedures may also contribute to failure by promoting cracks and fractures. Endodontic procedures such as the condensation of gutta-percha may produce stress, the consequences of which cannot be determined but are certainly undesirable [23]. The previous treatment procedures therefore have a cumulative weakening effect on the tooth and in the absence of any firm data on the essential effects of removing the pulp, the most helpful concept to bear in mind is one of restoring an extensively damaged tooth. In such cases, there is a need to:

1. Preserve and protect useful remaining tooth structure.
2. Minimize stress within both tooth and restoration.

Timing the restorative procedure

It is essential that endodontic treatment is part of an overall strategy for treatment of the patient. It may be better to consider extraction and construction of a fixed prosthesis when the condition of the tooth to be root-canal-treated makes it unrestorable. When the costs of the endodontic treatment and restoration are compared with those of a bridge and reviewed in the light of the prognosis for the tooth, extraction and replacement may be preferable to preservation. However, once the decision to root-treat and restore has been taken, a further decision will need to be made as to how long to wait after root canal treatment before placing the final restoration. There is no set answer to this and the following factors need to be considered:

1. The pre-existing endodontic status.
2. The quality of the root canal filling.
3. The site of the tooth in the mouth.
4. The type of restoration to be placed.

Given a satisfactory technical result on the final radiograph of the root-filled tooth and an absence of symptoms, where the pulp had previously been vital, it would be reasonable to proceed immediately to placement of the final restoration. In contrast, if there had been an apical radiolucency prior to treatment associated with an unsatisfactory root canal filling, the placement of a satisfactory root canal filling would not give the same chance of success. In such cases, it would be sensible to delay final restoration until evidence of periradicular healing is seen radiographically. This is particularly true if further endodontic treatment is made more complicated or even impossible once the final restoration has been placed. For example, the placement of a post in the palatal root of a maxillary molar makes further root canal treatment difficult. However, where the decision is taken to wait for evidence of healing, little will be seen radiographically for at least 6 months. During this time, the remaining tooth structure must be protected by an adequate interim restoration which must also be capable of preventing coronal leakage that would otherwise adversely influence the outcome.

Anterior teeth

Conservative restoration of anterior teeth

On many occasions, the restorative procedure required following endodontic treatment is simple and under such circumstances there is nothing to be gained by delay. Should further endodontic treatment become necessary, the restoration can easily be removed to allow access to the root canal filling. This is true for many anterior teeth where there has been little previous restoration. Such teeth may be restored using a combination of composite resin placed over a base of glass ionomer cement. Composite resin is the most appropriate material for restoring the access cavity, given its physical properties and a high-quality surface finish, together with a good seal achieved by acid-etching enamel. Care must be taken to ensure that the root canal filling is removed from the crown of the tooth if discoloration of the dentine due to endodontic sealers containing eugenol is to be prevented.

Tooth reinforcement

There is no indication for the placement of a post within the root canal of a relatively intact anterior tooth. The idea that such a post can reinforce a tooth and therefore protect against fracture has been shown to be untrue. A clinical study has shown that posts have no reinforcing effect [33]. In an *in vitro* study of extracted teeth where those which were root-treated were compared with those that had additionally received a post, the results showed no difference in their resistance to fracture whilst, in the group with posts, the fractures occurred further apically near the end of the post [8]. Translating this into clinical practice indicates that the presence of the post not only confers no advantage but in the event of fracture may make the tooth more difficult to restore.

With the increased range of adhesive techniques available for restoring anterior teeth, together with the lack of benefit of placing posts, there is every indication for a conservative approach to the restoration of even extensively damaged root-canal-treated anterior teeth. Figure 14.1 shows a root-treated anterior tooth which had discoloured some time following treatment. This was successfully treated by internal bleaching using a combination of sodium perborate and 30% hydrogen peroxide sealed within the access cavity for 1 week – the so-called walking bleach technique. Sometimes the tooth is relatively immature with a wide root canal (Figure 14.2); post placement not only has little to offer under such circumstances but

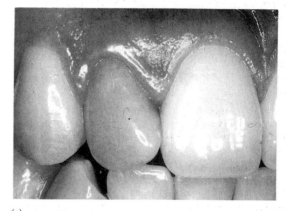

(a)

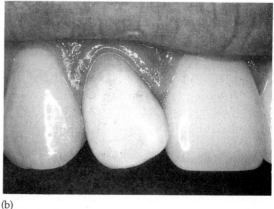

(b)

Figure 14.1 (a) Maxillary lateral incisor discoloured following root canal treatment. (b) Maxillary lateral incisor following 'walking bleach' treatment.

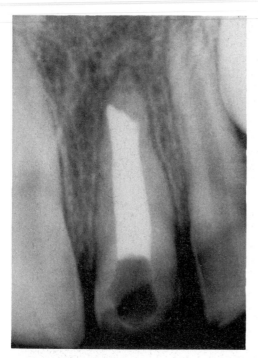

Figure 14.2 Periapical radiograph of a tooth with an immature root for which a post crown is not indicated.

would be clearly damaging. If bleaching of such a discoloured tooth were unsuccessful, it could be restored using a combination of composite resin in the access cavity together with a labial porcelain veneer.

Once it is accepted that posts do not strengthen teeth, there are good reasons to avoid post placement in anterior teeth, particularly in younger patients where wide root canals mean that there is little radicular dentine. Figure 14.3 shows tetracycline-discoloured incisors of a 16-year-old whose maxillary left central incisor had received a vital pulpotomy at the age of 10 years. The dimensions of the root canal made post placement inadvisable and there was further-more no indication for root canal treatment as the pulp was vital. This tooth was restored with a directly placed composite resin; and 7 years later this was in turn replaced with a porcelain veneer. The restoration continues to perform well and the pulp of the tooth remains vital 20 years after the initial pul-potomy. It could be argued that had a post been placed when the patient was 10 years

old, the tooth might by this time have been lost. The worst outcome for any of the con-servative restorative procedures that were undertaken would have been fracture of the remnants of the coronal tooth tissues with loss of the restoration. This would have still left the opportunity for placement of a post-retained crown but to date this has not been necessary.

Anterior crowns without posts

There are obviously occasions when a crown is necessary for a root-canal-treated anterior tooth but it is certainly not necessary that in all instances the tooth will require placement of a post. Where anterior teeth are in normal occlusion, it is the palatal wall of dentine in maxillary anteriors and the labial wall for mandibular anteriors which are particularly important in providing retention and resis-tance form, and in the root-filled tooth, resis-tance to fracture of the remaining coronal tooth structure.

The labiolingual dimension of mandibular incisors at the junction between the crown and the root is small. The combination of the loss of tooth structure produced by the endo-dontic access cavity and the crown prepara-tion generally removes such a large per-centage of the coronal tissue that very often a post will be necessary to support a crown. Maxillary anterior teeth, particularly maxillary central incisors, are larger at the amelo-cemental junction. When the endodontic access cavity is sited carefully, there is very often sufficient coronal tissue remaining after crown preparation to allow the dentine core to support the crown without the need to place a post. The further incisally that the endodontic access cavity is placed, the more palatal dentine will remain. By making access to the pulp chamber through the incisal edge, or just palatal to it, dentine is preserved in this critical area. If it is intended that the tooth being root-canal-treated should also receive a crown then the access cavity should be cut on the labial side of the incisal edge. This is even more conservative of palatal den-tine whilst still allowing straight-line access into the root canal (Figure 14.4).

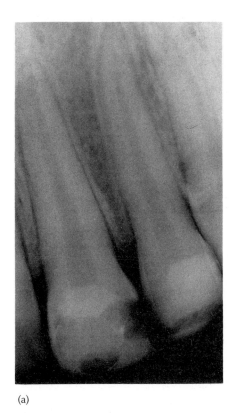

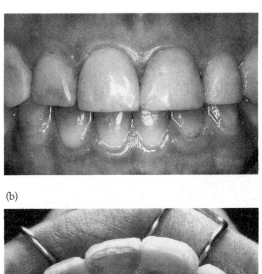

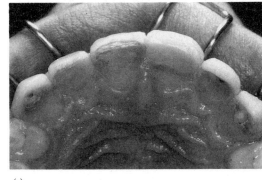

(a)

(b)

(c)

Figure 14.3 Anterior teeth discoloured due to tetracycline. (a) Radiograph showing maxillary central incisor that had had a coronal pulpotomy 6 years previously. (b) Labial view of completed direct composite resin restorations. (c) Palatal view of completed restorations.

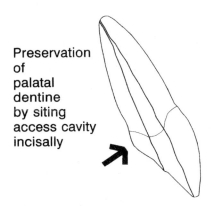

Preservation
of
palatal
dentine
by siting
access cavity
incisally

Figure 14.4 Diagram to show that incisally placed access cavity preserves palatal dentine.

Previously crowned anterior teeth

Not uncommonly, the pulp in a crowned maxillary anterior tooth becomes non-vital. A common error in making access through the crown and preserving the porcelain incisal edge of the tooth is to make the access too far palatal. After root canal preparation has been completed, there is very little palatal wall dentine remaining, and it is therefore not surprising that later fracture of the dentine core with loss of the crown is common.

Traditionally, the use of a cast dowel is recommended to provide coronal–radicular stabilization. This has little to commend it as the cast core is designed only to replace the missing coronal tissue and is unable to confer any degree of protection to the dentine which remains. Furthermore, it is not possible to make an assessment of the remaining coronal dentine, particularly the thickness of the walls. There is considerable benefit in removing the existing crown prior to root canal treatment after discussing the reasons with the patient (Figure 14.5). This allows the access cavity to be sited incisally or incisolabially, thereby preserving as much palatal dentine as possible (Figure 14.5a). It is important that the palatal finishing line is sited so as to cover a reasonable length of the axial wall (Figure 14.5b). Such an approach works well for single crowns but should be used with greater caution where the tooth is to be a bridge abutment where torsional and shear forces are increased.

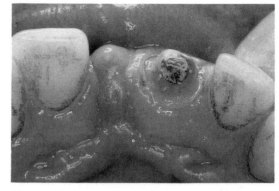

(a)

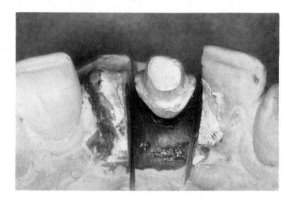

(b)

Posterior teeth

Conservative restoration of posterior teeth

The wider the isthmus in a class II cavity, the lower the resistance to fracture of the tooth [39]. The endodontically treated posterior tooth has lost the roof of its pulp chamber and both coronal and radicular dentine. Added to this is the loss of dentine associated with previous restorations. These teeth, even if previously lightly restored, can be considered to be very much weakened. Posterior teeth that have been endodontically treated require restorations that will:

1. Preserve and/or protect remaining tooth structure.
2. Maintain occlusal stability.

The reasons for protecting the remaining tooth structure are obvious, whilst stability in the occlusion is necessary to control the loads on the tooth and restoration. Where contacts between opposing teeth alter, there is risk of unwanted changes in the position of the restored tooth or its antagonists. Such changes in position may create interferences on mandibular movement which, particularly in the case of those on the non-working side, are associated with increased loads that may damage the teeth or restorations.

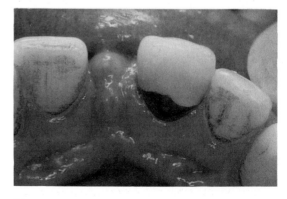

(c)

Figure 14.5 (a) The existing porcelain jacket crown on a maxillary central incisor was removed so that the access cavity could be made through the incisal edge; a cermet fills the access cavity. (b) The die of the new crown preparation. (c) Palatal view of the new metal–ceramic crown.

Adhesive restorations for posterior root-filled teeth

The endodontic access cavity in a posterior tooth not only removes the roof of the pulp chamber but also creates a wide occlusal isthmus. Consequently, even if both marginal ridges remain intact, the tooth must be considered at some risk from fracture. Much interest has centred in recent years on the ability of adhesive posterior restorations to reinforce the remaining tooth structure. Composite resin placed with an etched enamel technique increases the resistance to fracture of root-filled teeth compared with non-adhesive restorations [7].

An endodontically treated maxillary first premolar restored with a disto-occlusal composite restoration is shown in Figure 14.6. The reasons for this restoration being chosen are easy to understand, as given the nature of the occlusal contacts the only aesthetic alternative would be a metal–ceramic crown. Furthermore, the preparation for this type of crown would have removed much axial tooth tissue and this, coupled with the dentine lost in preparing the access cavity, would have necessitated the use of a post and core to support the crown. In addition, there is recession of the buccal gingival tissues which would have made aesthetic margin placement and its maintenance unpredictable. Whilst the reasons for this treatment decision are clear, the question remains as to whether it represents the best option, particularly in terms of protecting the remaining tooth structure and maintaining stability in the occlusion.

It can be argued that composite resin represents the best option when restoring small cavities in the occlusal surfaces of posterior teeth. The operative field can generally be well controlled, the margins of the cavity are all in enamel and a small restoration is not often required to replace a large number of occlusal contacts. However, all dentists are aware of the operative difficulties raised by using composite resin in larger cavities in posterior teeth, especially those involving approximal surfaces. In particular, isolation, control of matrices and the resultant approximal form are often difficult. From an occlusal standpoint, such restorations present problems when large because the ultimate

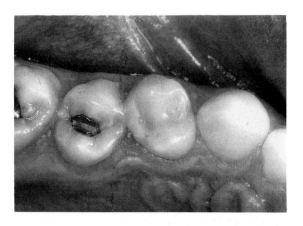

(a)

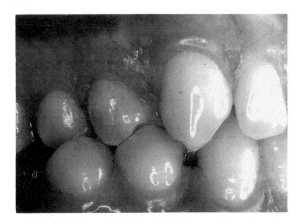

(b)

Figure 14.6 (a) Occlusal view of a disto-occlusal composite resin restoration in a root-filled maxillary first premolar. (b) Buccal view with the teeth in intercuspal position.

shaping and finishing of the occlusal surface have to be carried out with rotary instruments. Trying to produce precise occlusal functional form by such means is unlikely to be successful. A further factor affecting stability in the occlusion will be the resistance of the composite resin to wear and also its effect on the wear of opposing teeth. There is evidence to suggest that the further posterior the restoration in the mouth, the more it is likely to wear [17]. Figure 14.7 shows a moderately sized disto-occlusal composite resin restoration in a maxillary premolar; this restoration is only 5 years old and is of modern composite resin but it already displays wear both occlusally and approximally.

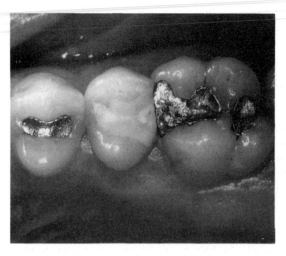

Figure 14.7 Maxillary premolar containing 5-year-old composite resin restoration.

It is generally conceded, although few data are available, that modern posterior composite resins are not as abrasive in respect of opposing natural tooth structure as their predecessors. Any strengthening effect of composite restorations will only be possible if the material is durably and effectively bonded to the dental tissues by means of an acid-etched enamel technique, perhaps enhanced by dentine bonding. The effects of the polymerization shrinkage are to induce stresses within the adjacent tooth structure. These lead to strains within the teeth and are also capable of producing cuspal displacement. These displacements cannot be prevented by modifying the technique of composite placement, nor are they relieved with time [21]. Their long-term effects are unknown but in teeth with vital pulps they have been associated with pain and cuspal fracture. In teeth already severely weakened by root canal treatment, additional stress would seem to be best avoided.

Indirect tooth-coloured adhesive restorations

The introduction of indirect posterior composite restorations was intended to address many of these problems. They provide an opportunity to improve physical properties by up to 30% through a greater degree of polymerization. The effects of polymerization shrinkage on the tooth structure are virtually eliminated by employing an indirect technique, and restorations can be made with accurate occlusal contacts. However, they are expensive and, compared with conventional techniques for gold and porcelain restorations, the precision of fit is disappointing. Any strengthening effect from these restorations will be reliant on the stability of the composite luting agent and there is little available evidence to confirm this. Ceramic inlays represent a further alternative (Figure 14.8). The long-term performance of such restorations, particularly in endodontically treated teeth, is as yet unknown. However, there does appear to be growing agreement that, where the isthmus is large, onlay, rather than inlay, construction is preferred for both composite resin and ceramic restorations.

Retrospective data covering a 20-year period of restoring root-treated posterior teeth with silver amalgam or composite resin have been reported [9,10]. At the 5- and 10-year points, there were fewer tooth fractures in the composite resin group than in the amalgam group. However, at the 20-year interval there was no difference between the two materials. Both showed that, without cuspal coverage, fracture of the teeth at the 10-year period was 16% for amalgam and 13% for composite resin. However, at the 20-year period the incidence of fracture was over 25% for both groups. It was concluded that the incidence of tooth fracture was so high that posterior endodontically treated teeth should be restored with cuspal coverage.

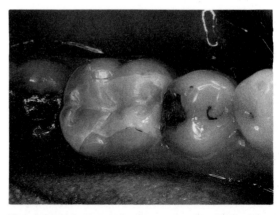

Figure 14.8 Cast ceramic inlay in a root-canal-treated mandibular first molar.

The production of extensive amalgam restorations combining cuspal coverage with good occlusal form is difficult. Where cusps are onlayed with amalgam, at least 2 mm of coverage must be used. It is difficult to create the appropriate occlusal form together with good axial contours. Such restorations are adequate to protect the remaining tooth structure and may also be considered as interim restorations when time is required to evaluate the success of root canal treatment or when financial considerations prevent placement of a crown. The principle of protecting the remaining tooth structure in a root-treated tooth using a restoration with an onlay component is fundamental. The fracture resistance *in vitro* of intact premolar teeth has been compared with those endodontically treated, those endodontically treated and restored with composite resin, and those endodontically treated and restored with onlays [40]. The teeth restored with traditional MOD onlay restorations in cast gold were the most resistant to fracture.

This review leads to two main conclusions regarding predictability in the restoration of endodontically treated posterior teeth:

1. Cuspal coverage is necessary to minimize the possibility of fracture.
2. Onlay restorations in cast metal are more likely to produce long-term occlusal stability than those made from composite resin or ceramic.

Cast restorations for extensively damaged teeth

A cast onlay provides a conservative method for restoring and protecting the root-treated posterior tooth. It is important not to regard a full ceramic-coverage metal–ceramic restoration in the same way, because heavy tooth reduction to create the necessary room is likely to remove the majority of remaining coronal dentine. Two three-quarter gold veneers on a maxillary premolar and molar, which appear unaesthetic through needing a comparatively large area of buccal wall covered with gold, are shown in Figure 14.9. This treatment decision was made after discussion with the patient because the only substantial wall of tooth structure remaining

in each tooth was the buccal cusp. Preparation of these teeth to receive full-coverage metal–ceramic restorations would have necessitated full buccal reduction and hence loss of these cusps. It was considered that this would have worsened the long-term prognosis for the teeth.

The use of partial and full-coverage restorations in yellow gold remains a very appropriate method for the restoration of endodontically treated posterior teeth where there is a reasonable quantity of coronal dentine remaining. The beneficial effect of crowns in preventing fracture of root-treated posterior teeth has been emphasized [33] in a study where an incidence of posterior tooth fracture of nearly 60% was recorded when crowns were not used.

Cores for cast restorations

The loss of coronal tissue by previous restorations and root canal treatment is frequently so great as to require a core to support the final crown. There is a need to provide adequate retention for the core. The general principles of core retention apply in the same way as for vital teeth, such as maximal use being made of the remaining tooth structure by providing boxes, rails and other retentive features within the bulk of dentine. However, there are virtually no indications for the use of self-threading pins in endodontically treated teeth. There is usually an inadequate bulk of dentine at the line angles of the teeth where pins would normally be placed as the access cavity will very often have reduced or undermined the dentine remaining in these areas. Furthermore, self-threading pins create stresses in both the tooth structure and the core [6,36]. The effect of these stresses within the reduced bulk of tooth structure is to enhance crack propagation, bringing with it the increased likelihood of tooth fracture or loss of core retention. Only if access cannot be gained to the root canals should pins be considered. If their use is absolutely necessary, they should be retained by a cement lute to avoid creating stresses in the tooth. However, they need to extend 4 mm into dentine to provide adequate retention, which can make them difficult to place safely.

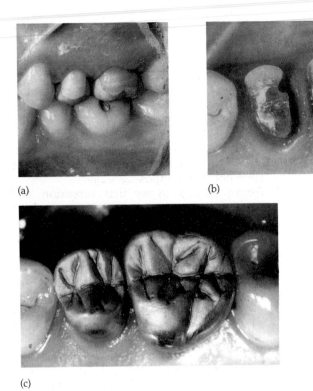

(a)

(b)

(c)

Figure 14.9 (a) Buccal view of partial-veneer crowns with extensive buccal coverage on maxillary second premolar and first molar. (b) Occlusal view of the preparations. (c) Occlusal view of the restorations (Courtesy of Mr A. Croysdill).

In contrast, the pulp chamber and root canals provide areas where retention and resistance for cores may be obtained relatively easily and with minimal generation of stress. As with anterior teeth, even if there has been considerable loss of coronal tooth structure it is not always necessary or advisable to place a post in order to retain a core. It may be said that the placement of a post is generally the last thing that is done to a tooth before it is finally extracted. Whilst this is not always true, it underlies an approach that places emphasis on the unpredictable nature of post crowns.

If root canal treatment fails and the root contains a post of good length, it is probable that the tooth will be lost unless the post can be removed or the site is accessible for surgery. It is therefore sensible to avoid a post where possible as such an approach allows access for root canal retreatment. Figure 14.10 shows a periapical radiograph of two molar teeth; the first molar is the abutment for a fixed bridge; it has a failed root canal treatment, signs of a possible perforation on the distal aspect of the mesial root and two

posts present. The chances of successful post removal and root canal retreatment are low. In contrast, the second molar is also root-canal treated but contains an amalgam core which extends 2–3 mm down each of the root canals. If this root canal treatment were to fail, there would be a reasonable chance of removing the core to allow access for root canal retreatment.

The amalgam core prior to cementation of the crown is shown in Figure 14.10b. It reveals the remaining buccal wall and the amalgam core which extends from the occlusal surface into the pulp chamber and the coronal 2–3 mm of the root canals for retention. This type of core is known as the *amalgam dowel core* [22].

Amalgam dowel core

This technique works well in posterior teeth where a minimum of one cusp with a good dentine base remains and will still be present following crown preparation [22]. If no cuspal dentine remains there is a danger that the amalgam core could fracture at the level of

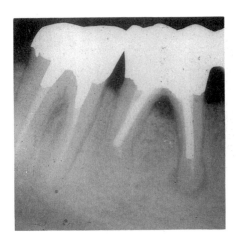

(a)

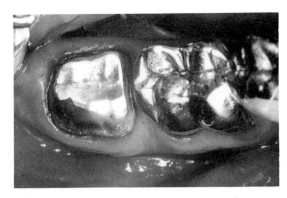

(b)

Figure 14.10 (a) Periapical radiograph of right mandibular first and second molars showing posts in the first molar and an amalgam dowel core in the second molar. (b) Crown preparation of mandibular second molar containing amalgam dowel core (mirror view).

the roof of the pulp chamber. The clinical technique is shown in Figure 14.11, in which an amalgam dowel core is placed in a maxillary first molar. The following points should be noted:

1. All the root canal filling material must be removed from the pulp chamber.
2. Gutta-percha is removed from the coronal 2–3 mm of the root canals using a Gates-Glidden drill, the dimensions of which are the same size or slightly larger than the coronal aspect of the root canal. This prevents the Gates-Glidden drill from penetrating the mass of gutta-percha and tearing it from the root canal. The Gates-

Glidden drill should be run at low speed and high torque to melt the gutta-percha ahead of the blunt tip.

3. Extension of the amalgam more than the recommended 2–3 mm will not improve the retention of the core but will make later removal of the amalgam much more difficult should root canal retreatment be required.
4. Optimal use should be made of the pulp chamber to make sure that it provides retention from opposing walls.
5. Figure 14.11b shows that retention and resistance form have been improved by the use of further auxiliary retentive features in the coronal aspect of the tooth. A groove has been placed in dentine palatal to the access cavity and the features of the distal box have been sharpened.
6. Condensation of the amalgam alloy into the coronal aspects of the root canals requires appropriately sized amalgam condensers.
7. Figure 14.11d shows the amount of coronal dentine which remains and the final preparation for a 7/8 gold veneer. The technique will not work consistently in the absence of coronal dentine.

Use of plastic core materials with prefabricated posts

The core takes on an increasingly structural role as the amount of coronal dentine decreases. Where there is considerable bulk of dentine, the mechanical demands placed on the core are of a generally low order and hence the choice of material is not critical. This is not the case where little dentine remains, as both the possibility of core failure and dentine fracture become more likely.

It is important that the clinician imagines the appearance of the crown preparation prior to preparation. The appropriate time to consider the final form of the preparation is when the core is placed.

Figure 14.12 shows a root-canal-treated maxillary second molar; the decision was made to place a cemented, serrated stainless-steel post in the palatal root canal and to place two amalgam dowels in the coronal 2–3 mm of the buccal root canals (Figure 14.12b). The reasons for this become clearer

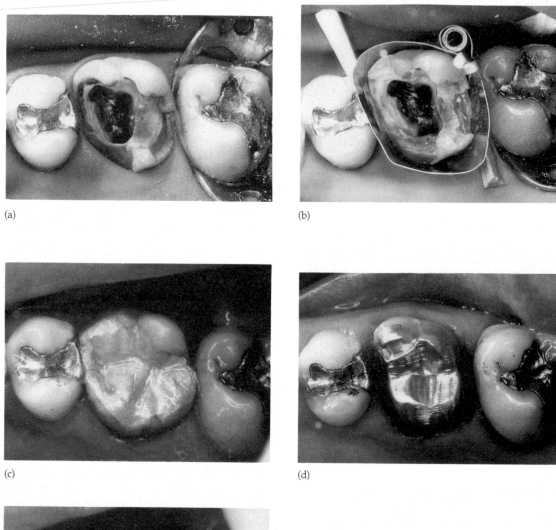

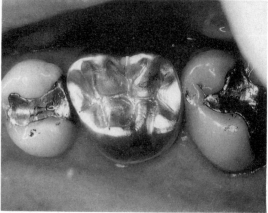

Figure 14.11 (a) Root-canal-treated maxillary first molar with gutta-percha removed from the pulp chamber and coronal 2–3 mm of root canals. (b) Matrix band in place; note the groove and distal box providing additional resistance form. (c) Completed amalgam dowel core. (d) Tooth prepared to receive 7/8 gold veneer crown. (e) Completed gold veneer crown.

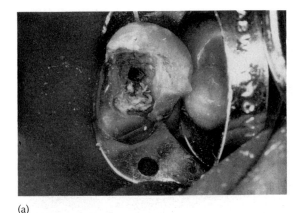

(a)

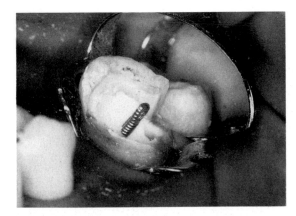

(b)

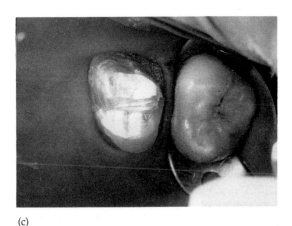

(c)

Figure 14.12 (a) Occlusal view of right maxillary second molar after removal of gutta-percha from palatal root canal. (b) Stainless-steel post cemented within palatal canal. (c) Completed preparation.

when the preparation for a metal–ceramic restoration is examined (Figure 14.12c). The only bulk of coronal dentine remaining is in the area of the palatal cusp. The tooth was to serve as an abutment for a fixed bridge to replace the maxillary first molar and would therefore receive greater loading. The cemented post was placed in order to increase the resistance of the tooth to *torsional and shear forces*. Prior to cementation the length of the post was adjusted to ensure that it was long enough to extend coronal to the pulp chamber but not so long as to be exposed by the subsequent crown preparation. Exposure of a pin or post during crown preparation weakens the core material. After the cement had set, all the excess was cleared from the pulp chamber so that the amalgam core was supported on a dentine base and could be well-condensed around the post and also into the coronal aspects of the two buccal root canals.

Choice of core material

The demands on the core vary depending on its size and also the loads it will receive. Where a large bulk of coronal dentine remains, the choice of core material is not critical, but it becomes increasingly so as the amount of dentine remaining decreases. The critical point is empirical but when less than one wall of a posterior tooth remains, the core can be assumed to have a considerable structural role. Under such circumstances, both composite resin and cermets are risky choices.

Composite resin has always performed well in tests *in vitro* of core materials [13], but more recently concerns have been expressed about its dimensional and hydrolytic stability [24]. These have added to the clinical impression of large composite resin cores tending to become loose beneath cast restorations.

Cermets, being glass ionomer cement derivatives, possess adhesive properties and this provides good resistance to microleakage. However, retentive values are low – approximately 25% of those obtained using composite resin on etched enamel. Consequently, their adhesion is of little use for retentive purposes. Furthermore, whilst these may be very useful materials for small cores, they are developments of glass ionomer cements and their compressive and tensile strengths are low compared with other core materials. They should be used with great caution when the core is large.

Silver amalgam as a core material remains popular because of its physical properties. Data are lacking regarding the clinical performance of core materials. However, in an interesting *in vitro* study, endurance testing of extracted root-treated premolar teeth restored with posts, cores of composite resin, cermet or amalgam, and then crowns showed failure of 60% in the composite resin group, 90% in the cermet group and 30% in the amalgam group [15]. It is often said that amalgam is not a practical core material as it cannot be prepared at the same visit as it is placed. However, if a fast-setting alloy is used, the bulk of the initial preparation can be made with an amalgam carver and completed using a turbine with light pressure under waterspray. There is evidence that this does not adversely affect the properties of the set amalgam. Silver amalgam remains the plastic material of choice for large cores in posterior teeth.

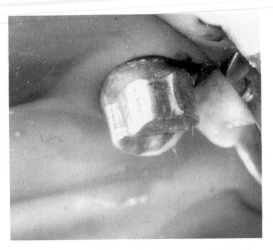

Figure 14.13 Buccal view of crown preparation to show position of margin extending well onto sound tooth. (This is the same tooth as in Figure 14.12.)

Position of the preparation margin

Whatever core material is used, the position of the axial margins of the crown is important as it is a site of stress concentration [3]. This is also likely to be true for the margin of a core. One aim of the crown preparation must be to position the margin so that stresses received by the crown are transferred to the root of the tooth; this helps to minimize the loads on the core. When different cores on extracted root-treated teeth were tested without final crowns covering them, there were quite marked differences in their resistance to failure [11]. However, when the tests were repeated with final crowns in place, and their margins were extended 2 mm onto sound tooth structure, there was little difference between groups. It is an important principle that to distribute loads and hence minimize stress concentration, the margins of the final preparation should extend well onto sound tooth structure (Figure 14.13). This may sometimes require that a surgical crown-

lengthening procedure is carried out after placement of the core prior to crown preparation to provide visible tooth structure apical to the margins of the core.

Posts

Selecting a post

It is clear that when the amount of coronal dentine is very much reduced, a large core may be required which needs a post placed within one of the root canals to retain it. The choice of post is important but there are few indicators as to what the best post may be. Indeed, looking in any dental catalogue will immediately reveal the enormous range of makes and types of post that are available. This indicates that there is not one post that is superior in all situations to any of the others. It is difficult to make an informed choice based on clinical data because such reports do not exist. The only information comes from studies which are necessarily *in vitro*, and a whole range of different tests have been used to evaluate their performance. This makes the results of different studies impossible to compare. A brief review is helpful in choosing a post.

Classical studies [2] of retention of posts have shown that:

1. The longer the post, the greater is the retention.
2. Parallel-sided posts have greater retention than tapered posts.
3. Roughening the post increases its retention.
4. Threaded posts are more retentive than posts with other surface finishes.

Many studies have examined the performance of posts and cores under angled compression as this has been regarded as more representative of the clinical situation. Variations in post design have been associated with different levels of resistance to failure. However, failure occurred in the tooth structure rather than in the post in one study *in vitro* [14]. The limiting factor in the performance of post systems is the amount of tooth structure remaining rather than the post itself [32]. The preservation of even small amounts of tooth structure is helpful. Further information has been derived from stress analysis studies using either photo-elastic or computer-generated finite element tests. The information from these can be summarized:

1. Increased post length leads to decreased stress.
2. Tapered posts produce greater stresses than parallel-sided posts.
3. Parallel-sided posts produce higher apical stresses [37].
4. Posts that are both tapered and threaded are associated with high levels of stress, particularly on insertion [5].
5. Posts have a role not only in retention but also in stress distribution [26].

Reasonable conclusions about the desirable characteristics of a post are that:

1. It should be of adequate length.
2. It should, if possible, be parallel-sided.
3. Its surface should be roughened or serrated.

Furthermore, posts that rely on the elasticity of dentine for their retention – self-threading posts – should be avoided.

How long should the post be?

A frequently asked question is: what is the appropriate length for a post? There are many recommendations:

1. As long as the crown.
2. Two-thirds the length of the root.
3. One-half root length surrounded by bone.
4. As long as possible.

To establish which of these is correct, further thought must be given to the functions of the post. These are:

1. Retention for the core.
2. Stress distribution.

Much of the research into posts has looked at their ability to distribute stress. The post distributes stresses not only into the dentine of the root but also into the surrounding alveolar bone via the periodontal ligament [26]. The most appropriate recommendation for the length of a post appears to be one that relates length to the level of alveolar bone surrounding the root. The distal root of a mandibular first molar that is an abutment for a fixed bridge is shown in Figure 14.14. The most worrying feature is the level of the alveolar bone in relation to the apical end of the post; they are virtually coincident and

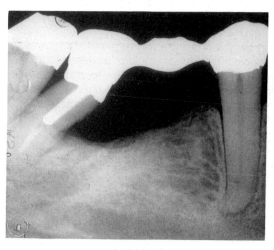

Figure 14.14 Periapical radiograph showing distal root of right mandibular first molar with the apical end of the post at the level of the alveolar bone.

consequently the ability of the post to distribute stresses via the root to the alveolar bone is very limited, increasing the chances of root fracture.

Preservation of the 'apical seal'

It is not appropriate to discuss post length without some consideration of the length of the root canal filling that must remain if the apical seal is to be preserved. The current recommendation for the minimum acceptable length of gutta-percha is 5 mm [18]. A maxillary central incisor may be 22 mm long with a crown that is 7 mm long. If allowance is made for the root canal filling being 1 mm short of the anatomical apex, this leaves 14 mm of root, 5 mm of which needs to be occupied by root canal filling material. This will allow 9 mm for the post which is adequate but the situation can radically change if:

1. The root canal filling is short of ideal length.
2. Periodontal bone levels are reduced.
3. The root is shorter than average.

Figure 14.15 shows root canal fillings in two mandibular premolars following preparation of post space. Both root canal fillings appear short of ideal position; in one tooth an adequate amount of root canal filling

remains, while in the other certainly less than the recommended 5 mm remains. If the alveolar bone levels are noted, these are reduced around the second premolar such that more root canal filling was removed to allow an appropriate length of post to be surrounded by root which was, in turn, surrounded by bone. This was done with the primary aim not of improving retention of the post but rather of helping stress distribution. The major reason for distributing such stresses is to prevent crack propagation and vertical root fracture.

It was assumed until comparatively recently that if slightly less than the optimal length of root canal filling remained, this would probably not be of great consequence if a post were subsequently cemented into the canal. Data from a retrospective study of root-canal-treated teeth restored with post crowns showed very clearly that, once the length of root canal filling fell below 3 mm, the incidence of periapical radiolucency increased significantly [16]. This does present a restorative dilemma – whether to compromise the length of root canal filling or the length of the post. At present there does not appear to be a satisfactory answer to this question, particularly when there is no detailed information on the performance of post-retained crowns.

Form of the post

Tapered versus parallel-sided

There is clear laboratory evidence that parallel-sided posts are better retained and distribute stresses more easily than those that are tapered [34]. However, this conclusion is simplistic. It is reasonable to suggest that if all other factors are equal the use of a parallel-sided post represents the better option. However, much will depend on the anatomy of the filled root canal. It is clearly unwise to widen a root canal that is already broad in its apical region in order to make it parallel-sided. To do so can often risk weakening the apical portion of the root. Stresses are concentrated at the apical end of the post and there would an increased risk of an apical root fracture. A clinical study reported superiority of parallel-sided over tapered posts [33]. However, teeth that were unsuitable for

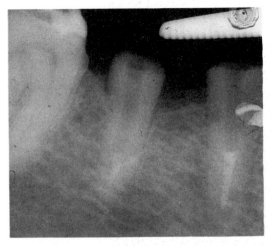

Figure 14.15 Periapical radiograph of mandibular first and second premolars. Note the amount of remaining root canal filling and the level of alveolar bone.

parallel-sided posts were provided with tapered posts. Such teeth would have tended to be those with relatively wide-tapering root canals: teeth of this type possess less dentine and would be more prone to root fracture. There is no doubt from a clinical point of view that tapered posts can function very well when there is adequate radicular dentine; the same is also true of parallel-sided posts. However, to choose to use a tapered post when both types are appropriate seems illogical.

Threaded posts

Self-threading designs. Earlier mention was made of self-threading posts which rely on dentinal elasticity for their retention, exerting high stresses on the root of the tooth [5]. Posts of this design are generally very retentive; however, they may also lead the user to believe that retention is the only important requirement. Some of these types of post display the characteristics of being short, markedly tapered and relatively coarsely threaded (Figure 14.16). Such posts screwed into somewhat undersized root canals will produce high stresses. The form of the threads may also serve to concentrate stresses, whilst their relative lack of length makes them of limited benefit in terms of stress distribution throughout the root and alveolar bone.

A number of improved variants of self-threading posts are available. Some resemble the traditional self-threading post but have been refined to reduce their taper and coarseness of thread, whilst also matching them to appropriately sized twist drills (Figure 14.17). An alternative design consists of a self-threading post with a longitudinal incomplete split (Figure 14.18). The intraradicular portion of the post compresses on insertion, thereby reducing the stress. Additionally, the post is tapered only at its tip, being parallel-sided over the rest of its length. However, concerns have been expressed that it may concentrate stresses coronally because it is not well adapted inside the canal [1]. One further design recognizing the stresses induced by tapered posts uses a matched system of twist drills and parallel-sided self-threading posts (Figure 14.19).

There are few data on the performance of these posts. However, what few there are suggest that they should be used with great caution if at all. Meta-analysis showed that they have a higher failure rate than cast gold posts and cores [4]. Comparison of teeth restored with Dentatus screws, Unimetric posts and Radix Anchors found a higher failure rate than anticipated [20]. However, the data are inconclusive as there was no information about how the teeth for restoration were chosen. It may have been that only those teeth with a poor prognosis were

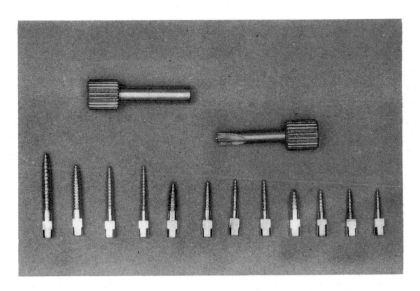

Figure 14.16 Dentatus screws and hand wrenches.

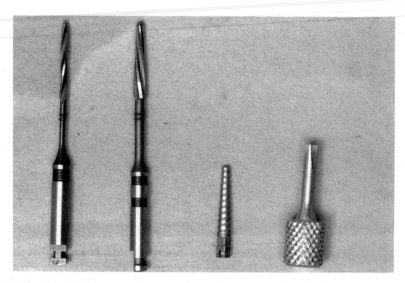

Figure 14.17 Unimetric post (second from right), reamers and wrench.

selected to be restored with the screw posts, perhaps on the grounds that this was a less expensive technique and the teeth did not have a good enough prognosis to warrant a cast-gold post and core.

Threaded posts used with taps. A number of threaded posts are designed for use in con-

junction with a thread previously tapped into dentine. Such posts have been shown to distribute stresses well following placement and to be retentive even over shorter lengths [38]. Care is required in tapping the thread within the root when high stresses can be generated if instructions about regular cleaning of the tap and removal of the swarf are not

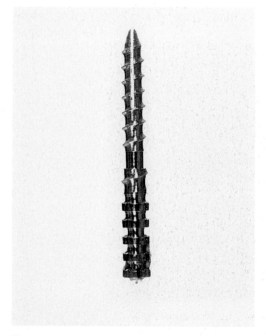

Figure 14.18 Flexipost.

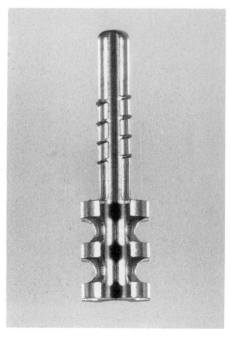

Figure 14.19 Radix Anchor.

observed [29]. Threaded posts of this type do carry the advantage of being well-retained, but their resistance to torsional forces which tend to unscrew them is a continued problem, particularly if the design incorporates a prefabricated core. There is a further potential problem: as retention is good, there can sometimes be a tendency to compromise post length. This must be avoided so that the post distributes stress. Another factor is that these prefabricated posts very often require the use of a plastic core material. This does not present great difficulty in large teeth where coronal dentine remains. However, in anterior teeth where the root diameters are less and if little coronal dentine remains the size of the head of the post may prevent room for an adequate bulk of core material. If the core material does not completely cover the head of the post, the strength of the core is reduced.

Metal posts with cast cores

Prefabricated posts designed to be used with a core 'build-up' material are unsuitable for the majority of anterior teeth or for posterior teeth where no coronal tissue remains. Therefore, the treatment of choice is the provision of a post and core that are integral with one another – either a cast post and core or a wrought post with a cast-on core. There are clear advantages in using one of the commercial systems, which provide a matched system of twist drills, impression posts, pattern posts and, in some instances, temporary posts (Figure 14.20). The important features of such systems are that they provide a useful range of sizes and are easy to use, whilst at the same time allowing a correctly designed post and core to be made.

Tooth preparation

The principles of preparation for a post and core are that:

1. All useful tooth structure should be preserved.
2. The apical seal is maintained.
3. Stress is minimized within the tooth and post and core.

The stages in preparation are:

1. Establishing post length.
2. Primary coronal preparation.
3. Complete post preparation, both length and width.
4. Develop antirotation features.
5. Finishing procedures.

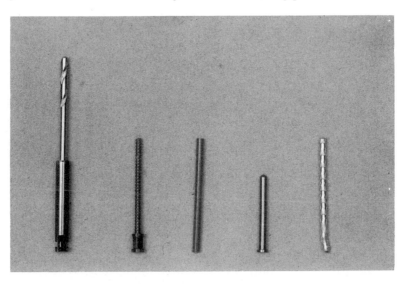

Figure 14.20 Part of a matched parallel-sided post system: Whaledent's Parapost. Left to right: twist drill, burn-out pattern, impression post, temporary post and wrought post.

Establishing post length

This should be carried out once the temporary restoration has been removed from the tooth. At this stage, the coronal landmarks remain; these will previously have provided the reference points used for the root canal treatment. As previously discussed, the length can only be determined from a clinical examination and reference to a good-quality postoperative endodontic radiograph from which can be determined:

1. The overall shape of the root, particularly its width in the apical third.
2. The apparent width of the root canal.
3. The length of the clinical crown.
4. The level of alveolar bone surrounding the root.
5. The approximate length of the root itself.

The shape of the root and the width of the root canal will determine whether the post can be parallel-sided or whether a tapered design should be used. The post should occupy no more than one-third of the radiographic width of the root at the apical end of the post. If the width of the root canal apically is such that this proportion would be exceeded, then a tapered post should be used. The other factors (points 3–5 above) will also influence the decision regarding the size of the post.

Removal of the root canal filling

A root canal filling of gutta-percha can be removed either immediately following root canal filling or at the time of preparation for the post if this takes place at a subsequent visit. This is a matter of convenience for the operator. Some studies show that there is damage to the apical seal by immediate removal, while others show no increased leakage. A number of techniques for removing gutta-percha have been described using heat, solvents or rotary instrumentation. Solvents are best avoided as they have the potential to damage the root canal filling material that remains. Heat is a safe and effective way of removing gutta-percha but it

is rather slow. Rotary instrumentation is quick, but has the potential to risk root perforation if carried out incorrectly. A number of instruments are available for this purpose but the commonest are the Peeso Reamer and the Gates-Glidden drill. The initial diameter of the Gates-Glidden drill should be approximately the diameter of the canal in the mid-portion of the root canal (Figure 14.21).

Coronal preparation

This is the second stage and the coronal preparation should be completed apart from final finishing. Under no circumstances should the coronal preparation ever consist of simply cutting off the clinical crown of the tooth. The concept of an elective 'roof-top' preparation is outdated and represents bad practice. The object of coronal preparation is to create the appropriate amount of space for the final coronal restoration. This requires that full occlusal and axial reduction should be carried out at this stage and not left until the post and core has been cemented. This is to ensure that a full evaluation of the remaining tooth structure can be made prior to post cementation as, once this has taken place, evaluation cannot be accurate. Any axial wall of dentine that is taller than wide may be considered weakened, and should be reduced.

Exact rules are not possible or appropriate and clinical judgement is of major importance. The axial tooth structure will require further evaluation and finishing once the intraradicular preparation has been completed. However, axial reduction should be completed, and also the site of the finishing line for the crown should have been established; this has a considerable bearing on the axial reduction.

Completion of post preparation

The operator should have made the decision about the length and diameter of the post at the beginning of the preparation. The factors affecting its length have already been discussed and broadly it has been suggested that the apical part of the post should occupy no more than one-third the width of the root. There are distinct limits imposed by

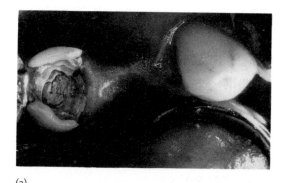

(a)

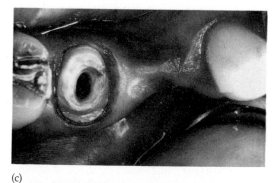

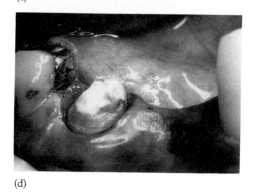

(c)

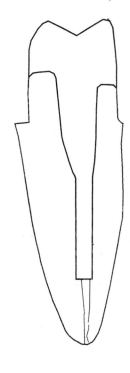

(b)

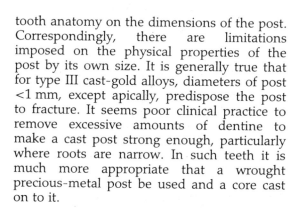

(d)

Figure 14.21 (a) Root-treated mandibular second premolar following removal of the coronal temporary restoration. (b) Diagram to represent ideal preparation of a mandibular second premolar for a cast post and core (digitized tooth outline – copyright P. Setchell). (c) Occlusal view of completed preparation. (d) Buccal view of the completed preparation.

tooth anatomy on the dimensions of the post. Correspondingly, there are limitations imposed on the physical properties of the post by its own size. It is generally true that for type III cast-gold alloys, diameters of post <1 mm, except apically, predispose the post to fracture. It seems poor clinical practice to remove excessive amounts of dentine to make a cast post strong enough, particularly where roots are narrow. In such teeth it is much more appropriate that a wrought precious-metal post be used and a core cast on to it.

The form of the post preparation is important if dentine is to be preserved and stresses within the tooth and the post are to be minimized.

A *tapered post* will reflect the essential anatomy of the root canal. It will be widened coronally in order to increase the bulk of the post, particularly at the point where the post joins the core. The widening will reflect the normal anatomy of the root canal and will be carried out buccolingually in the coronal half of the root. This flaring of the canal should not be overemphasized to avoid unnecessary dentine loss. Such enlargement of the canal may best be achieved by use of an appropriately sized Gates-Glidden drill. These instruments will not produce sharp angles and thus will minimize stress concentration.

Where the post is to be *parallel-sided*, it should be tapered in its coronal portion, reflecting the normal anatomy of the root canal. There is little to commend an intraradicular preparation that has sharp internal form. Rapid changes in bulk of material and consequently sharp line angles will promote stress concentration and will increase the possibility of fracture of either the tooth or post (Figure 14.21b).

The apical portion of the post preparation should be completed before the coronal part. If previous preparation has been carried out with Gates-Glidden drills, little extra work is required to complete this part. The final apical preparation is made with a parallel-sided twist drill which cuts on its tip. It should therefore be used by hand to minimize the chances of perforating the root and with a safety device to protect the patient. This part of the preparation is quick to complete by hand and rotary instrumentation is best avoided. When using twist drills, they should be withdrawn from the canal at frequent intervals and cleaned of swarf. Accurate depth markers are required. The original coronal reference point will probably have been removed during extracoronal preparation, therefore establish the new working length by measuring with the last Gates-Glidden drill to have been used to the full length.

The coronal part of the root canal is then prepared and blended into the radicular portion, such that sharp changes in direction are avoided and stress minimized. As for the tapered post, resistance to torsional forces is gained by removing dentine to emphasize further the normal anatomy of the root canal. This provides all the necessary *antirotation* and there is absolutely no indication for notching of the root canal or root face, both of which will be detrimental in terms of stress concentration. Care should be taken to ensure that the canal is clean of debris following preparation and that the internal walls are smooth. Visual and tactile inspection are required to ensure that no gutta-percha remains on the axial walls of the post preparation. The preparation of the root canal will have thinned the walls of remaining coronal dentine, which need to be re-evaluated.

Finishing procedures

The axial walls of the preparation are then bevelled coronally using a flame-shaped diamond, a finishing carbide or a friction-grip white stone. The aim is to create a *ferrule effect* around the coronal aspect of the preparation. In order to achieve this, the bevel should be reasonably long, i.e. cut at a relatively obtuse angle to the long axis of the preparation. However, such acute angles of metal are only sensible where the thickness of the coronal axial wall dentine is relatively large. In most circumstances, the bevel is necessarily not greater than approximately 45° so as to avoid producing a coronal spike of tooth structure which would be difficult to reproduce on a die and would be prone to fracture (Figure 14.21).

The other important area for finishing is at the coronal aspect of the root canal in cases where there is little or no coronal dentine remaining. In such circumstances, the junction between the root canal and the root face is a virtual right angle. This should be gently rounded using either a finishing instrument or even a large Gates-Glidden drill. This, once again, helps both die construction and stress distribution.

A final reassessment is then made of the whole preparation, checks being made for undercut, smoothness of finish and the overall final form. Particular attention should be given to the positioning and width of the finishing line for the final crown as this should not be significantly altered after the core has been placed.

Construction of the post and core

After preparation has been completed, a decision is required as to whether the post and core should be made either from a *direct pattern* or alternatively by an *indirect technique* on a cast made from an impression. The decision is only of relevance where the post and core is treated as a separate procedure from

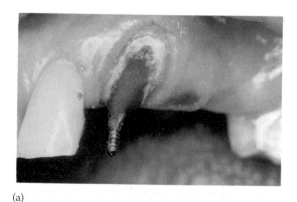

(a)

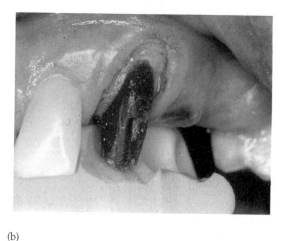

(b)

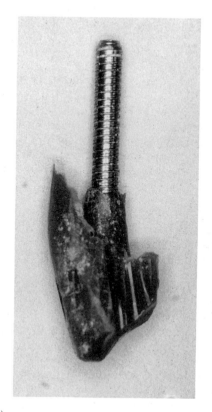

(c)

Figure 14.22 (a) Root-canal-treated maxillary canine with wrought precious metal post and Duralay intraradicularly. (b) Completed pattern (with contour matrix in position). (c) Completed pattern on removal from the tooth.

the crown. The shape of the core should not be the responsibility of the dental technician. A post and core will very rarely seat as well following cementation as it did at the try-in stage. The difficulties in cement escape from the apical portion of the post preparation make this improbable, and such failure to seat is likely to affect the seating of the final restoration. Furthermore, making a direct pattern gives an opportunity to assess accurately the intraradicular portion of the post and gives control over the final form of the core.

Direct technique

Non-residual self-curing acrylic resin is the material of choice. It is easy to use, trimmable with rotary instruments and sufficiently sturdy and dimensionally stable to withstand being transported to a dental laboratory for investing and casting. It is used with the proprietary pattern post or wrought precious post from the system chosen.

The post should be tried in to check whether it seats to the full depth of the preparation. If not, the most likely cause is debris within the post hole and the twist drill should be used to remove this, before washing, drying and rechecking. Lubricant is provided with the self-curing acrylic resin and can be applied to the walls of the post preparation with a paper point.

The resin is carried to the preparation using a paintbrush and a standard Nealon technique. With the post fully seated, resin is applied to the intraradicular portion of the post: the resin should not be too dry and the plastic pattern post may be bent gently to one side to allow the tip of the brush to reach the base of the antirotation feature. Once this is filled, further resin is added to ensure that it is well anchored to the post. However, no attempt is made to build up the coronal aspect of the core. The resin should be allowed to polymerize (Figure 14.22). The resin exposed directly to air will cure more rapidly than that in the depths of the preparation. Once hardened, the post is withdrawn and the intraradicular portion of the pattern checked for completeness. Gross deficiencies demand a remake; very minor deficiencies can be rectified by adding a small amount of soft wax, e.g. green occlusal indicator wax, after the coronal portion of the pattern has been completed. If the post cannot be withdrawn from the tooth, it is a sign that there may be an undercut intraradicularly. Careful checks on alignment and path of withdrawal will usually demonstrate where this is.

The coronal portion is formed by further additions of resin once the post has been reseated. The paintbrush is again used to carry the resin and to help form it in the desired shape. Once cured, the pattern is not withdrawn but is trimmed using a diamond stone in a high-speed handpiece. Generous waterspray must be used to avoid local heating of the pattern, which will cause the bur to snag. The final form of the coronal preparation is created before removing the pattern and once again checking for completeness (Figure 14.22). Once satisfied with the pattern, it should be placed in a small plastic box or similar container and sent to the laboratory to be cast in a hard precious alloy.

Once the arguments for making the post and the final crown separately are accepted, there are occasions on which a direct technique is appropriate and others when it may not be so. Creation of a direct pattern maintains the dentist's control over the procedure; however, it is necessary that the margins of the post preparation are visible and accessible. Subgingival margins on the coronal aspects of the cast core are a contraindication to the direct technique.

Indirect technique

This is indicated when the margins of the core are not easily visible, perhaps due to their being subgingival or when the design of the post and core is complicated such that a direct technique would be time-consuming or even impossible. Figure 14.23 shows a maxillary canine that has fractured subgingivally: the post and core are better made using an indirect technique as verification of the margins is possible (Figure 14.23b).

The stages in the preparation are identical to those for direct techniques. However, in

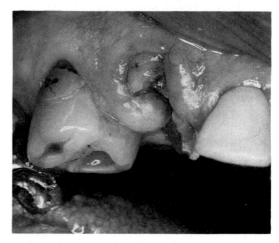

(a)

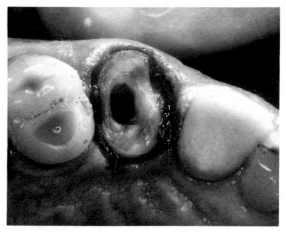

(b)

Figure 14.23 (a) Fractured crown of root-canal-treated maxillary canine with gingival proliferation. (b) Following electrosurgery to expose the margins and preparation for a post and core.

commercial systems an impression post is often substituted for the pattern post, as it is generally slightly wider to facilitate the laboratory procedures. Dentists who favour all-cast tapered posts sometimes make impressions of the root canal without the use of an impression post matched to the size of the prepared canal. This may appear to have the benefit of being quick and simple, and indeed it is, in relation to the clinical technique. However it may make difficulties for the technician as the impression will record the full detail of the inside of the root canal. The resultant die will reflect this and should the shape be unusual or undercut, release of the pattern may not be possible without distortion. The resultant cast post may then only seat in its die by abrasion of the stone; such abrasion will not happen inside the root canal of the tooth, and difficulties in seating may therefore be encountered clinically. Systems which use standardized impression and pattern posts minimize such potential difficulties.

The impression post generally requires modification. It should not protrude beyond the level of the adjacent teeth, otherwise it may contact the impression tray, leading to possible distortion; it should also have a retentive head. Both may be accomplished by using a heated wax knife to create a retentive button at one end whilst at the same time shortening the post. Additionally, the post should be coated with impression tray adhesive prior to use, with adequate time being allowed for it to dry.

Some operators argue that the post should be placed in the preparation before the impression material is syringed around it; others prefer to do it in the reverse order. There appears to be logic in having the post fully seated before placing impression material as it avoids the risk of having a small amount of impression material trapped beyond the end of the impression post. This small plug of material may be lost on its way to, or at, the dental laboratory.

It seems more sensible to seat the post fully before syringing the impression material into the preparation. If the post is bent gently to one side and material injected into the space between it and the internal walls of the post preparation, then the post may be pushed gently the other way and the syring-

ing repeated on the other side; good detail will result.

On removal of the impression, detail is checked. It is often said that, because only the post is to be made, marginal detail is not important. This is only partially true because the technician must have sufficiently well-defined margins to be able to visualize the form of the final restoration if errors in contour are to be avoided. On occasions voids will be found on the intraradicular portion of the impression corresponding to the anti-rotation feature within the preparation. If these are small it is reasonable to ask the technician to block these with soft wax or to do this before the impression is sent to the laboratory. If the void is larger the impression should be retaken. Indirect techniques require that the technician has sufficient occlusal information to create an accurate core: most commonly, full-arch impressions will be necessary.

Try-in and cementation

If a casting has been made from a direct pattern, it should need minimal finishing. The fitting surface should be inspected under magnification for 'blows', and if present these should be removed using a small round bur under magnification.

The temporary post crown is removed and the preparation cleaned of temporary cement. This will generally require use of the final twist drill used to prepare the root canal to ensure that no cement remains apically. The preparation must also be thoroughly washed and dried before being inspected to ensure that no debris remains. The fitting surface of the post should be lightly sandblasted to provide a matt surface, so that if it binds on seating a burnished area will result that can be seen more easily, thereby facilitating adjustment. A small in-surgery sandblaster is invaluable for this purpose. The post should be seated using only light finger pressure, as heavy seating forces may cause root fracture. The first thing to check if the post does not seat is whether debris remains in the root canal: the importance of thorough debridement must not be overlooked.

The core should require no great adjustment. Any finishing that is necessary is most easily carried out after cementation. The tooth itself and the core should need little further preparation, and if this is not the case there must have been a previous error. The thickness of the axial walls of dentine was evaluated prior to final finishing of the preparation. Any further axial reduction will thin these further; and there exists the possibility of making them too weak to support the core properly. This further emphasizes the need to complete the preparation before the pattern or impression is made.

Cements and cementation

There is a choice between using the more traditional acid–base cements such as zinc phosphate, polycarboxylate or glass ionomer, and a resin cement. Higher retentive values can be obtained with resin cements, particularly when there is some form of dentinal adhesion [19]. However, this has not been a universal finding and tests *in vitro* may not replicate the conditions found within the root canal intraorally, particularly in relation to the moisture content of radicular dentine and its contamination with materials used in root canal treatment. Furthermore, too great an emphasis placed on retentive values is unhelpful. Small gains in retention where posts are of reasonable dimensions have no particular clinical benefit, whereas if post length is lacking, improvements in retention do not improve stress distribution, which is arguably the most important function of the post. The case for resin cements for luting posts has not been clearly established.

The aims of post cementation are to ensure as complete seating as possible with minimal stress being applied to the root. The post is unlikely to seat completely because of the difficulties of venting the cement over the entire length of the post. Consider the distance over which the cement must travel from the end of the post to the coronal part of the preparation before it can escape. Added to this is the need to avoid heavy seating pressures that might increase the risk of root fracture. Complete seating is aided by the post having a vent longitudinally; some posts have these as a design feature but this will not be present when an antirotation feature has been added to the post. It is good practice to pro-

vide a vent by making a longitudinal groove in the post using either a fine cut-off disc or bur. Prior to cementation the post should be lightly sandblasted again to provide a clean surface to enhance micromechanical retention with the cement.

Complete seating will also be enhanced by correct mixing of the cement to provide maximal working time. Cements with longer working times are to be preferred: zinc phosphate cement still has much to commend it. A cold slab and incremental mixing provide good working time. It is important to take active steps to fill the canal with cement if voids in the film are not to result. The post preparation should be clean and dry; once the cement is mixed, the post is coated with cement and placed on the cold slab. Cement is then carried to the post preparation and the internal walls coated using a long probe, a cold endodontic heat carrier or a spiral paste filler. This must be carried out quickly and the post placed using only light finger pressure. The pressure must be maintained until the cement begins to set, otherwise the post may rebound out of the preparation.

If for any reason the cementation procedure using zinc phosphate cement needs to be aborted, the post and preparation should be swabbed immediately with a concentrated solution of sodium bicarbonate, which will break down the cement; this does not work with other cements. The cement should be left until fully set before excess is removed, the coronal preparation reevaluated and any final finishing carried out.

Cast cores and posts for multirooted teeth

On occasions there may be such a lack of coronal dentine in a posterior tooth that the demands placed on a plastic core material become unrealistic. Dentists understandably like to have a 'rule of thumb' for when this point is reached. However, it is not possible to be entirely prescriptive as the decision depends on:

1. The quantity of remaining coronal tooth structure.
2. The quality of dentine.

3. The loads that will act on the tooth and restoration.

As a broad guide, when the amount of dentine is less than one cusp, there is a significant indication for a cast core.

Number of posts

The availability of more than one root canal has traditionally often meant that more than one post is placed. Many of the techniques described reflect more the ingenuity of the dentist and technician rather than necessarily being of benefit to patients [25]. Certainly, in terms of loss of dentine, such an approach is not always valid. Additional posts may help to distribute stresses to those roots in which they are placed, but this needs to be balanced against the knowledge that posts do not provide reinforcement. Where a post is required, it should be placed in the largest root available and the post should be of appropriate length.

Antirotation features

Resistance to rotation is generally more easily achieved in multirooted than single-rooted teeth as the frequent availability of a definite pulp chamber naturally provides the basis for this feature. Where this needs to be enhanced internally, it should be carried out where a bulk of dentine is present. It hardly needs to be stated that such enhancement of the resistance form should not undermine useful remaining coronal dentine, nor should the floor of the pulp chamber be modified to any significant extent as the dentine is often thin and its bulk in this area is important to resist longitudinal fracture.

Indications for multiple posts

Two situations arise when more than one post may be required. These are:

1. When the root selected for the post is short or when the anatomy of the root prevents it being used to the required length.

2. When there is little in the way of pulp chamber to provide antirotation.

Two techniques are available. The first uses a separate post and core for each canal, which interlock on placement. In the second technique, one post is cast to be integral with the core, whilst the core is designed to permit further posts to be placed through it into additional root canals. The first method is able to make better use of the internal form of the pulp chamber, as each interlocking post and core has its own path of insertion; whilst in the second technique, the path of insertion of the post that is integral with the core also determines the path of insertion of the core itself. There is often a need to remove dentine to ensure that there is no conflict in the path of insertion. However, in terms of simplicity and practicality the second method is superior. Where the secondary post is being placed primarily for antirotation, the post need only extend into the root canal 2–3 mm. Figure 14.24 shows a maxillary first molar where there was a relatively deep subgingival fracture on the palatal aspect of the tooth. A cast core was considered advantageous, and the post in the palatal canal was cast with the core, whilst provision was made to pass the additional post through the core into the distobuccal canal at the time of cementation.

Impressions and cementation

Impression procedures require no particular precautions, even if the posts are significantly divergent. Modern polyvinyl siloxane materials have low permanent deformation and consequently distort little on removal from deep undercuts. If a problem were to arise, it would most likely be associated with tearing of the impression which would be obvious. At a practical level this is not a problem.

The cementation procedure follows that described above: the core with its integral post is placed first, followed immediately by the additional post. The cement will have been placed within both post preparations immediately prior to seating the main post and its core. The cement is allowed to set completely before the excess is removed and the supplementary post trimmed at its junction with the coronal aspect of the core. The protruding post is best held with a pair of fine curved haemostats before the excess length is cut off with a bur in a turbine handpiece.

Such posts and cores are attractive for their impression of solidity. However, their prognosis may not be so good, as the amount of tooth structure that remains is very much reduced. Figure 14.25 shows one such example, where 8 months following cementation of a multiple post casting, it became uncemented. On removal of the posts and core by sectioning, no evidence of root frac-ture was seen. Subsequent remaking of the post and core resulted in a further failure of cementation 9 months later. Once again, no evidence of root fracture or dental caries was evident. The tooth functioned thereafter as an overdenture abutment. The precise reason for the recurrent loss of cementation can only be a matter of conjecture, possibly either a lack of resistance form in the preparation or perhaps flexibility in the tooth leading to damage to the cement film. However, it is undoubtedly related to a lack of tooth structure for which synthetic materials are unable to compensate.

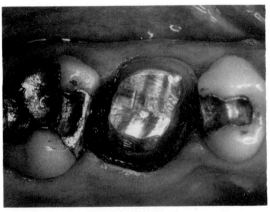

(a)

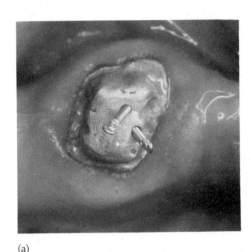

(a)

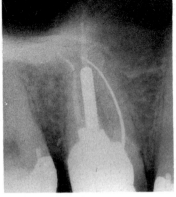

(b)

Figure 14.24 (a) Cast gold post and core with an auxiliary post in the distobuccal canal of a maxillary first molar. (b) Periapical radiograph showing integral post within the palatal canal and a shorter auxiliary post in the distobuccal canal.

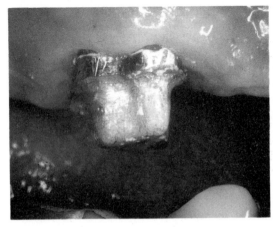

(b)

Figure 14.25 (a) Occlusal view of a cast post and core with two auxiliary posts. (b) Buccal view of the cast core, which later became uncemented.

Endodontically treated teeth as abutments

The root-treated tooth may be required to act as the abutment for a fixed or removable prosthesis. Abutments show an increased level of failure compared with other endodontically treated teeth [35], whilst in one of the very few studies of bridge retainers, post-retained crowns had a higher failure rate than partial or full-veneer retainers on teeth with vital pulps [28].

The higher rate of failure is probably due to the increased loads acting on teeth where the quantity of dentine is reduced. Such information should influence both the use of such teeth as abutments and also the prognosis that the patient is given for the lifespan of the prosthesis. Where the tooth is to be the major abutment for a fixed prosthesis or a strategic abutment for one that is removable, little can be done to protect the tooth other than not to provide the bridge or to change the design of the denture: either option may on occasions be correct. When there is an endodontically treated tooth acting as an abutment for a fixed bridge, consideration should be given to the consequences of losing the tooth. The strategic use of movable connectors within the design of the prosthesis may allow some provision for failure without the entire prosthesis being lost.

If the endodontically treated tooth is the minor abutment for the bridge, the design of the connector can sometimes be modified to reduce the lateral loads on the endodontically treated tooth. A movable connector distributes loads equally between abutments only when the two parts of the connector are fully engaged. Where the parts are not wholly engaged the loads are apportioned more to the major abutment than the minor. A movable connector is only fully engaged under direct axial loading whilst at all other times the two parts will be incompletely mated and the load distribution between the abutments will be dependent on the area of connector in contact at any one time. When incompletely seated, parallel-sided connectors will remain in more intimate contact than those that are tapered; and the greater the taper, the less is the contact between the two parts. This allows a proportionately

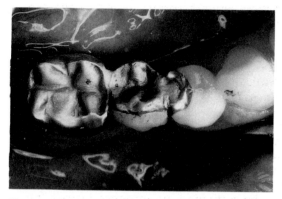

Figure 14.26 Three-unit bridge replacing a mandibular second premolar. The hand-cut movable connector in the first premolar reduces load on the abutment.

greater load to be distributed to the major abutment with less being transmitted to the endodontically treated minor abutment. This principle can only be applied to short-span bridgework in the posterior part of the mouth, otherwise the loads on the major abutment become excessive.

Figure 14.26 shows a three-unit fixed–movable bridge where this principle has been applied and a hand-cut tapered connector provided in the distal of the minor retainer to reduce the non-axial loading of the root-canal-treated minor abutment.

Elective devitalization

This procedure is sometimes incorrectly employed as a technique for improving retention of the final restoration. Its use is a symptom of a lack of crown height, and the solution is to increase the height available and use axial grooves, rather than employ the root canal for retention.

Its use has been recommended in teeth where the existing intracoronal restoration is deep and the tooth is to act as an abutment for a fixed bridge [27]. The suggestion was made because a small number of teeth suffered loss of pulpal vitality subsequent to the bridges being placed. These teeth were generally those that had previously shown signs of pulpal inflammation or had deep carious lesions. When root canal treatment through the retainer became necessary, this was followed by fracture of the remaining coronal dentine in a number of instances. The reason for these fractures was considered to be due to the endodontic access cavity removing much of the core dentine, and no estimate of what remained could be made. It was therefore suggested that in instances where long-term pulpal vitality was in doubt and the tooth was to be used as a bridge abutment, elective devitalization prior to bridge construction should be carried out.

Such suggestions need to be seen against the success of endodontically treated teeth as abutments. If the history and diagnostic tests are suggestive of chronic pulpitis, there may be merit in discussing with the patient the advantages of elective root-canal treatment prior to bridge construction. However, this should be considered against the significant loss of dentine that will occur.

Conclusions

There have been advances in the methods available for restoring endodontically treated teeth. Many of these are adhesive in nature; however, there is an improved understanding of the behaviour of endodontically treated teeth in response to continued loading within the mouth. Two major conclusions can be drawn:

1. Stress within the tooth and restoration must be kept to a minimum.
2. The preservation of useful tooth structure should be seen as a prime obligation. This applies as much to the endodontic procedures as it does to the subsequent restoration.

References

1. BURNS DA, KRAUSE WR, DOUGLAS HB, BURNS DR (1990) Stress distribution surrounding endodontic posts. *Journal of Prosthetic Dentistry* **64**, 412–418.
2. COLLEY IT, HAMPSON EL, LEHMAN ML (1968) Retention of post crowns. An assessment of the relative efficiency of posts of different shapes and sizes. *British Dental Journal* **124**, 63–69.
3. CRAIG RG, FARAH JW (1977) Stress analysis and design of single restorations and fixed bridges. *Oral Sciences Reviews* **10**, 45–74.
4. CREUGERS NHJ, MENTINK AGB, KAYSER AF (1993) An analysis of durability data on post and core restorations. *Journal of Dentistry* **21**, 281–284.
5. DEUTSCH AS, CAVALLARI J, MUSIKANT BL, SILVERSTEIN L, LEPLEY J, PETRONI G (1985) Root fracture and the design of prefabricated posts. *Journal of Prosthetic Dentistry* **53**, 637–640.
6. DHURU VB, MCLACHAN K, KASLOFF Z (1979) A photoelastic study of stress concentrations produced by retention pins in amalgam restorations. *Journal of Dental Research* **58**, 1060–1064.
7. EAKLE WS (1986) Fracture resistance of teeth restored with class II bonded composite resin. *Journal of Dental Research* **65**, 149–153.
8. GUZY GE, NICHOLLS JI (1979) *In vitro* comparison of intact endodontically treated teeth with and without endo-post reinforcement. *Journal of Prosthetic Dentistry* **42**, 39–44.
9. HANSEN EK, ASMUSSEN E (1990) *In vivo* fractures of endodontically treated posterior teeth restored with enamel–bonded resin. *Endodontics and Dental Traumatology* **6**, 218–225.
10. HANSEN EK, ASMUSSEN E, CHRISTIANSEN NC (1990) *In vivo* fractures of endodontically treated posterior teeth restored with amalgam. *Endodontics and Dental Traumatology* **6**, 49–55.
11. HOAG EP, DWYER TG (1982) A comparative evaluation of three post and core techniques. *Journal of Prosthetic Dentistry* **47**, 177–181.
12. HUANG TJG, SCHILDER H, NATHANSON D (1991) Effects of moisture content and endodontic treatment on some mechanical properties of human dentin. *Journal of Endodontics* **18**, 209–215.
13. KANTOR ME, PINES MS (1977) A comparative study of restorative techniques for pulpless teeth. *Journal of Prosthetic Dentistry* **38**, 405–412.
14. KING PA, SETCHELL DJ (1990) An *in vitro* evaluation of a prototype CRFC prefabricated post developed for the restoration of pulpless teeth. *Journal of Oral Rehabilitation* **17**, 599–609.
15. KOVARIK RE, BREEDING LC, CAUGHMAN WF (1992) Fatigue life of three core materials under simulated chewing conditions. *Journal of Prosthetic Dentistry* **68**, 584–590.
16. KVIST T, RYDIN E, REIT C (1989) The relative frequency of periapical lesions in teeth with root canal-retained posts. *Journal of Endodontics* **15**, 578–580.
17. LEINFELDER KF, WILDER AD, TEIXEIRA LC (1986) Wear rates of posterior composite resins. *Journal of the American Dental Association* **112**, 829–833.
18. MATTISON GD, DELIVANIS PD, THACKER RW, HASSELL KJ (1984) Effect of post preparation on the apical seal. *Journal of Prosthetic Dentistry* **51**, 785–789.
19. MENDOZA DB, EAKLE WS (1994) Retention of posts cemented with various dentinal bonding cements. *Journal of Prosthetic Dentistry* **72**, 591–594.

20. MENTINK AGB, CREUGERS NHJ, MEEUWISSEN R, LEEM-POEL PJB, KAYSER AF (1993) Clinical performance of different post and core systems – results of a pilot study. *Journal of Oral Rehabilitation* **20,** 577–584.

21. MEREDITH N (1992) An *in vitro* analysis of stresses induced in natural and restored human teeth. PhD Thesis. London, UK: University of London.

22. NAYYAR A, WALTON RE, LEONARD LA (1980) An amalgam coronal-radicular dowel and core technique for endodontically treated posterior teeth. *Journal of Prosthetic Dentistry* **43,** 511–515.

23. OBERMAYR G, WALTON RE, LEARY JM, KRELL KV (1991) Vertical root fracture and relative deformation during obturation and post cementation. *Journal of Prosthetic Dentistry* **66,** 181–187.

24. OLIVA RA, LOWE JA (1986) Dimensional stability of composite used as a core material. *Journal of Prosthetic Dentistry* **56,** 554–561.

25. PAMEIJER JHN (1985) *Periodontal and Occlusal Factors in Crown and Bridge Procedures,* p. 217. Amsterdam, the Netherlands: Dental Center for Postgraduate Courses.

26. REINHARDT RA, KREJCI RF, PAO YC, STANNARD JG (1983) Dentin stresses in post-reconstructed teeth with diminishing bone support. *Journal of Dental Research* **62,** 1002–1008.

27. REUTER JE, BROSE MO (1984) Failure in full crown retained dental bridges. *British Dental Journal* **157,** 61–63.

28. ROBERTS DH (1970) The failure of retainers in bridge prostheses. An analysis of 2,000 retainers. *British Dental Journal* **128,** 117–124.

29. ROSS RS, NICHOLLS JI, HARRINGTON GW (1991) A comparison of strains generated during placement of five endodontic posts. *Journal of Endodontics* **17,** 450–456.

30. SEDGLEY CM, MESSER HH (1992) Are endodontically treated teeth more brittle? *Journal of Endodontics* **18,** 332–335.

31. SJOGREN U, HAGGLUND B, SUNDQVIST G, WING K (1990) Factors affecting the long-term results of endodontic treatment. *Journal of Endodontics* **16,** 498–504.

32. SORENSEN JA, ENGELMAN MJ (1990) Ferrule design and fracture resistance of endodontically treated teeth. *Journal of Prosthetic Dentistry* **63,** 529–536.

33. SORENSEN JA, MARTINOFF JT (1984) Intracoronal reinforcement and coronal coverage: a study of endodontically treated teeth. *Journal of Prosthetic Dentistry* **51,** 780–784.

34. SORENSEN JA, MARTINOFF JT (1984) Clinically significant factors in dowel design. *Journal of Prosthetic Dentistry* **52,** 28–35.

35. SORENSEN JA, MARTINOFF JT (1985) Endodontically treated teeth as abutments. *Journal of Prosthetic Dentistry* **53,** 631–636.

36. STANDLEE JP, CAPUTO AA, COLLARD EW (1971) Retentive pins installation stresses. *Dental Practitioner and Dental Record* **21,** 417–422.

37. STANDLEE JP, CAPUTO AA, COLLARD EW, POLLACK MH (1972) Analysis of stress distribution by endodontic posts. *Oral Surgery, Oral Medicine, Oral Pathology* **33,** 952–960.

38. STANDLEE JP, CAPUTO AA, HANSON EC (1978) Retention of endodontic dowels: effects of cement, dowel length, diameter and design. *Journal of Prosthetic Dentistry* **39,** 400–405.

39. VALE WA (1956) Cavity preparation. *Irish Dental Review* **2,** 33–41.

40. WENDT SL, HARRIS BM, HUNT TE (1987) Resistance to cusp fracture in endodontically treated teeth. *Dental Materials* **3,** 232–235.

Index